EMERGENCY DERMATOLOGY

A RAPID TREATMENT GUIDE

Alan B. Fleischer, Jr., MD
Associate Professor, Co-Director
Westwood-Squibb Center for Dermatology Research
Wake Forest University School of Medicine
Winston-Salem, North Carolina

Steven R. Feldman, MD, PhD
Professor of Dermatology
Wake Forest University School of Medicine
Winston-Salem, NC

Charity F. McConnell, MD
Franklin Dermatology
Franklin, TN

Asha G. Pardasani, MD
Columbia Skin Clinic
Columbia, SC

Mark R. Hess, MD
Assistant Professor of Emergency Medicine
Wake Forest University School of Medicine
Winston-Salem, NC

Marco Petrazzuoli, MD
Granite Medical Group
Quincy, MA

EMERGENCY DERMATOLOGY
A RAPID TREATMENT GUIDE

Alan B. Fleischer, Jr., MD

Steven Feldman, MD

Charity F. McConnell, MD

Marco Petrazzuoli, MD

Asha Pardasani, MD

Mark R. Hess. MD

The McGraw-Hill Companies
MEDICAL PUBLISHING DIVISION

New York   Chicago   San Francisco   Lisbon   London   Madrid   Mexico City   Milan
New Delhi   San Juan   Seoul   Singapore   Sydney   Toronto

McGraw-Hill

*A Division of The **McGraw-Hill** Companies*

EMERGENCY DERMATOLOGY: A Rapid Treatment Guide

1234567890 IMA IMA 098765432

This book was set in 9/11 Times Roman by Techbooks.
The editors were Darlene Cooke, Susan Noujaim, and Regina Brown.
The production supervisor was Richard Ruzycka.
The designer was Marsha Cohen/Parallelogram Graphics.
Printed and bound in China by Imago.
This book is printed on acid-free paper.

Library of Congress Cataloging-in-Publication Data
Emergency dermatology: a rapid treatment guide / Alan B. Fleischer, Jr. ...[et al.].
    p.; cm.
  Includes bibliographical references and index.
  ISBN 0-07-137995-9
  1. Dermatology—Handbooks, manuals, etc. 2. Medical emergencies—
    Handbooks, manuals, etc. I. Fleischer, Alan B.
  [DNLM: 1. Skin Diseases—therapy—Handbooks. 2. Emergencies—
    Handbooks. WR 39
  E53 2002]
  RL72. E446 2002
  616.5025—dc21
                                        2001056274

NOTICE

Medicine is an ever-changing science. As new research and clinical experience broaden our knowledge, changes in treatment and drug therapy are required. The authors and the publisher of this work have checked with sources believed to be reliable in their efforts to provide information that is complete and generally in accord with the standards accepted at the time of publication. However, in view of the possibility of human error or changes in medical sciences, neither the authors nor the publisher nor any other party who has been involved in the preparation or publication of this work warrants that the information contained herein is in every respect accurate or complete, and they disclaim all responsibility for any errors or omissions or for the results obtained from use of the information contained in this work. Readers are encouraged to confirm the information contained herein with other sources. For example and in particular, readers are advised to check the product information sheet included in the package of each drug they plan to administer to be certain that the information contained in this work is accurate and that changes have not been made in the recommended dose or in the contraindications for administration. This recommendation is of particular importance in connection with new or infrequently used drugs.

SPECIAL ACKNOWLEDGEMENT

Mr. Mario P. DeMarco was instrumental in the final assembly of this manuscript. Without his dedication and devotion, this work could not have come to fruition.

CONTENTS

P R E F A C E

Emergency physicians and other emergency healthcare provides are faced with an increasing workload of patients that present with either true emergencies and non-emergencies. Dermatologic disease constitutes a large proportion of outpatient care, and this is also reflected in emergency practice. Recognizing the increasing time pressures on all healthcare providers, this brief guide to dermatologic emergencies was designed to be a rapid reference.

This text is sparse on detailed discussion of pathphysiology and histopathology and there is no discussion of diseases that are exceptionally rare. Rather, the diagnoses chosen are all commonly seen, or are dermatologic emergencies that demand rapid intervention. The authors worked on this project as a team, and we hope that this text will swiftly guide the clinician to the best diagnosis and treatment. Illustrations are essential for dermatologic texts, and this collection includes many published elsewhere in other fine McGraw-Hill more comprehensive reference texts and from our own collections. We hope that this work helps provide better care for your patients with skin diseases.

CUTANEOUS ANTHRAX

HISTORY

- This infection is caused by the contact of an abrasion or a laceration with soil or material containing the gram positive organism, *Bacillus anthracis,* an encapsulated, non-motile, non-hemolytic bacillus
- Although contact with contaminated wool, hides, leather or hair products (especially goat hair) of infected animals have historically been the infection sources, bioterrorist activities have changed the entire risk spectrum so that mail handling is now considered a risk factor
- Patients may present with a history of a rapidly growing painless but possibly pruritic papule arises after contact in three to seven days, with the range from one to fifteen days
  - After the papule arises, a vesicle forms within 24 to 36 hours, with subsequent central necrosis and black eschar formation
  - Patients hay have a history of fever, malaise and/or headache

PHYSICAL EXAMINATION

- The malignant pustule is a rapidly growing well-circumscribed papule that quickly develops into a 1 to 3 cm papule with central necrosis, often surrounded by brawny, non-pitting erythematous edema (Figs. 1 and 2)
  - The border of the necrotic area may show vesiculation
  - The edema may be marked, especially on the head and neck
  - Regional lymphadenopathy is common

DIAGNOSIS

- The diagnosis should be considered in any susceptible patient and confirmatory investigations should occur to establish this diagnosis with certainty
- The clinician should obtain three skin biopsies including:
  - A skin biopsy for routine histopathology (preserved in formalin)
  - Two skin biopsy specimens in a sterile cup: one for gram stain and culture and a second for PCR, culture, and immunohistochemistry staining at the Centers for Disease Control and Prevention (CDC)
    - Acute *B. anthracis* ELISA testing may be performed by the CDC if the disease has been present less than five days and convalescent testing at 14 to 21 days
  - A blood culture and blood gram stain should be ordered, with blood for PCR testing

DIFFERENTIAL DIAGNOSIS

- Arthropod assault: the earliest erythematous papule may be indistinguishable from an typical arthropod bite reaction, and the

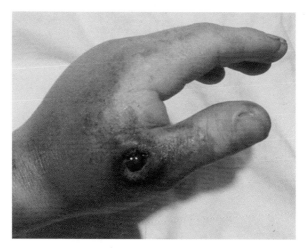

Figure 1: *Cutaneous anthrax with malignant pustule*

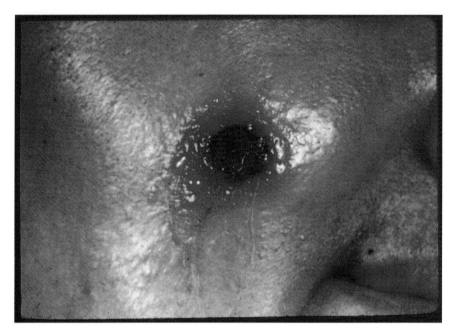

Figure 2: *A second cutaneous anthrax patient with a malignant pustule*

necrotic-appearing malignant pustule could mimic a necrotizing spider bite reaction

- Pyoderma gangrenosum: This condition is found most commonly in patients with inflammatory bowel disease or other autoimmune diseases, and presents as an erythematous to violaceous papule, which over weeks may centrally ulcerate. Constitutional symptoms such as fever are almost always absent
- Ecthyma gangrenosum: This infection with *Pseudomonas aeruginosa* most commonly occurs in immunocompromised patients, and one sees edematous, well-circumscribed erythematous plaques that rapidly become hemorrhagic, leading to bulla and eschar formation. This process from erythematous plaque to necrotic eschar may occur in 12 hours and most patients have profound systemic symptoms
- Tularemia: In ulceroglandular tularemia, which results from the handling a contaminated carcass or following an infective arthropod bite, a local cutaneous papule appears at the inoculation site at about the time of onset of systemic symptoms (fever, headache, chills, and coryza), becomes pustular, and becomes a tender ulcer within a few days of its first appearance. Lymphadenopathy may be present
- Orf: This virus infection is caused by the parapox virus and is acquired through direct innoculation by contact with infected lambs and goats. Following innoculation generally on the hand or forearm, within 5 or 6 days patients develop a small, tender, firm, erythematous papule that enlarges to form a flat-topped, blood-tinged pustule or bulla as large as 5 cm. Lymphadenopathy and fever may be present
- Rickettsialpox: Rickettsialpox is a bacterial disease caused by *Rickettsia akari,* a bacteria transmitted to humans by mouse mites from mice, in which patients develop a painless papule that subsequently ulcerates and forms an eschar 0.5–3.0 cm in diame-

ter. Three to seven days later, the patient may experience the fever and mild constitutional symptoms, and may develop a generalized exanthem

TREATMENT

- Treatment of cutaneous anthrax is an emergency
  - The mortality rate approaches 20% for untreated patients, but is less than 1% for treated patients
  - Consultation with an infections diseases specialist and/or the CDC should be considered
  - Doxycycline
    - > 45 kg: 100 mg po BID for 60 days
    - < 45 kg: 2.5 mg/kg/d po for 60 days
  - Ciprofloxacin 20 to 30 mg/kg/d po for 60 days
  - Although their efficacy is unknown, other possibly effective antibiotics could include chloramphenicol, clindamycin, rifampin, clarithromycin, and vancomycin

MANAGEMENT/FOLLOW UP

Follow up recommended within one day or hospital admission should be considered

ICD-9-CM code: 022.0

CPT code: skin biopsy 11100, subsequent skin biopsy 11101
Figure 1: Fitzpatrick's Dermatology in General Medicine, fifth edition, figure 200-1, p. 2258.
Figure 2: enclosed as a slide
Special source: Ray TL: Cutaneous Anthrax, A Primer for Dermatologists. Internet site accessed 11/05/01 <http://tray.dermatology.uiowa.edu/BT/sld001.htm>
Figure 2 courtesy of Drs. James and Gloria Graham

EMERGENCY DERMATOLOGY

A RAPID TREATMENT GUIDE

CHAPTER 1

ABRASIONS

HISTORY

- Patient often presents with "sores" and a history of minor trauma to the skin

PHYSICAL EXAMINATION

- Superficial irregularly shaped (suggesting exogenous source) erosion, which is defined as partial or complete loss of the epidermis (Fig. 1-1)

- In some cases, a very shallow ulcer that extends to the most superficial aspect of the dermis occurs
- Evidence of foreign body, such as dirt, may be noted superficially within open lesions

DIAGNOSIS

- Usually made clinically by history and physical exam

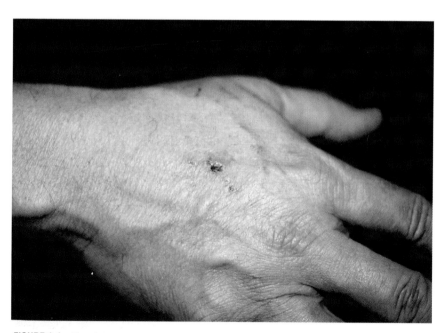

FIGURE 1-1 *Abrasion.*

DIFFERENTIAL DIAGNOSIS

- Since history and physical exam are usually diagnostic, no specific differential diagnosis is warranted

TREATMENT

- The primary goal of treatment is to make certain that cleansing is sufficient to remove any obvious foreign body
- Subsequently, a bland ointment (e.g., Vaseline®) or topical antibiotic preparation (e.g., Polysporin®) may be applied to accelerate healing and prevent infection
- Keeping the wound moist and covered will accelerate healing
- For deeper lesions, oral antibiotics may be prescribed in an attempt to prevent infection
  - Choice of antibiotic should be based on the environment in which the wound occurred

MANAGEMENT/FOLLOW-UP

- No specific follow-up required

ICD-9-CM Codes

910.0   Abrasion without infection of face, neck, and scalp except eye

910.1   Infected abrasion of face, neck, and scalp except eye
911.0   Abrasion without infection of trunk
911.1   Infected abrasion of trunk
912.0   Abrasion without infection of shoulder and upper arm
912.1   Infected abrasion of shoulder and upper arm
913.0   Abrasion without infection of elbow, forearm, and wrist
913.1   Infected abrasion of elbow, forearm, and wrist
914.0   Abrasion without infection of hand(s) except finger(s) alone
914.1   Infected abrasion of hand(s) except finger(s) alone
915.0   Abrasion without infection of finger(s)
915.1   Infected abrasion of finger(s)
916.0   Abrasion without infection of hip, thigh, leg, and ankle
916.1   Infected abrasion of hip, thigh, leg, and ankle
917.0   Abrasion without infection of foot and toe(s)
917.1   Infected abrasion of foot and toe(s)
918.0   Abrasion of eyelids and periocular area
919.0   Abrasion without infection of other, multiple, and unspecified sites
919.1   Infected abrasion of other, multiple, and unspecified sites

CPT Code

None

ABSCESS, FURUNCLE, AND CARBUNCLE

HISTORY

- Very painful, tender papules, pustules, or nodules presenting on any skin region, particularly hair-bearing sites
- Usually arise over a period of a few days
- Foul-smelling discharge
- Occasionally low-grade fever and malaise

PHYSICAL EXAMINATION

- Abscess
  - May arise on any cutaneous surface (Fig. 2-1)
  - Initially presents as a tender nodule that becomes fluctuant; develops a central pustular area within a few days to weeks

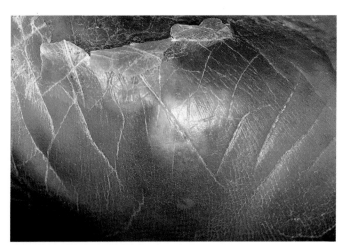

FIGURE 2-1 Staphylococcus aureus: *abscess.*

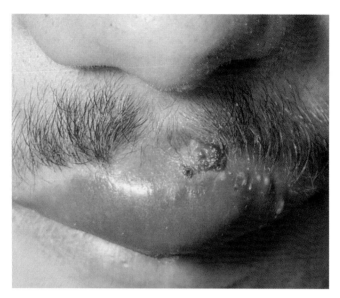

FIGURE 2-2 *Furuncle of the upper lip.*

- Furuncle
  - ○ Usually arises on hair-bearing sites (e.g., beard, posterior scalp) as a firm, tender nodule with a central necrotic plug (Fig. 2-2)
  - ○ Nodule becomes fluctuant with an abscess formation below it

- Carbuncle
  - ○ Comprises several coalescing furuncles (Fig. 2-3)
  - ○ Forms loculated abscesses, necrotic plugs, and superficial pustules

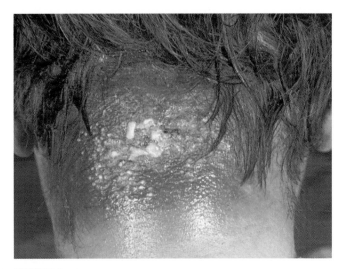

FIGURE 2-3 *Carbuncle.*

- Most commonly caused by *Staphylococcus aureus*
- Diagnosis based on clinical findings, which can be confirmed by Grams stain and culture

DIFFERENTIAL DIAGNOSIS

- Ruptured epidermal inclusion (sebaceous) cyst: erythematous, firm, tender plaque with foul-smelling drainage; patient may report a history of a gradually enlarging, tender, recurrent cyst
- Pseudofolliculitis barbae and acne keloidalis nuchae: multiple papules, pustules, and keloids occurring on the beard area and posterior scalp areas, respectively; commonly seen in African-American males
- Hidradenitis suppurativa: draining sinus tracts associated with ulcerations occurring on hair-bearing sites

TREATMENT

- Treatment of abscesses, furuncles, and carbuncles is nonemergent
- Incision and drainage plus systemic antimicrobial therapy appropriate for *Staphylococcus* coverage
  - Dicloxacillin: 500 mg bid for 10 days (adults); 12.5 to 25 mg/kg/day (children <40 kg)
  - Cephalexin (Keflex®): 500 mg bid for 10 days (adults); 25 to 50 mg/kg/day (children)
  - *Penicillin-allergic*: erythromycin 500 mg bid for 10 days (adults); 40 mg/kg/day for 10 days (children)
- Application of heat to the lesions often promotes drainage; warm wet towel compresses 2 to 3 times daily for 10 minutes each time
- Recurrent furunculosis: benzoyl peroxide wash for prophylaxis; examples include Benzac AC 5% wash and Brevoxyl 4% creamy wash

MANAGEMENT/FOLLOW-UP

- Those patients who have isolated lesions can follow up with a primary care physician or a dermatologist as needed
- Those patients who have recurrent lesions should be seen every 3 to 4 months by either their primary care physician or a dermatologist

ICD-9 Codes

682.9 Abscess
680.9 Furuncle, carbuncle

CPT Code

10060 Incision & drainage cyst or abscess

CHAPTER 3

ACNE VULGARIS

- Teenage and adult males and females with chronic or recurrent inflammatory skin lesions of the face and trunk
  - These lesions may be painful but are usually asymptomatic
  - Males tend to have more severe involvement than females
- Exacerbating factors include systemic use of corticosteroids, androgenic steroids, or lithium, as well as topical exposure to certain industrial compounds such as coal tar derivatives, cutting oils, and chlorinated hydrocarbons
- Females with other symptoms of virilization (hirsutism, husky voice, increased muscle mass, irregular menses, etc.) should be evaluated for hyperandrogenic state
- Acne fulminans is a rare acute febrile ulcerative acne that is highly inflammatory. This is almost exclusively seen in young males
  - Explosive onset of fever, malaise, polyarthralgias, tender nodules, and cysts

PHYSICAL EXAMINATION

- Involvement of the face/neck and sometimes trunk with characteristic lesions (Fig. 3-1)
- Open and closed comedones are blackheads and whiteheads, respectively (Fig. 3-2)
- Red papules, pustules, and nodules are all common types of skin lesions
- Inflammatory lesions often result in post-inflammatory hyperpigmentation in patients with dark skin
- Scarring is characteristic of the very inflammatory forms of acne

DIAGNOSIS

- Clinical exam

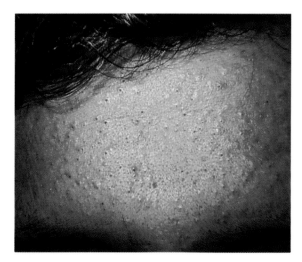

FIGURE 3-1 *Acne vulgaris.*

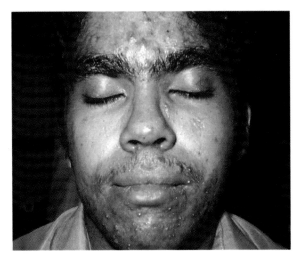

FIGURE 3-2 *Cystic acne.*

- Folliculitis: folliculitis and acne vulgaris can have identical morphology, but folliculitis is less likely to be located on the face, superior chest, and superior back and is usually more monomorphous in appearance
- Rosacea is generally located almost exclusively on the central face and nose and displays not only papules and pustules but also striking erythema
- Perioral dermatitis has erythema and brightly erythematous papules but is located circumorally

TREATMENT

- Treatment of acne is nonemergent
- Treatment is dependent on the type of lesion—multiple modalities of treatment are often required
  - Comedones
    - Topical tretinoin (Retin A®) or adapalene (Differin®) cream or gel qhs as tolerated
    - Topical salicylic acid or glycolic acid cleansers qd to bid as tolerated
  - Superficial inflammatory papules or pustules
    - Topical antibiotics such as 1% clindamycin (Cleocin®, Clindets®) or erythromycin (Emgel®) bid
    - Topical benzoyl peroxide 4% to 10% (e.g., Benzac AC® or Brevoxyl®) in gel or wash form bid
  - Numerous deep papules or nodules
    - Systemic tetracycline (Sumycin®) or erythromycin (Emycin®) 250 to 500 mg bid
    - Systemic minocycline (Minocin®) or doxycycline (Dynacin®) 50 to 100 mg bid
    - Systemic oral contraceptives for women such as Tricyclen® or Yasmin® have a modest effect
    - For treatment-resistant disease, isotretinoin (Accutane®) 0.5 to 1.0 mg/kg/day for 15 to 20 weeks
    - Appropriate use requires a minimum of two forms of birth control, pregnancy and teratogenicity counseling with informed consent, depression counseling with informed consent, and initial and subsequent blood monitoring

MANAGEMENT/FOLLOW-UP

- Patients should follow up with their primary care physician or dermatologist

ICD-9 code

706.1

ACQUIRED ACANTHOSIS NIGRICANS

- Localized development of hyperpigmented, velvety textured skin
- Patients may describe it as having a "dirty" appearance
- May report recent increase in weight
- May have history of obesity, diabetes mellitus, or malignancy
- Obtain review of systems to screen for malignancy-associated acanthosis nigricans

and a drug history to rule out drug-induced acanthosis nigricans

PHYSICAL EXAMINATION

- Velvety, hyperpigmented plaques most commonly located on axillae or neck; other body folds may be involved (Figs. 4-1 to 4-3)
- Surface may become mammillated

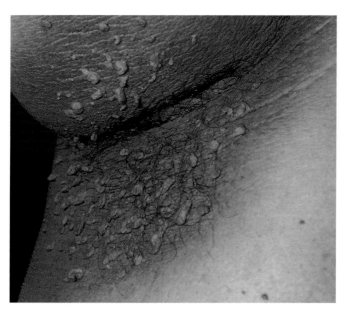

FIGURE 4-1   *Acanthosis nigricans of the axilla.*

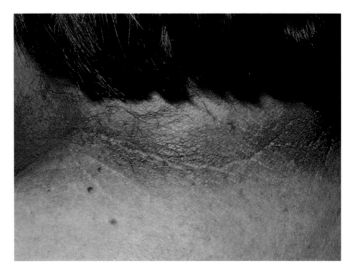

FIGURE 4-2   *Acanthosis nigricans of the neck.*

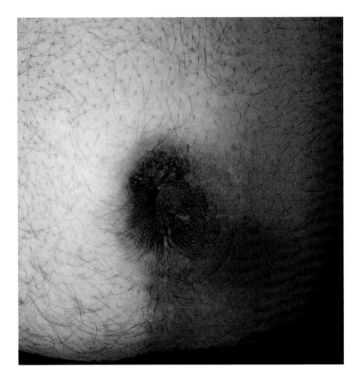

FIGURE 4-3 *Acanthosis nigricans of the umbilicus.*

- May have associated skin tags within the plaques
- Mucous membranes may be involved; if so, usually less pigmented and more hypertrophic, with velvety texture

- Clinical examination suggests diagnosis; biopsy rarely needed
- Most common cause is obesity; however, other underlying causes may be suggested by history and physical examination
  ○ Hereditary benign acanthosis nigricans: no associated underlying cause
  ○ Endocrinopathies: include various disorders associated with insulin resistance, such as diabetes mellitus, acromegaly, Addison's disease, and Cushing's disease
  ○ Malignancy: the acanthosis nigricans tends to be more extensive and involves mucosal surfaces; most common associated malignancies are adenocarcinomas, usually gastric in origin
  ○ Drugs: nicotinic acid, diethylstilbestrol, oral contraceptives, glucocorticoids and others

DIFFERENTIAL DIAGNOSIS

- Confluent and reticulated papillomatosis: in this rare condition, patients have velvety brown plaques in a reticulated pattern over the back and chest

TREATMENT

- Treatment of acanthosis nigricans is nonemergent
- If an underlying cause is present, it should be identified and treated
  ○ Obese patients can reverse skin changes with weight loss
  ○ Malignancy-associated acanthosis nigricans may regress following effective treatment of the underlying cancer
- Topical lactic acid (Lac-Hydrin® lotion or cream 12%) or glycolic acid (Aqua Glycolic® body lotion) applied 1 to 2 times daily may be of benefit
  ○ Patients should be forewarned that these agents may irritate the skin

MANAGEMENT/FOLLOW-UP

- These patients should be seen by their primary care physician if further diagnostic or management issues need to be addressed regarding the underlying etiology of the acanthosis nigricans
- Follow-up as needed for the skin condition

ICD-9 Code

701.2

ACQUIRED KERATODERMAS

HISTORY

- Thickening of the skin over the palms and/or soles that has not been present since birth or early infancy
- The skin thickening may or may not be associated with other skin complaints

PHYSICAL EXAMINATION

- Thickening of the skin is observed over the palms and/or soles (Fig. 5-1)
- One of three distinct clinical patterns may be present
  - Diffuse: symmetric and even hyperkeratosis over the entire palm and/or sole
  - Focal: thick masses of keratin over pressure sites or sites of recurrent friction
  - Punctate: tiny raindrop-shaped keratoses over the palms and/or soles
- Other associated skin findings may be present as well, depending on the etiology of the keratoderma

DIAGNOSIS

- The diagnosis of acquired keratoderma is usually made by history and physical examination; however, there are several known causes for acquired keratoderma that need to be explored in these patients
- The initial approach to the patient should focus on determining whether the keratoderma is part of a more generalized disorder (e.g., psoriasis), a sign of internal disease (malignancy, diabetes), or a secondary reaction to external forces (calluses)
  - If the keratoderma is thought to be associated with a more generalized skin condition, a skin biopsy may be required to confirm the primary diagnosis
  - If the keratoderma is thought to be a sign of internal disease, history and physical exam should guide any further testing that may be required

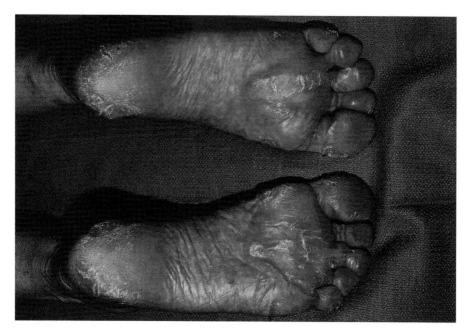

FIGURE 5-1 *Keratoderma.*

- Keratodermas associated with a generalized skin condition: can present with either diffuse or focal thickening
  - Psoriasis: usually psoriasis has significantly more erythema, and psoriatic disease may be displayed in typical locations such as the elbows, knees, scalp, and other locations
  - Pityriasis rubra pilaris: has the rapid onset of a near-total body erythroderma with wax-dipped–appearing palms and soles
  - Reiter's syndrome (keratoderma blennorrhagicum): one finds red to brown papules, pustules, and vesicles with peripheral scaling and central erosion that occurs on the palms and soles
  - Secondary syphilis: one sees individual scaling lesions that are round to oval on the palms and soles, with a scaly eruption on the trunk
- Keratoderma as a sign of internal disease: most commonly presents with a diffuse keratoderma
  - Diabetes mellitus
  - Acquired immunodeficiency syndrome (AIDS)
  - Malignancy
  - Myxedema
- Keratoderma as a reactive process
  - Callus: one sees thickened noninflammatory skin in sites of greatest trauma
- Miscellaneous
  - Keratoderma climactericum: this keratoderma is characterized by hyperkeratotic plaques on the palms and soles in women at menopause, commonly at pressure-bearing sites

- The treatment of acquired keratoderma is nonemergent
- Treatment of any underlying cause should be initiated, which may help to improve the keratoderma
- Local therapy
  - Hydration followed by application of an unscented moisturizer (e.g., Moisturel®, Lubriderm®, Eucerin®, Vaseline®, Cetaphil®) is an important supplement to treatment
  - Generous use of moisturizers should be encouraged on a daily basis

- Keratolytic agents
  - Topical keratolytic agents can be used to decrease the thickness of the skin
  - Patients can be told to soak the affected areas in water prior to application to enhance penetration of the substance
  - Patients should also be warned that these agents may be very irritating to normal or diseased skin and should only be applied to the thickened areas
  - The agents are as follows:

Salicylic acid: Keralyt® gel; MG 217® Sal-Acid ointment or solution
Lactic acid: Lac-Hydrin® 12% cream or lotion
Urea: Carmol® 10% to 40% cream or U-Lactin® cream

- Systemic therapy
  - Oral retinoids, such as acitretin (Soriatane®), may play a significant role in the treatment of refractory keratoderma
  - Immunosuppressive agents, such as methotrexate, have also been used in refractory keratoderma with some success
  - These systemic agents require close laboratory monitoring, informed consent when needed, and appropriate follow-up
  - Thus they should be administered in an outpatient setting rather than the emergency department

MANAGEMENT/FOLLOW-UP

- Any patient with an acquired keratoderma needs to follow up with either a primary care physician or a dermatologist for further evaluation of possible causes of the condition, as well as for continued therapy

ICD-9 Code

701.1

ACTINIC KERATOSIS

HISTORY

- These occur most commonly in middle-aged to elderly whites with a light complexion who gradually develop scaly lesions on habitually sun-exposed skin
- Patients have a history of chronic sun exposure through occupational or recreational activities
- Lesions may last for months to years and may be tender or asymptomatic
  - Lesions may spontaneously disappear or may give rise to squamous cell carcinoma in a small percentage of cases
- Immunosuppressed individuals such as transplant recipients, AIDS patients, and albinos are at increased risk

PHYSICAL EXAMINATION

- Most commonly patients have one or more skin-colored to reddish brown or yellowish ill-defined macules or papules with a characteristic dry, adherent scale located on sun-exposed skin of arms, face, scalp, and upper chest (Fig. 6-1)
- Lesions vary in size from a millimeter to several centimeters

- The diagnosis is often better recognized through palpation or lesional roughness than visually
- Lesions may be hypertrophic with a horn-like projection (cutaneous horn) (Fig. 6-2)
- Occasionally actinic keratoses are pigmented
- The condition may involve the lower lip in actinic cheilitis and is sometimes seen in association with oral leukoplakia

DIAGNOSIS

- Clinical exam is usually sufficient
- A biopsy may be necessary to differentiate from an invasive squamous cell carcinoma

DIFFERENTIAL DIAGNOSIS

- Invasive squamous cell carcinoma: these lesions have a feeling of induration on palpation, may or may not be ulcerated, and are generally larger than actinic keratoses
- Chronic cutaneous lupus erythematosus: patients have discrete, indurated plaques on sun-exposed skin that show atrophy, erythema, and telangiectasia

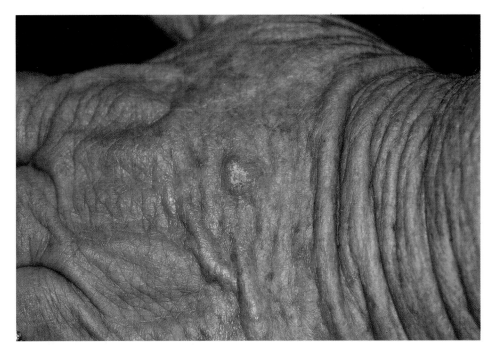

FIGURE 6-1 *Actinic keratosis of the hand.*

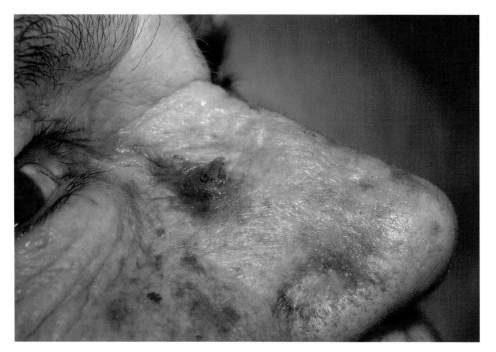

FIGURE 6-2 *Actinic keratosis.*

- Seborrheic keratosis: these common, benign lesions have a pebbly, scaly appearance
- Lentigo: this hyperpigmented macule has no scale visibly and no palpability and is also located on sun-damaged skin

TREATMENT

- All treatment is nonemergent
- Cryotherapy with liquid nitrogen is a practical method for limited numbers of lesions
- Topical chemotherapy
  - 5-Fluorouracil cream or solution (0.5% to 5%) bid for 3 weeks for the head and neck, 4 to 6 weeks for other areas such as the forearms
  - Tretinoin cream and imiquimod may also be used
- Miscellaneous treatments used include:
  - Photodynamic therapy with topical application of 20% aminolevulinic acid followed by exposure to red light is an emerging treatment
  - Electrodessication and curettage
  - Dermabrasion for extensive actinic keratoses
  - Chemical peels with alpha hydroxy acids, Jessner's solution and 35% trichloroacetic acid have all been used successfully

- Carbon dioxide laser therapy has been used for extensive actinic keratoses
- Systemic retinoids (e.g., isotretinoin) have been used in patients with widespread actinic keratoses

MANAGEMENT/FOLLOW-UP

- Hats, protective clothing, and sunscreens are preventatives
- Patients with actinic keratoses are at increased risk for development of subsequent skin cancers and frequent skin checks are warranted
- It has been calculated that over a 10-year period, there is approximately a 10% chance of a single actinic keratoses on a patient evolving into a squamous cell carcinoma

ICD-9-CM Code

702.0

CPT Codes

17000   Destruction of one actinic keratosis
17003   Destruction of each additional actinic keratosis up to 13
17004   Destruction of 15 or more actinic keratoses

CHAPTER 7

ALOPECIA AREATA

HISTORY

- Patchy or generalized hair loss on scalp, face, or body occurring gradually over a period of weeks to months
- New patches of alopecia may appear while others resolve
- No pain, itching, or burning
- May report a similar history of hair loss in the past that may or may not have spontaneously improved
- May report a family history of alopecia areata and/or a personal history of other autoimmune conditions

PHYSICAL EXAMINATION

- Well-circumscribed round to oval patches of hair loss is the most common pattern, but occasionally the hair loss may be more generalized (Fig. 7-1)
  - Alopecia totalis: complete loss of scalp hair
  - Alopecia universalis: complete loss of scalp and body hair
- Examination reveals normal scalp without erythema, scale, scarring, or atrophy

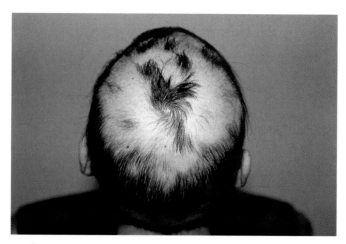

FIGURE 7-1   A. Extensive patchy alopecia areata.

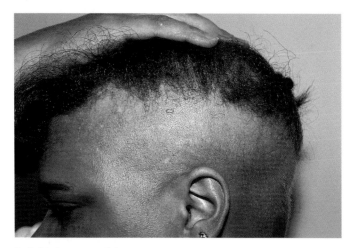

B. Ophiasis pattern of alopecia areata.

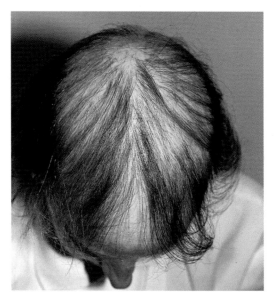

C. Diffuse pattern of loss in alopecia areata.

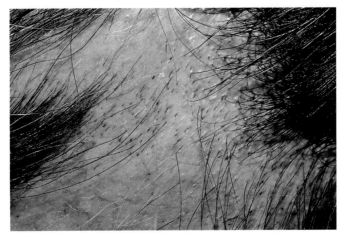

FIGURE 7-2 *Exclamation mark hairs of alopecia areata.*

- "Exclamation point" hairs, short, broken hairs with distal ends broader than proximal ends, are noted at periphery of alopecia (Fig. 7-2)
- Fingernail pitting (tiny depressions in the nail) or other nail changes may be noted

DIAGNOSIS

- "Exclamation point" hairs are pathognomic
- Pull test may be positive, depending on activity of disease
- A skin biopsy is rarely needed

DIFFERENTIAL DIAGNOSIS

- Tinea capitis: usually a single area of alopecia with a scaly, erythematous scalp; perform KOH preparation to rule out tinea, especially in children
- Anagen effluvium: diffuse and generalized hair loss such as that induced by chemotherapy
- Telogen effluvium: diffuse and generalized hair loss on scalp 2 to 3 months after a "physiologic stress" to body

- Trichotillomania: short, broken, uneven hairs caused by patients pulling or twisting their own hair
- Secondary syphilis: patchy "moth-eaten" hair loss of scalp and beard area

TREATMENT

- Treatment of alopecia areata is nonemergent
- Local treatment
  - Intralesional corticosteroids
    - Can inject with triamcinolone acetonide (Kenalog®) 2.5 to 5.0 mg/ml to treat small areas of alopecia
    - Inject around periphery as well as in center of the alopecia, using about 0.1 ml with each injection
    - Areas with positive pull test should be treated as well
  - Topical corticosteroids
    - Available as a solution, cream, lotion, ointment, gel, foam, or oil; for areas bearing some hair, a solution vehicle is most suitable for the patient; for areas of complete alopecia, ointments may be used

- Should use medium- to high-potency topical corticosteroid bid up to 4 weeks on the area of alopecia, at which time the patient should be followed up by a primary care physician or a dermatologist

Mid-potency: prednicarbate (Dermatop®) 0.1% ointment or cream; triamcinolone acetonide (Aristocort®) 0.1% ointment or cream

High-potency: fluocinonide (Lidex®) 0.05% ointment or cream; clobetasol propionate (Temovate®) 0.05% ointment or cream; halobetasol propionate (Ultravate®) 0.05% ointment or cream; betamethasone dipropionate 0.05% in optimized ointment (Diprolene®)

- Emphasize side effects of prolonged use of topical corticosteroids including skin atrophy
- Topical tacrolimus (Protopic®) 0.1% ointment may be use for prolonged periods without risk of atrophy

- Systemic treatment: corticosteroids
  ○ Generally reserved for those patients with extensive disease who have either had hair loss for less than 6 months or hair loss refractory to topical measures
  ○ May induce regrowth, but risk of long-term side effects precludes prolonged use
  ○ Taper over 4 to 6 weeks with the dose depending on age and weight; generally 0.5 to 1.0 mg/kg/day can be used as the starting dose
- Other systemic treatments available for refractory patients include topical irritants and topical immunotherapy

MANAGEMENT/FOLLOW-UP

- Follow-up recommended with either a primary care physician or a dermatologist within 2 weeks if alopecia not treated and within 4 weeks if treatment has been initiated

ICD-9 Code
704.01

CPT Code
11900   Intralesional injection ≤7 sites

APHTHOUS STOMATITIS (CANKER SORES)

- The patient may report the sudden appearance of one or more painful oral ulcers
- Acidic or spicy food consumption intensifies the pain
- Often there is a history of recurrent oral ulcers that spontaneously resolve within 2 weeks
- Recurrences may or may not be associated with precipitating factors, such as menses, stress, trauma

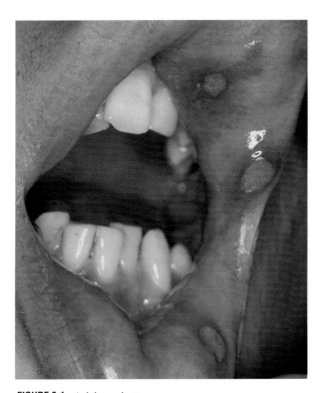

FIGURE 8-1 *Aphthous ulcers.*

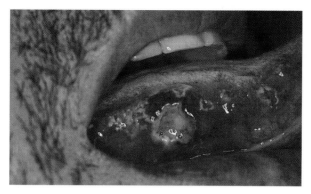

FIGURE 8-2 *Aphthous ulcer of the tongue.*

- Well-circumscribed, shallow ulcers with a gray or white fibrinous base and an erythematous rim on the lining mucosa of the oral cavity in an otherwise healthy-appearing patient (Figs. 8-1 to 8-3)
- Lesions usually occur singly and not in groups, although many lesions may be present at one time

DIAGNOSIS

- The diagnosis is a clinical one, but the clinician should carefully consider other diagnoses in the differential diagnosis below

DIFFERENTIAL DIAGNOSIS

- Primary or recurrent herpes simplex virus (HSV)
  - In primary HSV, the patient usually appears ill and may have constitutional symptoms such as fever and malaise
  - In recurrent oral HSV, lesions usually occur in groups and almost always involve only the vermilion of the lip rather than intraoral areas
- Hand-foot-and-mouth disease: viral disease in children associated with vesicles and papules on hands, feet, and occasionally the buttocks area, along with constitutional symptoms
- Erythema multiforme: oral ulcerations associated with constitutional symptoms, a typical rash or targetoid lesions, and involvement of other mucosal sites such as the genitalia and conjunctivae
- Behçet's disease: recurrent oral and genital ulceration associated with eye disease, arthritis, vasculitis, and other skin lesions
- Autoimmune bullous diseases: bullous pemphigoid, pemphigus vulgaris, and cicatricial pemphigoid
- Rarely, persistent forms of aphthae may be secondary to systemic problems, such as iron deficiency, vitamin B_{12} deficiency, human immunodeficiency virus (HIV) infection, or gluten-sensitive enteropathy

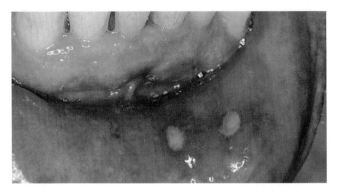

FIGURE 8-3 *Aphthous ulcers of the labial mucosa and vestibule.*

TREATMENT

- Treatment of oral aphthous ulcers is nonemergent
- Local treatment
  - Topical corticosteroids
    - A gel or Orabase® form is usually suitable for oral lesions. Examples include clobetasol propionate (Temovate®) gel 0.05%, augmented betamethasone dipropionate gel (Diprolene®) 0.05%, or triamcinolone 0.1% (Kenalog in Orabase®)
    - These agents may be used for up to 5 times a day prn for lesions
  - Intralesional corticosteroids may be of some immediate benefit for patients; triamcinolone acetonide 3 to 5 mg/ml can be used to inject individual sites, using 0.1 to 0.2 ml/site
  - Local anesthetic (benzocaine, lidocaine, and similar agents) solutions for symptomatic treatment
- Systemic treatment (these agents are reserved for those patients refractory to topical therapy)
  - Oral corticosteroids
  - Colchicine and/or dapsone
  - Immunosuppressive agents such as methotrexate, azathioprine (Imuran®), or cyclosporin (Neoral®)
  - Thalidomide
  - Treat for superimposed candidal infections with oral fluconazole (Diflucan®) 100 mg once a week for 3 weeks (adults) and/or clotrimazole troches up to 5 times daily (adults)

- These patients should be followed by a primary care physician or a dermatologist within a week if no treatment is initiated
- Patients who have been started on therapy should follow up in a month

ICD-9-CM Code

528.2

CPT Code

11900   Intralesional injection ≤7 sites

CHAPTER 9
APHTHOUS VULVITIS

HISTORY

- Sudden appearance of painful genital ulcers
- History of recurrent ulcers that spontaneously resolve within 2 weeks
- Recurrences may or may not be associated with precipitating factors, including menses, stress, or trauma
- May or may not be associated with oral ulcers

PHYSICAL EXAMINATION

- Presents as either small, punched-out ulcers with a gray-white, fibrinous base or as larger, irregular ulcers with central granulation tissue (Fig. 9-1)

- Ulcerations most often located within the vulvar vestibule of females

DIAGNOSIS

- Diagnosis is one of exclusion

DIFFERENTIAL DIAGNOSIS

- Primary or recurrent herpes simplex virus (HSV)
  - In primary HSV, the patient usually appears ill and may have constitutional symptoms such as fever and malaise
  - In recurrent genital HSV, lesions often occur and the ulcers are found in groups

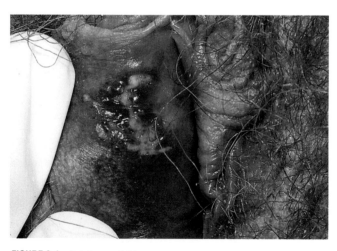

FIGURE 9-1 *Aphthous vulvitis.*

- Other infections, such as syphilis, chancroid, and granuloma inguinale, should be excluded
- Erythema multiforme: ulcerations associated with constitutional symptoms, a typical rash of targetoid lesions, and involvement of other mucosal sites such as the oral mucosa and conjunctivae
- Behçet's disease: recurrent oral and genital ulceration associated with eye disease, arthritis, vasculitis, and other skin lesions
- Crohn's disease: usually present with draining sinus tracts and fistulas from the bowel to the skin; ulcers are usually linear and resemble lacerations
- Hidradenitis suppurativa: draining sinus tracts associated with ulcerations occurring on hair-bearing areas of the vulva as well as on the mucosal surfaces
- Rarely, persistent forms of aphthae may be secondary to systemic problems, such as iron deficiency, vitamin B_{12} deficiency, HIV infection, or gluten-sensitive enteropathy

TREATMENT

- Treatment of aphthous vulvitis is non-emergent
- Local treatment
  - Topical corticosteroids
    - A gel or ointment form is usually suitable for vulvar lesions
    - Examples include clobetasol propionate (Temovate®) gel or ointment

0.05% or augmented betamethasone dipropionate (Diprolene®) gel or ointment 0.05%; these agents may be used for up to 5 times a day prn for lesions for short periods
  - Intralesional corticosteroids may be of some immediate benefit for patients; triamcinolone acetonide (Kenalog®) 3 to 5 mg/ml can be used to inject individual sites, using 0.1 to 0.2 ml/site
- Systemic treatment (these agents are reserved for those patients refractory to topical therapy)
  - Oral corticosteroids
  - Colchicine and/or dapsone
  - Immunosuppressive agents such as methotrexate, azathioprine, cyclosporine, and thalidomide
  - Treat for superimposed candidal infections with oral fluconazole 100 mg once a week for 3 weeks

MANAGEMENT/FOLLOW-UP

- These patients should be followed up by a primary care physician or a dermatologist within 1 to 2 weeks

ICD-9-CM Code

616.10

CPT Code

11900   Intralesional injection ≤7 sites

ARTHROPOD ASSAULT (INSECT BITES AND STINGS)

HISTORY

- The patient may or may not recall exposure to biting bugs and may deny that such exposure could have occurred
- Lay terminology for types of arthropods may not be consistent with accepted scientific speciation

PHYSICAL EXAMINATION

- Each type of arthropod produces different types of reaction patterns including single or multiple erythematous macules, papules, wheals, small vesicles to large bullae, necrotic ulcers (Fig. 10-1)

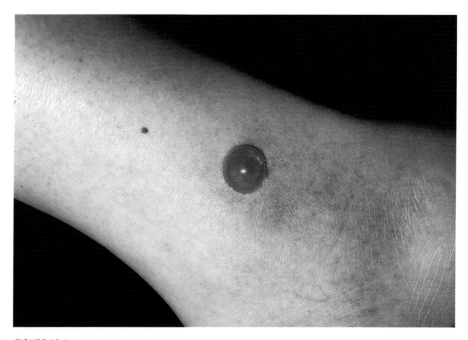

FIGURE 10-1   *Ballons insect bite*

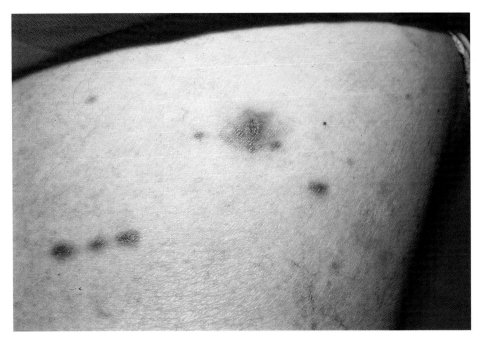

FIGURE 10-2 *Flea bites*

- The reponse to the identical bite or sting will differ in each affected individual
- Fleas: flea bites are generally on the lower legs and present with multiple pruritic erythematous macules and papules (Fig. 10-2)
- Mites: mite bites occur wherever the mites contact the patient and the most common location and appearance is erythematous papules are on the lower legs
- Spiders: most spider bites cause local pain with small erythematous papule or wheal formation
  ○ Black widow (*Lactrodectus mactans*) bites can produce severe muscle spasms, headache, sweating, and nausea
  ○ Brown recluse bites (*Loxosceles reclusa*) can produce small, nondescript bites that progress to develop necrotic centers, which can rapidly spread to cover small to large areas, resulting in impressive full thickness necrosis (Fig. 10-3)
- Ticks: local bite reactions are most commonly include urticarial or erythematous papules to persistent bite reactions, but rarely patients can develop tick paralysis by toxin injection
- Mosquitoes: local bite reactions most commonly include urticarial or erythematous papules
- Hymenoptera (bees, hornets, and wasps): these produce painful papules or localized wheals, with uncommon but serious generalized urticaria and/or angioedema
  ○ Patients may present with bronchospasm, shock, or respiratory arrest
- Fire ants: patients may develop simple wheals, or the well-known pattern of a circular distribution of erythematous papules to pustules surrounding tiny petechial puncta
- Scorpions: stings usually produce local pain, erythema, and edema
  ○ Systemic symptoms may include central nervous system activation, respiratory distress, bradycardia, pancreatitis, and other effects

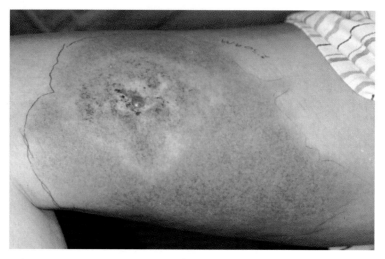

FIGURE 10-3 *Typical brown recluse spider bite*

DIAGNOSIS

- The history and physical examination establish the diagnosis of bites and stings

DIFFERENTIAL DIAGNOSIS

- Arthropod assaults can mimic viral exathems, autoimmune blistering diseases, pyoderma gangrenosum, and other conditions.

TREATMENT

- Nonvenemous reactions
  - Local pruritic bites can be treated with potent topical corticosteroid agents such as fluocinonide (Lidex®) 0.05% ointment or cream; clobetasol propionate (Temovate®) 0.05% ointment or cream; halobetasol propionate (Ultravate®) 0.05% ointment or cream, betamethasone dipropionate 0.05% in optimized ointment (Diprolene®)
  - Extensive numbers of pruritic bites may require systemic corticosteroids such as prednisone 1.0 mg/kg/day tapered over 1 week
  - If secondary infection is present, mupirocin (Bactroban®) cream topically can be helpful
  - Recommend prevention using DEET-containing agents
- Venemous reactions
  - Hymenoptera (bees, hornets, and wasps) reactions are treated similarly to other venomous reactions with fire ants, scorpions, and other arthropods

Minor reactions may require wound cleansing with stinger removal, elevation, ice, and systemic antihistamine agents such as diphenhydramine (Benadryl®): adults: 25 to 50 mg QHS; kids 0.3 mg/kg/day of 10 mg/5 ml suspension

  - Severe reactions acutely require stabilization of the patient including, but not limited to epinephrine, intravenous corticosteroids, antihistamines, and supportive intravenous fluid hydration

Adults: subcutaneous epinephrine (1:1000), 0.4 to 0.5 ml or intravenous epinephrine (1:1000) 0.25 ml in a 0.01% solution, injected slowly

Kids: 0.15 ml or 0.01 ml/kg

Patients should be carefully observed and doses may need to be repeated within 30 minutes

Any patient that has had a severe bite reaction should carry an AnaKit® or EpiPen® and should be instructed in the appropriate use; they should also consider a desensitization program

- Spider bites
  - Black widow (*Lactrodectus mactans*) bites may require supportive care with wound cleansing, ice, and analgesics

Severe muscle spasms can be treated with calcium gluconate (10 mL of 10% solution in adults)

  - Brown recluse bites (*Loxosceles reclusa*) can be treated with local wound cleansing, prevention of secondary infection with mupirocin (Bactroban®) cream, and allowing the eschar to develop, and general supportive care

Dapsone 100 to 200 mg per day has an unproven role in treating acute bite reactions, but caution must be exercised since this can cause rapid hemolysis in patients with glucose-6-phosphate deficiency

MANAGEMENT/FOLLOW-UP

- Follow up with their primary care physician is recommended for all patients with severe reactions within 1 week

ICD-9-CM Code
Nonvenemous Assaults

910.4   Insect bite, Nonvenemous, without infection of face, neck, and scalp except eye
910.1   Insect bite, Nonvenemous, Infection of face, neck, and scalp except eye

911.4   Insect bite, Nonvenemous, without infection of trunk
911.5   Insect bite, Nonvenemous, Infection of trunk
912.4   Insect bite, Nonvenemous, without infection of shoulder and upper arm
912.5   Insect bite, Nonvenemous, Infection of shoulder and upper arm
913.4   Insect bite, Nonvenemous, without infection of elbow, forearm, and wrist
913.5   Insect bite, Nonvenemous, Infection of elbow, forearm, and wrist
914.4   Insect bite, Nonvenemous, without infection of hand(s) except finger(s) alone
914.5   Insect bite, Nonvenemous, Infection of hand(s) except finger(s) alone
915.4   Insect bite, Nonvenemous, without infection of finger(s)
915.5   Insect bite, Nonvenemous, Infection of finger(s)
916.4   Insect bite, Nonvenemous, without infection of hip, thigh, leg, and ankle
916.5   Insect bite, Nonvenemous, Infection of hip, thigh, leg, and ankle
917.4   Insect bite, Nonvenemous, without infection of foot and toe(s)
917.5   Insect bite, Nonvenemous, Infection of foot and toe(s)
918.0   Abrasion of eyelids and periocular area
919.4   Insect bite, Nonvenemous, without infection of other, multiple, and unspecified sites
919.5   Insect bite, Nonvenemous, Infection of other, multiple, and unspecified sites

Venemous Assaults

989.5   Venemous insect bites

ASTEATOTIC DERMATITIS (ECZEMA CRAQUELÉE)

HISTORY

- Usually an elderly man or woman presents complaining of dry, itchy skin, generally on the extremities but may also be on the trunk
- Usually exacerbated in the winter, especially by low-humidity environments, frequent bathing with hot water, and lack of use of moisturizers
- Most patients with asteatotic eczema have a history of xerosis (dry skin)

PHYSICAL EXAMINATION

- On the extremities and trunk, one can see very dry, fissured, scaling skin with poorly defined, erythematous lesions that have a "cracked river bed" appearance

DIAGNOSIS

- Usually made clinically by history and physical exam

DIFFERENTIAL DIAGNOSIS

- Allergic or irritant contact dermatitis: patients often have a history of topical application of potential irritants or allergens, and the dermatitis is limited to these areas of exposure
- Nummular eczema: patients present with round to ovoid scaling macules rather than diffuse erythema and scale, as is seen in asteatotic dermatitis (Fig. 11-1)
- Atopic dermatitis: patients tend to be younger, and there is more likely to be disease present on the antecubital and popliteal fossae, neck, and face
- Mycosis fungoides: this is a chronic lymphomatous condition of scaling patches, plaques, and tumors that starts localized and becomes generalized over the course of months to decades

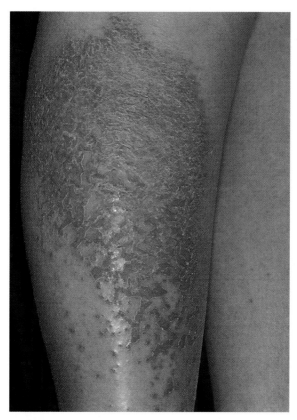

FIGURE 11-1 *Asteatotic dermatitis.*

- The best treatments include avoidance of frequent bathing, using tepid water for bathing, using frequent moisturizers (e.g., Moisturel®, Lubriderm®, Eucerin®, Vaseline®, Cetaphil®), and adding a humidifier to the bedroom
- For more severe disease, mid-potency corticosteroid agents such as triamcinolone 0.1% cream or ointment used bid for 1 to 2 weeks at a time may be helpful
  - An alternative is the use of tacrolimus (Protopic®) 0.1% ointment bid, which is safe for prolonged use

- This may be a chronic problem and almost always is exacerbated during the winter months
- Follow-up with a primary care physician or a dermatologist may be needed if patients do not respond to treatment

ICD-9-CM Code

706.8

CHAPTER 12

ATOPIC DERMATITIS

HISTORY

- Acute, subacute, or chronic pruritic eruption that often starts between early infancy and age 12, but can occasionally have onset in adulthood
- Lesions have usually been present for months to years at the time of presentation

- Patients usually complain of dry, itchy skin as well as a "rash"
- Patients or their family may have a history of asthma and/or allergic rhinitis (atopic diathesis)

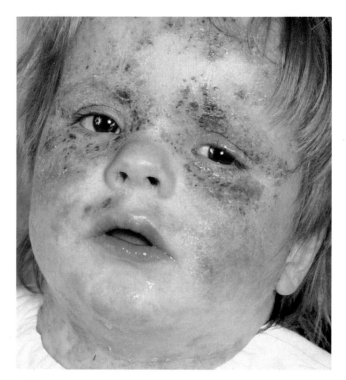

FIGURE 12-1 *Childhood atopic dermatitis.*

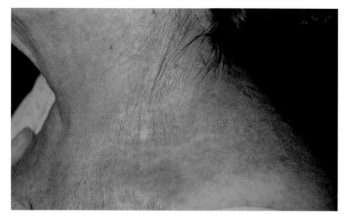

FIGURE 12-2 *Lichenification of the neck and shoulders with atopic dermatitis.*

- Acute lesions are erythematous patches, papules, and plaques that may have scales
- The skin often appears edematous and lesions are often excoriated and have superficial crusts (Fig. 12-1)
- In chronic disease, lichenified plaques (thickening of the skin and accentuated skin markings) are seen; in darker patients postinflammatory hyperpigmentation or hypopigmentation may be seen (Fig. 12-2)
- Lesions are most commonly located on flexures, front and sides of the neck, eyelids, forehead, cheeks, wrists, and dorsa of feet and hands (Fig. 12-3)
- Infected lesions may have hundreds or thousands of pustules present throughout the eczematous areas (Fig. 12-4)
- Background areas of the skin are often very scaly

- The diagnosis based on history and clinical findings
- Culture can be performed if secondary infection is suspected

- Dermatophyte infection: scaly erythematous plaques affecting the skin of the body that can be diagnosed by KOH preparation examination
  - Majocchi's granuloma is a deep fungal infection that involves the hair follicles
- Seborrheic dermatitis: a chronic dermatosis associated with redness and scaling on areas where sebaceous glands are prominent, such as the scalp ("dandruff"), face, and chest; lesions are yellowish red, greasy scaling macules and papules of various sizes

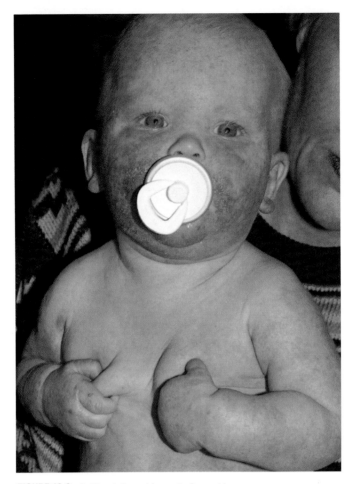

FIGURE 12-3 *Itching infant with atopic dermatitis.*

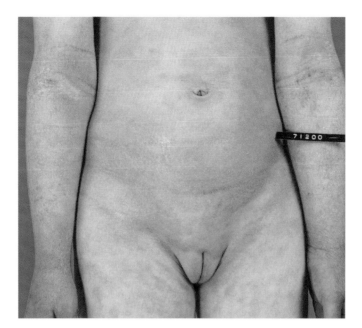

FIGURE 12-4 *Childhood atopic dermatitis.*

- Contact dermatitis (allergic or irritant): acute or chronic inflammatory reaction to agents that come into contact with the skin
  - Acute: well-demarcated plaques of erythema, edema, and vesicles often with superimposed erosions and crusting
  - Chronic: erythematous and lichenified (thickened skin with accentuation of skin markings) plaques with scale
  - Arranged in linear or bizarre patterns, indicating an exogenous etiology
- Mycosis fungoides: a chronic, scaling lymphoma presenting with scaly patches and plaques that may be located on any cutaneous surface
  - Lesions have usually been present longer than those of nummular eczema and are more resistant to treatment
- Psoriasis: inflammatory skin disease characterized by thick, erythematous papules and plaques with silvery scale; pruritus is common; sites of predilection include elbows, knees, scalp, ears, umbilicus, and gluteal cleft
- Pityriasis rosea: erythematous to pink scaly papules and plaques classically in a "Christmas tree" distribution over the trunk; begins with a "herald patch," which is slightly larger than the other lesions; self-limited eruption that spontaneously regresses in 6 to 12 weeks
- Secondary syphilis
  - Erythematous and hyperkeratotic scaly plaques located on trunk, extremities, palms, and soles
  - Patient may report a history of a chancre (ulcer of primary syphilis) in the previous 2 to 10 weeks
  - Condyloma lata: soft, flat-topped pink to tan papules on the perineum and perianal areas

TREATMENT

- The treatment of atopic dermatitis is nonemergent
- Education regarding the need to avoid scratching and/or rubbing and the need to use skin moisturizers (e.g., Moisturel®, Lubriderm®, Eucerin®, Vaseline®, Cetaphil®)
- Localized lesions can be treated with topical tacrolimus or topical corticosteroid agents bid
  - Corticosteroid agents cause less burning when applied to the skin but do cause atrophy when repeatedly applied over months or years
    - Mid-potency: triamcinolone acetonide (Kenalog®) 0.1% ointment or cream bid to affected skin, hydrocortisone valerate (Westcort®) 0.2% cream or ointment
    - Low-potency: hydrocortisone 0.5% to 2.5% ointment or cream bid; Desonide (DesOwen®) 0.05% cream or ointment bid; or fluocinolone oil (Derma-Smoothe/FS® Atopic Pak) bid to affected skin
  - Corticosteroid-sparing agents such as tacrolimus (Protopic®) 0.1% ointment has no known ability to cause skin atrophy even when applied chronically
    - Apply bid to affected skin areas, but note that a burning sensation is occasionally felt at the site of application
    - Although somewhat less effective but equally as safe, some clinicians recommend that children should only be prescribed the tacrolimus 0.3% ointment

- Sedating oral antihistamines can be used to improve patients' sleep and decrease the amount of time they scratch during the night
  - Hydroxyzine (Atarax®, Vistaril®): adults: 10 to 50 mg qhs; children: 0.3 mg/kg/day of 10 mg/5 ml suspension
  - Diphenhydramine (Benadryl®): adults: 25 to 50 mg qhs; children 0.3 mg/kg/day of 10 mg/5 ml suspension
- Skin hydration by bathing followed by application of an unscented moisturizer is an important supplement to the above treatments
- Harsh soaps should be replaced with no soaps or mild cleansers such as Cetaphil®, Aquanil®, or Dove®
- Treat any secondary infections (*Staphylococcus aureus* most common cause)
  - Dicloxacillin: 500 mg bid for 10 days (adults); 12.5 to 25 mg/kg/day in children <40 kg
  - Cephalexin: 500 mg bid for 10 days (adults); 25 to 50 mg/kg/day (children)
  - *Penicillin-allergic*: erythromycin 500 mg bid for 10 days (adults); 40 mg/kg/day for 10 days (children)
- Severe cases of atopic dermatitis that are nonresponsive to conventional therapy may require more complex forms of therapy, such as ultraviolet light therapy or oral immunosuppressive agents

MANAGEMENT/FOLLOW-UP

- Patients who are treated with topical or systemic agents should be followed up by a primary care physician or a dermatologist in 4 weeks to assess progress

ICD-9 Code

691.8

CHAPTER 13

BASAL CELL CARCINOMA

HISTORY

- Most common in fair-skinned middle-aged to elderly adult with a slowly growing tumor on sun-exposed skin
  - Rarely found in darker skinned persons
  - Males are more at risk than females
  - Can occur in younger patients with significant solar exposure
  - Exposure to arsenic or therapeutic radiation increases risk
  - Rare syndromes make development more common including nevoid basal cell carcinoma syndrome, albinism, xeroderma pigmentosum, Bazex's syndrome, Rasmussen's syndrome, and Rombo's syndrome
- Lesions are asymptomatic except when bleeding or infected

PHYSICAL EXAMINATION

- Round or oval, pink or red, firm, translucent, or pearly dome-shaped papule or nodules, often with a depressed center (Fig. 13-1)
  - Such papules or nodules may ulcerate centrally, maintaining a rolled border with hemorrhagic crust in some cases
  - Fine telangiectasias may be seen within the papule
- Eighty percent develop on the head and neck
- Pigmented variants appear brown or black and can be mistaken for malignant melanoma

- More common in darker-skinned individuals
- Morpheaform variant appears as an ill-defined, whitish, sclerotic patch or plaque
- Superficial variant appears as red, slightly scaly plaques, often with a pearly, rolled border
  - These are more often located on the trunk or limbs and can therefore be mistaken for tinea corporis, eczema, or psoriasis

DIAGNOSIS

- Clinical exam
- Skin biopsy for histology

DIFFERENTIAL DIAGNOSIS

- Fibrous papule: these lesions appear as firm papules, usually less than 2 mm in diameter, that lack translucency and telangiectasia
- Nevus: melanocytic nevi appear to be dome-shaped, may or may not be pigmented, and lack translucency and telangiectasia
- Sebaceous hyperplasia: these are papules, often umbilicated, that lack translucency and telangiectasia
- Dermatofibroma: these rarely appear in the face, are slowly growing, often have a peripheral rim of uniform hyperpigmentation, and lack translucency and telangiectasia

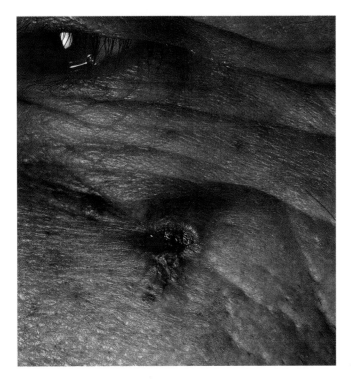

FIGURE 13-1 *Typical nodular basal cell carcinomas.*

- Malignant melanoma: generally these are pigmented and display asymmetry, border irregularity, and color variation; they are usually larger than 6 mm
- Molluscum contagiosum: these often are rapidly growing
- Skin adnexal tumors
- Deep fungal infection

TREATMENT

- Treatment of basal cell carcinoma is nonemergent
- The carcinoma may be removed by excision, electrodesiccation one 's' two 'c' s curettage, cryosurgery, and external beam radiation
- Mohs micrographic surgery is indicated for basal cell carcinomas with indistinct margins, for recurrent tumors, for which tissue conservation is critical (e.g., eyelids, nasal ala), and for the morpheaform (sclerosing) variant of basal cell carcinoma

MANAGEMENT/FOLLOW-UP

- Patients should follow up with their primary care physician or dermatologist
- Half of the patients with primary basal cell carcinoma develop another basal cell carcinoma within 5 years
- Thus close clinical follow-up with frequent exams is recommended

ICD-9-CM Codes

173.0   Skin of lip
173.1   Eyelid, including canthus
173.2   Skin of ear and external auditory canal
173.3   Skin of other and unspecified parts of face
173.4   Scalp and skin of neck
173.5   Skin of trunk, except scrotum
173.6   Skin of upper limb, including shoulder
173.7   Skin of lower limb, including hip
173.8   Other specified sites of skin
173.9   Skin, site unspecified

BULLOUS PEMPHIGOID

HISTORY

- This is an uncommon autoimmune blistering disease that generally occurs in an elderly person who develops few to hundreds of bullae associated with marked pruritus
- This condition rarely occurs in young adults
- The condition may be relatively rapid in onset
- Bullous pemphigoid is an autoimmune disorder of autoantibodies to basal keratinocytes

PHYSICAL EXAMINATION

- Large, tense bullae on normal skin or an erythematous base, usually on lower abdomen, inner or anterior thighs, and flexor forearms (Fig. 14-1)
- One may also see urticarial plaques with very few, if any, bullae (Fig. 14-2)
- The most common sites are lower abdomen, inner or anterior thighs, and flexor forearms, although bullous pemphigoid may occur anywhere on the body
- Bullous pemphigoid lesions heal without scarring, but patients may be with left with postinflammatory hyperpigmentation
- Lesions occur on mucous membranes in 10% to 35% of people

DIAGNOSIS

- The diagnosis is based on both clinical and histopathologic and immunohistopathologic findings
- To confirm the diagnosis, a skin biopsy and direct immunofluorescence biopsy should be performed (direct immunofluorescence requires a special medium called Michel's medium) to distinguish from other bullous diseases
- A salt-split skin test may be required to distinguish bullous pemphigoid from epidermolysis bullosa acquisita

DIFFERENTIAL DIAGNOSIS

- Other bullous disorders
- Need histopathology and immunofluorescence to distinguish from linear IgA disease, chronic bullous disorder of childhood, dermatitis herpetiformis, pemphigus vulgaris/foliaceus, erythema multiforme, epidermolysis bullosa acquisita, stasis bullae, and cicatricial pemphigoid, since these may all have a similar clinical appearance

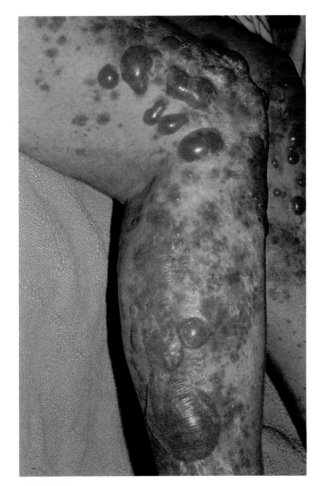

FIGURE 14-1 *Bullous pemphigoid.*

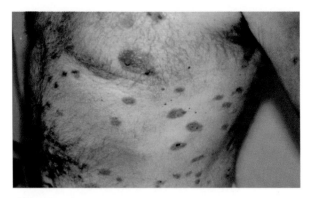

FIGURE 14-2   *Urticarial lesions of bullous pemphigoid.*

- Epidermolysis bullosa acquisita: can be difficult to distinguish from bullous pemphigoid clinically, but usually tense blisters develop over pressure points, such as feet, hands, elbows, knees, etc.
- Cicatricial pemphigoid: usually involves the head and neck area, particularly the mucous membranes, and is scarring, which causes significant morbidity
- Pemphigus vulgaris/foliaceus: flaccid vesicles or bullae that are Nikolsky positive are seen
- Stasis bullae: usually found on the lower extremities of person with massive pitting edema of the extremities; not usually associated with pruritus or an erythematous base

- Although the prognosis is relatively good, bullous pemphigoid can be a potentially fatal disease in elderly people
- Localized disease
  - One may attempt potent topical corticosteroid application if the patient has only a few localized lesions
    - High-potency: fluocinonide (Lidex®) 0.05% ointment or cream; clobetasol propionate (Temovate®) 0.05% ointment or cream; halobetasol propionate (Ultravate®) 0.05% ointment or cream, betamethasone dipropionate 0.05% in optimized ointment (Diprolene®)

- Extensive disease
  - The mainstay of treatment is oral prednisone; however, since this is usually a disease of the elderly, one must be mindful of the complications of steroid use, such as osteoporosis, diabetes, immunosuppression, cataracts, etc.
  - Doses of prednisone often start in the range of 1 to 1.5 mg/kg/day and are tapered over several weeks, once control is obtained
- May require an additional immunosuppressive agent to allow use of a lower dose of prednisone, such as azathioprine, cyclophosphamide, or methotrexate

- This condition requires close monitoring by the primary care physician in concert with a dermatologist due to the potential adverse effects of immunosuppressive medications, certainly in frail elderly people

ICD-9-CM Code

694.5

CPT Code

11100   Biopsy

CALCIPHYLAXIS

HISTORY

- Patients most commonly are dialysis patients
- The lesions begin as areas that look and feel like painful bruises
- Painful skin nodules and ulcers over the abdomen, buttocks, or lower extremities
- Patients often have hyperparathyroidism
- This is a systemic condition characterized by widespread small and medium-sized vessel calcification leading to a panniculitis and progressive cutaneous necrosis

PHYSICAL EXAMINATION

- Initial lesions present as erythematous to purpuric, tender nodules and plaques overlying a livedoid (lace-like) pattern of erythema on abdomen, buttocks, and/or lower extremities (Figs. 15-1 and 15-2)
- Eventually, extensive ischemia that progresses to necrosis, ulceration, and gangrene occurs
- An eschar often overlies the subcutaneous lesions
- Ulcers often become secondarily infected, causing cellulites and sepsis

DIAGNOSIS

- The diagnosis is based on history, clinical findings, and skin histologic confirmation
- Patients should have their levels of calcium, phosphorus, and parathyroid hormone assessed

DIFFERENTIAL DIAGNOSIS

- Any panniculitis can present with a subcutaneous lesion, such as erythema nodosum, nodular vasculitis, and polyarteritis nodosa
- Vasculitides: Wegener's granulomatosis, Goodpasture's syndrome
- Infection, including bacterial, deep fungal, and atypical mycobacteria
- Pyoderma gangrenosum: borders of ulcer are violaceous, boggy, and undermined
- Venous stasis ulcers

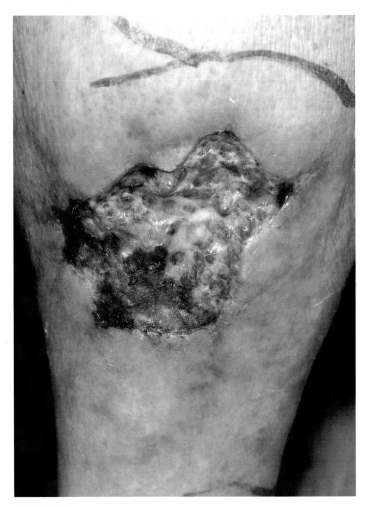

FIGURE 15-1 *Calciphylaxis.*

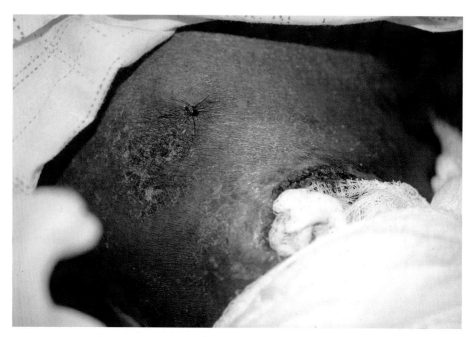

FIGURE 15-2 *Calciphylaxis.*

- Calciphylaxis is best managed by early diagnosis
  - Calciphylaxis requires prompt treatment to prevent systemic complications as well as secondary infection and gangrene
- Phosphate-binding agents may be used to lower the phosphate levels to prevent disease progression
- Treatment of renal failure should be maximized
- Debridement of any necrotic tissue should be performed to aid wound healing
- Treatment of the hyperparathyroidism via total or subtotal parathyroidectomy may be required if extensive skin necrosis has occurred
- Clinicians should identify any secondary infections and treat appropriately

- If there is no sign of necrosis, cellulitis, or sepsis, patients may be managed on an outpatient basis
  - Patients need follow-up with their nephrologist within 1 to 2 days to assess progress
- Any concern about necrosis, cellulitis, or sepsis should prompt admission

ICD-9 Code

729.30   Panniculitis

CALLUSES

HISTORY

- Patients complain of thickened areas of skin that have been present for months to years and are usually located on the hands or feet
- Patients often have a history of repeated friction and/or pressure to the site of the lesions, such as from manual labor, weight lifting, holding a tennis racket, etc.

PHYSICAL EXAMINATION

- Ill-defined thickened, waxy, yellowish plaque of skin with indistinct skin margins that commonly occurs over the metacarpophalangeal joints and/or the metatarsal heads of the hands and feet, respectively (Fig. 16-1)
- Lesions are usually asymptomatic

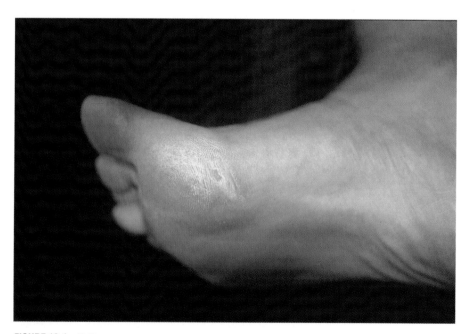

FIGURE 16-1 *Callus.*

DIAGNOSIS

- The diagnosis of calluses is usually made through history and physical examination

DIFFERENTIAL DIAGNOSIS

- Verrucae vulgaris (warts): skin-colored lesions that vary in size and shape and can appear on any cutaneous surface; after paring the lesion, "black dots" representing thrombosed capillaries may be seen on the surface of the lesions
- Corns: small, painful hyperkeratotic lesions that are also usually present on the feet and are secondary to focal pressure; very painful when pressed vertically to the skin, as opposed to warts, which are usually more painful when squeezed between the finger and thumb
- Prurigo nodularis: keratotic flesh-colored to erythematous papules or nodules that occur secondary to chronic picking or scratching of the skin

TREATMENT

- The treatment of calluses is nonemergent
- The primary goals of treatment are attempting to alleviate the mechanical problem and providing symptomatic relief

- Symptomatic relief can be achieved through careful and regular paring of the skin lesions with either a blade, a pumice stone, or another abrasive device
- Salicylic acid preparations that are available over the counter can be used as a keratolytic agent and should be applied once to twice daily as needed; patients should be instructed to apply the acid only on the affected areas of skin, and they should be told that it may cause some irritation; examples include Compound W®, Dr. Scholl's, and DuoFilm®

MANAGEMENT/FOLLOW-UP

- Patients can follow up with either a primary care physician, podiatrist, or dermatologist if they have lesions refractory to the above-mentioned treatments

ICD-9 Code

700

CANDIDIASIS

- Found in immunocompromised, young, or severely debilitated patients, with a characteristic oral or skin eruption
- Predisposing factors include recent antibiotic use, obesity, and diabetes mellitus
- Poorly fitting dentures, vitamin deficiency, and malocclusion may predispose to oral candidiasis, which may present with tender mouth
- Vaginal and vulvovaginal candidiasis may present with thick vaginal discharge along with burning or itching and/or dysuria
  - Rarely, systemic candidiasis may occur with spiking fevers and chills
  - Patients may also have myalgias, arthralgias, bone pain, diarrhea
  - With central nervous system involvement, altered mental status, blurred vision, papilledema, meningismus, nuchal rigidity, and focal neurologic deficits

- Oral candidiasis
  - Oral involvement may consist of acute pseudomembranous candidiasis (thrush) in which discrete white patches resembling milk curds, which become confluent, develop on the buccal mucosa, tongue, palate, and gingival
    - These white patches can be scraped off with a tongue blade, revealing a bright red, sometimes ulcerated, mucosal surface
  - Oral involvement may be in the form of candidal cheilosis or perleche, in which there is erythema and maceration at the angles of the mouth
  - Oral involvement may be in the form of candidal leukoplakia in which an adherent, firm, white plaque with surrounding erythema develops on the buccal mucosa or tongue
  - Oral involvement may be in the form of medial rhomboid glossitis that affects the dorsal surface of the tongue, with atrophy of the central papillae
- Superficial skin candidiasis (Figs. 17-1 and 17-2)
  - Genital involvement may be in the form of vaginal and vulvovaginal candidiasis, in which thick vaginal discharge and white plaques on the vaginal mucosa with surrounding erythema are present
  - Genital involvement may be in the form of balanitis in which small papules or papulopustules develop on the glans penis or coronal sulcus, coalescing into superficial red erosions
  - Intertriginous involvement may present with bright red macerated areas of skin with satellite vesicopustules in the genitocrural, subaxillary, gluteal, or interdigital areas

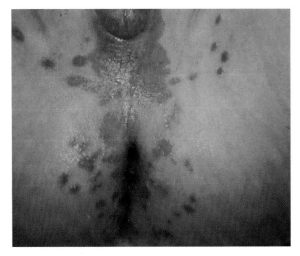

FIGURE 17-1 *Candidiasis.*

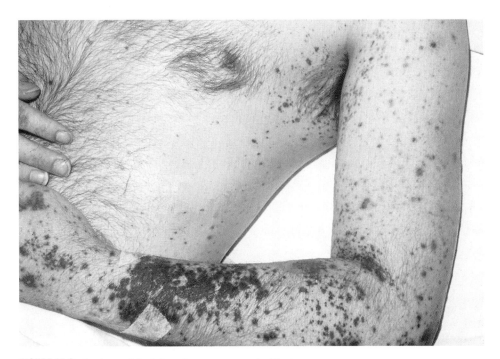

FIGURE 17-2 *Septic candidiasis in an immunocompromised host.*

- Involvement of the periungual tissues (candida paronychia) presents with redness, swelling, and tenderness of the periungual soft tissue, with retraction of the cuticle
  - Note that bacterial paronychia is much more common than candidal paronychia
  - Secondary nail plate alterations may be present in chronic cases
- In systemic candidiasis, 0.5- to 1.0-cm discrete maculopapules, pustules, and/or papulonodules that are often purpuric appear on the trunk and extremities
  - Lesions can be few or many in number, and patients may appear septic
  - Most patients are profoundly immunocompromised

DIAGNOSIS

- In superficial (nonsystemic) candidal infections, the diagnosis can be aided by clinical exam demonstrating characteristic eruption with satellite lesions
- A microscopic examination of vesicle or lesional contents with KOH or vaginal wet preparation demonstrating budding yeast forms with hyphae or pseudohyphae is confirmatory
  - Fungal culture can be performed, but results take days to weeks to obtain
- In systemic candidiasis, skin biopsy for histology and culture is indicated since blood cultures may be negative
  - Body fluids such as urine and cerebrospinal fluid may also be analyzed microscopically and for culture
  - Blood fungal culture

DIFFERENTIAL DIAGNOSIS

- Systemic candidiasis
  - Ecthyma gangrenosum usually presents as a single lesion that had a preceding history of trauma and has remarkable tenderness; patients are usually not immunocompromised

- Other causes of sepsis should be considered including bacterial sepsis, other fungal sepsis, and atypical mycobacterial sepsis
- Superficial candidiasis
  - Intertriginous involvement may present similarly to a number of conditions listed below
    - Dermatophyte (tinea) infections often present with erythematous patches with scale and central clearing
    - The erythema of dermatophyte infections is usually more subtle than candidiasis and lacks satellite pustules
  - Erythrasma is usually found in similar locations of the groin, axillae, or inframammary skin; there are well-marginated irregularly shaped red to brown patches
  - Intertriginous dermatitis is an irritant disease that lacks candidal infection and is in sites of moistness, maceration, and friction and lacks the bright erythema and satellite pustules of candidiasis
  - Psoriasis can uncommonly present in intertriginous areas, has a much slower onset of disease, and lacks satellite pustules
    - Patients often have evidence of more typical plaques of psoriasis elsewhere, such as in their scalp, elbows, and knees
  - Hailey-Hailey disease is a rare, hereditary disease in which the skin in intertriginous areas gets easily superinfected and confluent shallow erosions occur
- Paronychial involvement
  - Bacterial paronychia is much more common than candidal paronychia and is essentially indistinguishable except by microscopic examination of pus or confirmation by bacterial and/or fungal culture

- Oral and genital involvement
  - Mucositis from chemotherapeutic drugs usually presents as multiple oral or anogenital erosions rather than the curd-like exudative lesions in candidiasis
  - Erythema multiforme has vesicles that often coalesce into confluent vesicles, and targetoid lesions are most commonly found as well on the palms, soles, and elsewhere
  - Lichen planus presents as subtle erythematous patches with a lacy appearance to the surface
  - Pemphigus
  - Secondary syphilis
  - Vitamin deficiencies may rarely present with nonspecific erosions that lack curd-like exudate
  - Leukoplakia is a chronic condition of the mouth in which one sees white patches with adherent scales that cannot be scraped away with a tongue blade

TREATMENT

- Systemic involvement should be managed by intravenous amphotericin B and requires hospital admission
- Paronychia
  - Topical antifungal solution
  - Four percent thymol in absolute alcohol
  - Oral ketoconazole or fluconazole
- Vaginal involvement
  - Topical antifungal creams and lotions (butoconazole, terconazole, tioconazole, miconazole, clotrimazole)

- Fluconazole 150 mg one dose
- Clotrimazole 500 mg vaginal suppository one dose
- Intertrigo
  - Topical antifungal creams and lotions (butoconazole, terconazole, tioconazole, miconazole, clotrimazole)
  - Miconazole or nystatin powder
- Oral involvement
  - Nystatin suspension (400,000 to 600,000 U) held in the mouth and then swallowed qid
  - Clotrimazole troches (10 mg dissolved in the mouth five times/day)
  - Itraconazole (Sporanox®) 200 mg/day for 1 to 2 weeks (adults)
  - Fluconazole (Diflucan®) 50 to 100 mg q day for 1 week (adults)

MANAGEMENT/FOLLOW-UP

- For skin or anogenital involvement, follow-up with a primary care physician or dermatologist in the next week is recommended
- All systemic candidal diseases require admission with appropriate treatment

ICD-9 Codes

112.0	Oral Candidiasis
112.1	Valvovaginal Candidiasis
112.2	Candidal balanitis
112.3	Skin and Nails
112.5	Systemic candidiasis

CAPILLARY HEMANGIOMA OF INFANCY

- A newborn presents with a caregiver complaining about a rapidly enlarging vascular nodule
- Lesions are present at birth in 25% cases and by 4 weeks in 88% cases
- Sixty percent of single lesions are on the head and neck, 25% on the trunk, and 15% on the extremities
- The natural history is for rapid growth lasting 3 to 9 months followed by a plateau phase for months to several years, followed by a phase of gradual involution
  - Complete resolution in 50% to 60% by 5 years of age, in 75% by age 7, and in 90% by age 9
  - More than 40% of patients experience irreversible cutaneous changes after involution including scarring, hypopigmentation, atrophy, telangiectasias, or fibrofatty tissue
- Large rapidly growing or involuting hemangiomas may ulcerate, bleed, or become infected
- Proliferating hemangiomas may obstruct or compromise critical structures
  - Nasal passage hemangiomas may obstruct the respiratory tract
  - Lesions of the oropharynx or subglottic areas may cause feeding and/or breathing difficulty
  - Obstruction of the orbit can lead to amblyopia
  - Lesions in the parotid area can cause conductive hearing loss
- Kasabach-Merritt syndrome can occur in large, rapidly growing hemangiomas, usually of the trunk or extremities, in which platelets become trapped within the hemangioma
  - The overlying skin may demonstrate petechiae and purpura, and patients may develop severe thrombocytopenia
- Associated structural abnormalities rarely occur
  - The acronym PHACE has been proposed to represent abnormalities associated with large cervicofacial hemangiomas, which include *p*osterior fossa malformations (including the Dandy-Walker malformations), *h*emangioma, *a*rterial abnormalities (persistent embryonic vessels and absence of ipsilateral carotid/vertebral vessels), *c*oarctation of (a right-sided) aortic arch, and *e*ye abnormalities (microphthalmia, congenital cataract, optic nerve hypoplasia)

- Soft, bright red to deep purple vascular nodule (Fig. 18-1)
- Superficial lesions are more red, whereas deeper tumors are more purple and lobulated and firmer
- Most commonly on the head and neck
- As the lesion ages, it changes color from bright crimson to dull faded red; as involution begins, graying is first noted in the center that spreads centrifugally

- Forty percent of patients are left with a skin abnormality after involution, including telangiectasia, atrophy, scarring, or hypopigmentation
- Large, tense hemangiomas should lead to suspicion of platelet trapping, especially if other signs of thrombocytopenia are present
- Patients with lumbosacral hemangiomas should be investigated by magnetic resonance imaging (MRI) for underlying spinal dysraphism

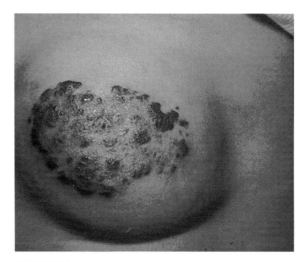

FIGURE 18-1 *Hemangioma.*

- Clinical exam
- MRI for distinction between hemangiomas and other neoplasms such as vascular malformations, meningoceles, and dermoid cysts

DIFFERENTIAL DIAGNOSIS

- Diffuse neonatal hemangiomatosis: presents as multiple cutaneous hemangiomas in association with visceral hemangiomas, usually the gastrointestinal tract and liver Serious systemic sequelae may result in a mortality rate of 80% of untreated cases
- Benign neonatal hemangiomatosis: presents as multiple cutaneous hemangiomas without systemic involvement and results in uncomplicated involution
- Lymphatic malformations: generally presents with nonerythematous growing papules or nodules
- Pyogenic granuloma: these lesions are rapidly growing and small (usually less than 1 cm), and they bleed easily

TREATMENT

- Treatment for all capillary hemangiomas is nonemergent unless there is uncontrolled bleeding
- Most hemangiomas spontataneously involute, so no treatment is necessary

- Flash-lamp pulse dye laser may decrease the proliferation of early capillary hemangiomas but does not help those lesions with a deep component
- Intralesional glucocorticoid (triamcinolone 3 to 5 mg/kg every 4 to 6 weeks) for small (1 to 2 cm) hemangiomas in critical areas such as the lip or nasal tip
  - Retrobulbar hematoma and microvascular embolism resulting in blindness has been reported from periocular intralesional injection
- Systemic corticosteroids may be used if coagulopathy, functional impairment, or involvement of vital structures are seen
  - Prednisolone or prednisone at 2 to 3 mg/kg per day is given orally and continued at a tapering dose for 1 to several months depending on the age of the patient
  - One-third of hemangiomas treated in this fashion do not respond
- Life-threatening lesions can be treated with subcutaneous injection of interferon-2α and -2β, 3 million units/m^2 per day, for 6 to 12 months
  - Spastic diplegia develops in 5% to 10% of treated infants
- Surgical excision for excess fibrofatty tissue after the involutional phase
  - Early surgical intervention is also warranted in certain situations

- The primary care physician needs to follow the progress of lesions in noncritical locations
- Any lesion obstructing a vital function requires follow-up with their primary care physician and specialist (e.g., ophthalmologist for eye involvement)

- Forty percent of patients are left with skin abnormality after involution, including telangiectasia, atrophy, scarring, or hypopigmentation

ICD-9 Code

228.01

CHAPTER 19

CELLULITIS AND ERYSIPELAS

HISTORY

- Patient reports localized pain, redness, and swelling in an area of skin arising over a period of a few days
- Patient may report systemic symptoms, including fevers, chills, nausea, vomiting, and/or malaise
- Patient may have had an underlying skin disease or recent trauma to the skin allowing for a portal of entry for various organisms causing cellulitis and erysipelas
- Cellulitis is an acute, spreading infection of dermal and subcutaneous tissues most commonly caused by *Staphylococcus aureus* and group A beta-hemolytic *Streptococcus pyogenes*
- Erysipelas is a distinct type of superficial cutaneous cellulitis caused by group A beta-hemolytic *Streptococcus pyogenes*

PHYSICAL EXAMINATION

- Erythematous, warm, edematous, tender areas of skin with borders that are more defined in erysipelas than in cellulitis (Fig. 19-1)

- Most common site in adults is the lower extremity and in children the head and neck
- The involved area of skin may have superimposed vesicles, bullae, erosions, hemorrhage, and/or necrosis; regional lymphadenopathy may be present (Fig. 19-2)
- A portal of entry may be evident, including sites of trauma, surgical wounds, and areas of underlying dermatoses (e.g., dermatophytosis; Fig. 19-3)
- Patient may appear ill, with fever, anorexia, and dehydration

DIAGNOSIS

- Diagnosis is usually made by history and physical exam
- White blood count may be elevated; blood cultures should be performed if patient appears ill
- Specific organism causing the infection may be identified via needle aspirate culture or tissue culture

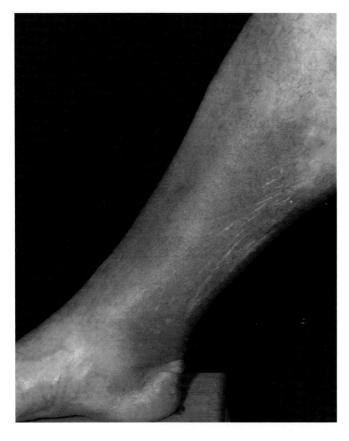

FIGURE 19-1 *Erysipelas.*

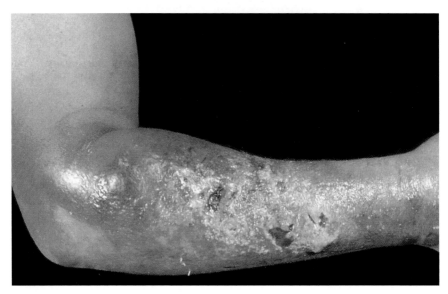

FIGURE 19-2 *Cellulitis following puncture trauma.*

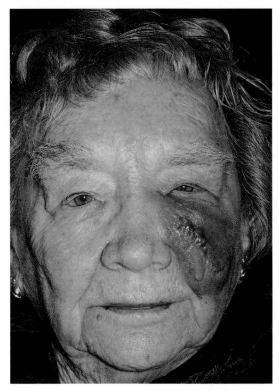

FIGURE 19-3 *Cellulitis at site of surgical excision.*

- Deep vein thrombosis: an acute thrombosis of a vein in the deep venous system that causes symptoms similar to those of a cellulitis, including pain, edema, and erythema; Doppler ultrasound should be performed if a deep vein thrombosis is suspected
- Stasis dermatitis: inflammation of the skin of the lower extremities occurring secondary to venous stasis and increased capillary pressure; associated with edema, erythema, hyperpigmentation, erosions/ulcerations, and chronic fibrotic changes of the skin and subcutaneous tissue (lipodermatosclerosis)

- Contact dermatitis (allergic or irritant): acute or chronic inflammatory reaction to agents that come into contact with the skin
  - Acute: well-demarcated plaques of erythema, edema, and vesicles often with superimposed erosions and crusting
  - Chronic: erythematous and lichenified plaques with scale
  - Arranged in linear or bizarre patterns, indicating an exogenous etiology
- Necrotizing fasciitis: starts with painful erythema and induration that rapidly develops overlying black eschar; malodorous necrotic tissue develops and surgical debridement

- Erysipelas and/or cellulitis should be treated promptly to prevent bacteremia and/or sepsis
- Treatment will depend on the infecting organism and the immune status of the patient
  - Erysipelas
    - Mild cases of erysipelas can be treated on an outpatient basis with oral penicillin V, 250 to 500 mg every 6 hours for 10 days; penicillin-allergic individuals can be treated with erythromycin 250 to 500 mg po every 6 hours
    - Patients with underlying medical problems such as diabetes mellitus or patients with more extensive streptococcal infections should be hospitalized and treated with intravenous aqueous penicillin G (600,000 to 2 million units every 6 hours); penicillin-allergic individuals can be treated with IV vancomycin
  - Cellulitis
    - Mild cases of cellulitis can be treated on an outpatient basis with oral antibiotics, as follows:

Non–penicillinase-producing *Staphylococcus aureus*: oral penicillin V or erythromycin, as discussed above
Penicillinase-producing *S. aureus*: oral dicloxacillin 500 mg bid for 10 days
Methicillin-resistant *S. aureus*: intravenous vancomycin

- For an ill patient in whom a staphylococcal etiology is suspected, a penicillinase-resistant semisynthetic penicillin, like nafcillin 1.0 to 1.5 g IV q4h, should be employed; penicillin-allergic patients can be treated with vancomycin, 1.0 to 1.5 g IV daily
- Other etiologies:

Haemophilus influenzae: common bacteria causing head and neck cellulitis in children under the age of 2; most common in periorbital area; treat with cefotaxime or ceftriaxone; in severely immunocompromised patients, organisms such as *Pseudomonas aeruginosa, Mycobacterium fortuitum* complex, *Cryptococcus neoformans, Pasteurella multocida, Proteus mirabilis,* and *Escherichia coli* should be considered

- Patients treated with antibiotics on an outpatient basis should be seen within a week by a primary care physician or a dermatologist for follow-up

ICD-9 Code

035 Erysipelas
682.9 Cellulitis

CHANCROID

- The chief complaint is a painful ulcer or ulcers usually occurring on the external genitalia
  - Patients may also complain of lesions that can occur at other sites of inoculation, such as the mouth, fingers, or breast
- Patients may report a history of unprotected sexual activity within a week of onset of the ulcer
- Patients may complain of symptoms of painful regional lymphadenopathy

- A tender erythematous papule first appears that evolves into a pustule, erosion, and then an ulcer (Fig. 20-1)
- The most common location is the external genitalia, but the vaginal wall, cervix, and perianal areas should be examined as well (Figs. 20-2 and 20-3)
  - Involvement of other sites occasionally occurs, including fingers, breast, oral mucosa, and thighs
- The or ulcers are tender and have sharp, undermined borders with a friable gray-yellow base of granulation tissue
- Ulcers often merge to form large ulcers with a serpiginous shape
- Painful inguinal unilateral lymphadenopathy occurs in 50% of patients within 1 to 2 weeks of the onset of the primary lesion

- The diagnosis is a clinical one, supported by laboratory evidence of the gram-negative bacillus *Haemophilus ducreyi*
- Gram's stain of exudates from the ulcer base may show parallel chains of gram-negative bacilli ("school of fish" pattern)
- Culture is required for definitive diagnosis; such cultures require special growth media

- Herpes simplex virus: tends to present with an erythematous base with grouped, painful, umbilicated vesiculopustules
- Primary syphilis: most commonly presents with an asymptomatic, indurated chancre
- Lymphogranuloma venereum: has a painless, nonindurated superficial ulcer in association with painful regional lymphedenopathy
- Granuloma inguinale: presents with one or more painless nodules in the genital areas
- Erythema multiforme: this reaction pattern is often associated with constitutional symptoms, a typical rash of targetoid lesions, and involvement of other mucosal sites such as the oral mucosa and conjunctivae
- Aphthous ulcers: these painful ulcers of the oral or genital mucosa can mimic chancroid, but aphthous ulcers tend to be shallower and have no associated lymphadenopathy

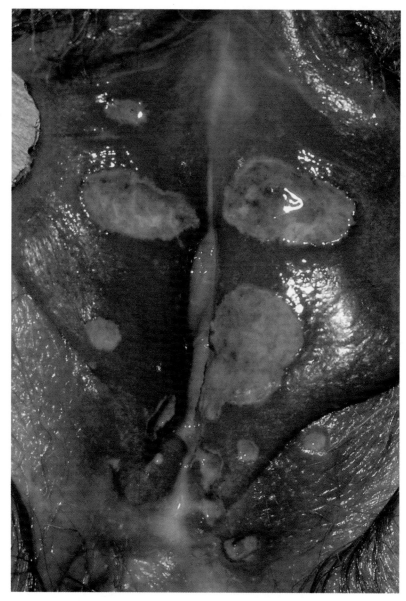

FIGURE 20-1 *Chancroid.*

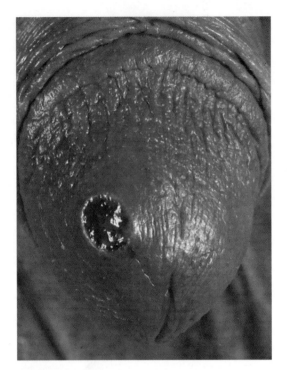

FIGURE 20-2 *Sharply circumscribed ulcer on the glans.*

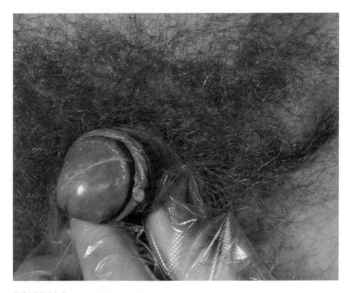

FIGURE 20-3 *Small chancroid ulcer*

CHANCROID

- Crohn's disease: this inflammatory bowel disease may present ulcers that are usually linear and resemble lacerations
- Hidradenitis supparativa: this chronic condition presents with multiple tender nodules associated with scarring and draining sinus tracts in the axilla, inframammary areas, and groin

- Patients should be treated promptly to prevent spread of the infection to others
- Antimicrobial therapy
  ◦ Azithromycin 1 g po in a single dose, or
  ◦ Ceftriaxone 250 mg IM in a single dose, or
  ◦ Erythromycin 500 mg po qid for 10 days

- Other factors
  ◦ Consider discussion of condom use to prevent spread of the infection to others
  ◦ Sexual partners should be seen for evaluation and treatment
  ◦ Consider testing the patient for HIV

- Patients should be seen by a primary care physician or dermatologist within 1 to 2 weeks of treatment

ICD-9 Code

099.0

CHAPTER 21

CHRONIC ULCERS OF THE LEG

- Venous ulcers
  - Patients complain of ulcers that have usually been present for weeks to months on the lower extremities
  - The ulcers are often found in a setting of stasis changes, and patients complain of chronic swelling and aching of their lower extremities that improve with elevation of the legs
  - Stasis dermatitis may also be present, with an itchy red rash over the affected extremities, as well as weeping vesicles
- Arterial ulcers
  - Patients complain of ulcers that have been present for weeks to months over the lower extremities
  - The ulcers are found in the setting of atherosclerotic disease, and patients complain of intermittent claudication and pain on exertion, with eventual development of pain at rest
  - The pain may worsen with elevation of the legs
- Neuropathic ulcers
  - Ulcers of the lower extremities found in the setting of peripheral neuropathy such as in a patient who has had diabetes mellitus for many years
  - Symptoms of peripheral neuropathy (paresthesias, pain, numbness) make patients unaware of trauma to their lower extremities; thus repeated injury leads to the ulcer

- Venous ulcers
  - The lower extremities may be either edematous (early disease) or fibrotic (chronic disease; Figs. 21-1 to 21-4)
  - The background skin often has changes of stasis dermatitis, with an erythematous eruption early in disease that then progresses to red-brown macules and papules
  - The ulcers are usually found on the medial side of the lower legs, although any portion of the lower legs may be involved
  - The ulcers begin superficially and may progress if left untreated
  - Cellulitis may complicate all leg ulcer diseases
  - Pedal pulses are usually strong and the feet are warm with good capillary refill
- Arterial ulcers
  - Ischemia for arterial disease leads to hair loss on lower legs and feet, shiny atrophic skin, cool extremities, and poor capillary refill of the digits
  - Pedal pulses are very weak
  - The ulcer appears as a punched-out, sharply demarcated lesion with minimal exudates
- Neuropathic ulcers
  - The feet are usually warm and dry with palpable pulses, but the area surrounding the ulcer and beyond is often numb
  - The ulcers are commonly surrounded by thick callus and are usually located at pressure sites, especially the heels, metatarsal head, and great toe

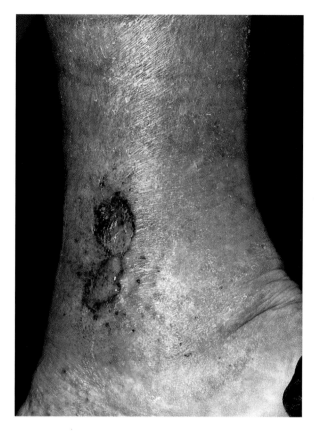

FIGURE 21-1 *Venous insufficiency.*

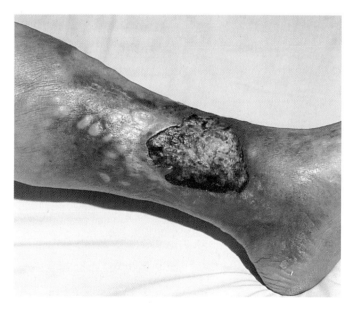

FIGURE 21-2 *Large venous ulcer.*

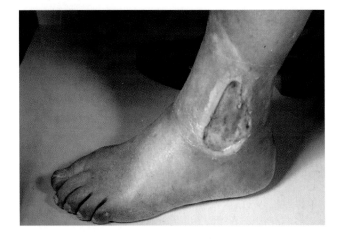

FIGURE 21-3 *Ischemic ulcer.*

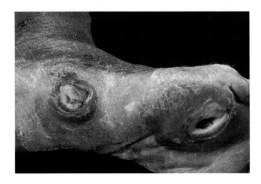

FIGURE 21-4 *Two neurotropic ulcers.*

- The diagnosis of the three types of leg ulcers can usually be made by history and physical examination

DIFFERENTIAL DIAGNOSIS

- Infections: bacterial, viral, fungal, and atypical mycobacteria can cause leg ulceration, but clues to the presence of such infection are readily gleaned by physical examination
- Tumors: squamous cell carcinoma, basal cell carcinoma, and lymphoma (skin biopsy to confirm)
- Pressure ulcer: ulcers that develop over bony prominences as a result of external pressure and/or friction on the skin causing tissue necrosis
- Vasculitis: ulcers found in an area of palpable purpura, necrosis, and/or a livedo reticularis pattern (violaceous discoloration of the skin in a net-like pattern); may be isolated to the skin or associated with systemic vasculitis
- Pyoderma gangrenosum: begins as a nodule or hemorrhagic pustule and rapidly evolves to form an ulcer; borders of the ulcer are characteristic, with undermined, raised, boggy edges; base of the ulcer displays hemorrhagic exudates
- Calciphylaxis: lesions present as erythematous, tender nodules and plaques overlying a livedo pattern of erythema on abdomen, buttocks, and/or lower extremities; extensive ischemia that progresses to necrosis, ulceration, and gangrene occurs; eschar often overlies the subcutaneous lesions

- General measures to improve wound healing should be taken, such as smoking cessation, treatment of diabetes, weight reduction, and correction of anemia or malnutrition
- Treat any secondary infections (*Staphylococcus aureus* most common)
  ○ Dicloxacillin: 500 mg bid for 10 days (adults); 12.5 to 25 mg/kg/day in children <40 kg
  ○ Cephalexin (Keflex®): 500 mg bid for 10 days (adults); 25 to 50 mg/kg/day in children
  ○ *Penicillin-allergic*: erythromycin 500 mg bid for 10 days (adults); 40 mg/kg/day for 10 days (children)
- Venous stasis
  ○ The treatment of venous stasis ulcers is nonemergent
  ○ However, infection is a common complication that can be reduced if prompt treatment is performed
  ○ The mainstay of treatment for underlying venous stasis is the use of elastic support stockings, which should be worn on a daily basis while the patient is awake
  ○ Ulcers are managed by applying dressings to cover the wound and to prevent external damage
    - DuoDerm® or similar hydrocolloid dressings can be applied to wounds with mild to moderate exudates

A second sticky dressing or tape is required for adhesion
The dressing and the wound exudates often create a foul-smelling odor and a yellow gel over the wound
The dressing should be changed approximately every 3 days

    - Lyofoam® can be applied to wounds with severe exudates

A second sticky dressing or tape is required for adhesion
The dressing should be changed approximately every 3 days

- The surrounding skin that is affected by stasis dermatitis changes should be treated with topical corticosteroids to decrease inflammation
    - A mid-potency topical corticosteroid may be applied to the affected area bid for 2 weeks; should not be applied to the ulcer itself, or the face, axillae, or groin
    - Mid-potency: triamcinolone (Aristocort®) 0.1% ointment or cream
    - Emphasize that the principal side effect of prolonged use of corticosteroids is skin atrophy
- Arterial ulcers
  ○ Methods to improve atherosclerotic disease should be taken, including cessation of smoking, hypertension and diabetes control, weight reduction, increasing exercise, and blood lipid control
  ○ Ulcers can be treated with dressings similar to those listed above
  ○ Surgical reconstruction and/or bypass of occluded arteries may be required for refractory ulcers
- Neuropathic ulcers
  ○ Special shoes and/or plaster casts can help to redistribute weight off of pressure points
  ○ Surgical debridement may be required
  ○ Imaging may be required to rule out osteomyelitis

MANAGEMENT/FOLLOW-UP

- Any patient with a chronic leg ulcer should be seen by either a primary care physician or a dermatologist within a few weeks to assess progress with treatment

ICD-9 Code

454.0 Stasis ulcer
707.9 Miscellaneous ulcer
707.0 Pressure ulcer

CHAPTER 22

CONDYLOMA ACUMINATUM (GENITAL WART)

- Genital warts that are usually asymptomatic and have been present for months to years
- Although they are commonly sexually transmitted, they may be transmitted to infants during delivery or through other nonsexual contact

- Verrucous, filiform, or flat-topped papules and tumors present on external genitalia and/or perianal area of both males and females (Figs. 22-1 to 22-3)
- Color is usually skin-colored, brown, or red
- May be solitary or grouped into cauliflower-like clusters
- One can examine the area after soaking it in 5% acetic acid solution to help visualize subclinical lesions; however, there are many false-positive results using this technique

- Diagnosis is usually made by clinical exam
- A skin biopsy is rarely required

- Condyloma lata (secondary syphilis): soft, flat-topped pink to tan papules on the perineum and perianal areas; the patient may or may not report a history of primary syphilis; the patient may have other features of secondary syphilis
- Pearly penile papules: small angiofibromas found on the glans penis; they appear as skin-colored to pink, 1-mm papules arranged circumferentially around the corona and are a normal variant
- Angiokeratomas: multiple small blood vessel tumors occurring on scrotum and labia majora; asymptomatic 1- to 2-mm violaceous papules that do not blanch; no therapy required
- Lichen planus: flat-topped violaceous polygonal papules or annular lesions; may be associated with oral mucosal lesions as well
- Molluscum contagiosum: dome-shaped papules with a central keratotic plug that may be located on external genitalia, suprapubic area, or inner thighs
- Other: squamous cell carcinomas, scabies, or skin tags

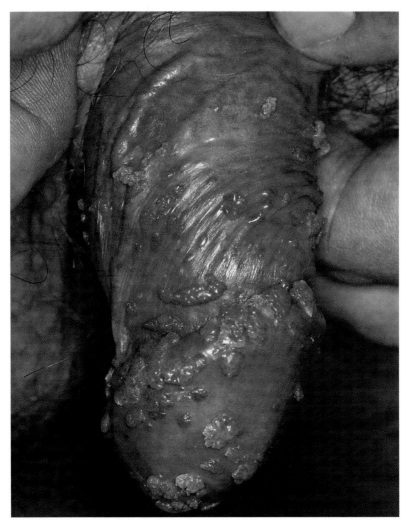

FIGURE 22-1 *Condylomata acuminata: penis.*

- Treatment of condyloma acuminata is non-emergent
- Prompt treatment and education are recommended to prevent the spread of infection to others
- Patient education
  - The cause of genital warts is the human papillomavirus (HPV), of which there are many types
  - Some types of HPV that cause genital warts are also known to cause cervical dysplasia and cervical, vulvar, penile, and anal squamous cell carcinoma
  - HPV infection probably persists throughout a patient's lifetime and becomes active and infectious intermittently
  - Treatment of condyloma acuminata generally is to remove the exophytic lesions, thus decreasing the chance of transmission

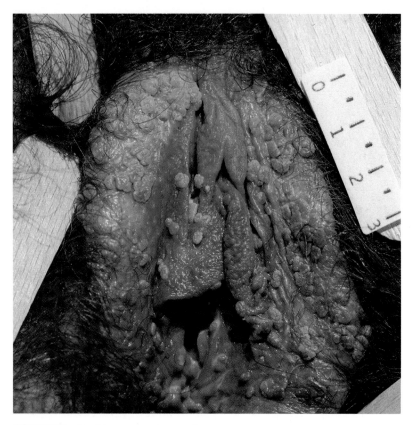

FIGURE 22-2 *Condylomata acuminata: vulva.*

- However, HPV is probably not eradi-
  cated; thus condom use is recommended to reduce the risk of transmission to others
- Medical/surgical treatment
  - Destruction by cryosurgery, trichloro-
    acetic acid, or excision
    - These are painful but effective ap-
      proaches
    - Patients should be forewarned that
      blistering, redness, and irritation are
      likely to occur following treatment
  - Podofilox (Condylox®)
    - A 0.5% solution or gel applied on an
      outpatient basis
    - Should be applied with a cotton swab
      to affected areas bid for 3 consecu-
      tive days of the week, repeating
      weekly as needed
    - May cause some irritation but is not
      painful when applied
  - This medication can be used in con-
    junction with destructive therapies
  - Contraindicated in pregnancy
  - Podophyllin
    - This solution is applied in the office
      by a physician; it is never prescribed
      for home use
    - The clinician applies the product di-
      rectly to the wart using a cotton swab
      and the patient washes the product
      off in 1 to 4 hours
    - This medication can be used in con-
      junction with destructive therapies
    - Patients may experience blistering,
      redness, and irritation after treatment
    - Contraindicated in pregnancy
  - Imiquimod (Aldara®)
    - A 5% cream that functions as an
      immune response modifier
    - Applied at home bid for 3 days per
      week for 1 to 4 months

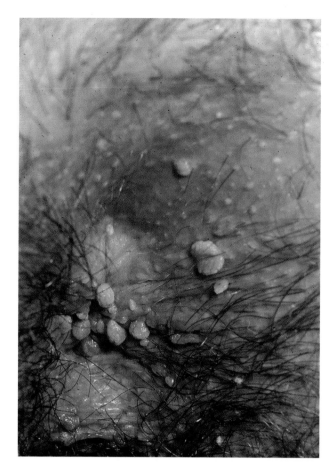

FIGURE 22-3 *Condylomata acuminata: perianal.*

- May cause local irritation, but the cream does not elicit pain when applied
- This medication can be used in conjunction with destructive therapies

MANAGEMENT/FOLLOW-UP

- Patients not treated for their genital warts should be encouraged to seek treatment with a primary care physician, gynecologist, or dermatologist within 1 to 2 weeks
- Treated patients should be followed up by a primary care physician, gynecologist, or dermatologist within 4 weeks of treatment
  - All patients undergoing treatment on an outpatient basis should be encouraged to follow up as well

- All women with genital warts should make an appointment with a primary care physician or gynecologist for a complete pelvic examination, including a Pap smear
- Consider testing patients for the human immunodeficiency virus

ICD-9 Code

078.11

CPT Codes.

46900	Anal chemical destruction
46916	Anal cryosurgical destruction
54050	Penis chemical destruction
54056	Penis cryosurgical destruction
54065	Penis destruction, any method
56501	Vulva destruction

CONTACT DERMATITIS

HISTORY

- Contact dermatitis is an acute or chronic inflammatory reaction to a substance that comes into contact with the skin and is either allergic or irritant in nature
- Both types of contact dermatitis can resemble each other clinically, so the history becomes critical in distinguishing the two conditions
- *Allergic* contact dermatitis is a delayed hypersensitivity response; thus, in the acute setting, lesions usually do not arise until 48 to 72 hours after exposure
- Acute *irritant* contact dermatitis often occurs within a few hours after exposure
- Acute contact dermatitis is characterized by pruritic lesions that have been present for days to weeks
- Chronic contact dermatitis is characterized by pruritic lesions that wax and wane or persist for months to years
- Patients may or may not recall a history of exposure to allergens or irritants that have come into contact with the skin

PHYSICAL EXAMINATION

- Lesions arranged in "artificial" patterns, indicate an exogenous etiology; linear streaks are often present (Figs. 23-1 to 23-3)
- Lesions may be localized to one area (e.g., from shoe dermatitis) or may be generalized (e.g., plant dermatitis)
- Acute contact dermatitis: well-demarcated erythematous and edematous plaques with superimposed vesicles, serum, and crust
  - Acute airborne contact dermatitis appears according to where the airborne contactant made contact with the skin, especially the face and neck
- Chronic contact dermatitis: lichenified papules and plaques (epidermal thickening with accentuated skin lines), often with superimposed excoriations
  - Postinflammatory pigment changes often present as well

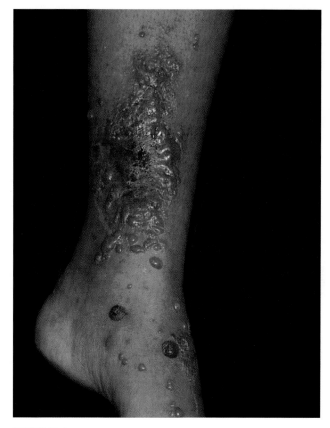

FIGURE 23-1 *Acute dermatitis due to poison ivy.*

- If an allergen is suspected of inducing an allergic contact dermatitis reaction:
  - There may or may not be a good history of exposure to plants, new cosmetics or toiletries, cleaning compounds, or other allergens
  - Some of these others include neomycin (contained within Neosporin® and other topical antibiotics), nickel (metals, jewelry), thiurams (rubber), and formalin (cosmetics and toiletries, plastics)
  - If the diagnosis is clear but the contactant cannot be identified, patch testing can be performed by an experienced physician who applies the allergen to any area of normal skin

DIFFERENTIAL DIAGNOSIS

- Herpes simplex virus: grouped vesicles on an erythematous base on either keratinized skin or mucosal surfaces
  - Patients with primary herpes often have constitutional symptoms; recurrent herpes presents with lesions similar to the primary infection but less intense

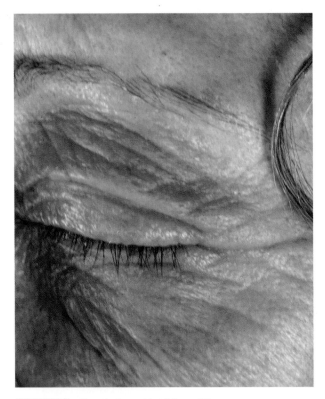

FIGURE 23-2 *Chronic dermatitis of the eyelids.*

- Atopic dermatitis: poorly defined erythematous patches and plaques that usually begin in early infancy; adult onset is rare
  - Acute lesions appear edematous; chronic lesions appear thickened with accentuation of skin markings (lichenified)
  - Often this condition is seen in association with hay fever and asthma
- Dermatophyte infection: scaly erythematous plaques affecting the skin of the body that can be confirmed by KOH preparation examination
- Seborrheic dermatitis: a chronic dermatosis associated with redness and scaling on areas where sebaceous glands are prominent, such as the scalp (dandruff), face, and chest
  - Lesions are yellowish red, greasy scaling macules and papules of various sizes

- Mycosis fungoides: a chronic cutaneous T-cell lymphoma that presents with scaly patches, plaques, and tumors that may be located on any cutaneous surface
- Psoriasis: inflammatory skin disease characterized by thick, erythematous papules and plaques with silvery scales; pruritus is common
  - Sites of psoriatic predilection include the elbows, knees, scalp, ears, umbilicus, and gluteal cleft
- Pityriasis rosea: erythematous to pink scaly papules and plaques classically in a "Christmas tree" distribution over the trunk
  - Pityriasis rosea begins with a herald patch that is slightly larger than the other lesions

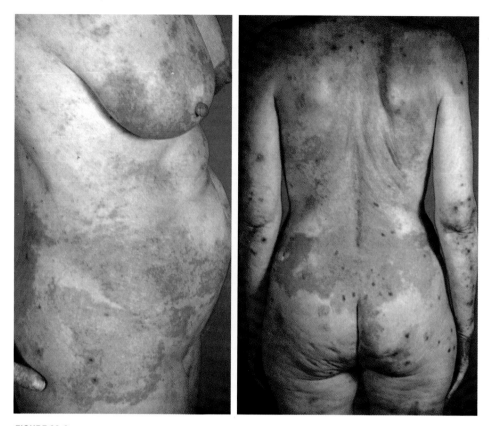

FIGURE 23-3 *Systemic contact dermatitis due to balsam of Peru. The eruption cleared when the patient was place on a balsam-free diet.*

- This is self-limited eruption that sponta-neously regresses in 6 to 12 weeks
- Secondary syphilis
  - Erythematous and hyperkeratotic scaly plaques located on trunk, extremities, palms, and soles
  - Patient may report a history of a "chan-cre" (ulcer of primary syphilis) in the previous 2 to 10 weeks
  - Condyloma lata: soft, flat-topped pink to tan papules on the perineum and perianal areas

TREATMENT

- The treatment of contact dermatitis is non-emergent; however, the itching associated with acute contact dermatitis can be quite devastating to the patient; thus treatment should be given promptly
- Identification and removal of the offending agent is most important
- Localized lesions can be treated with topical corticosteroids: a mid-potency to super-high-potency topical corticosteroid may be applied to the lesions bid for 2 weeks; should not be applied to the face, axillae, or groin
  - Mid-potency: prednicarbate (Dermatop®) 0.1% ointment or cream; triamcinolone acetonide (Aristocort®) 0.1% ointment or cream
  - High-potency: fluocinonide (Lidex®) 0.05% ointment or cream, clobetasol propionate (Temovate®) 0.05% ointment or cream; halobetasol propionate (Ultra-vate®) 0.05% ointment or cream
  - Although topical corticosteroids are indicated for use for a few weeks, em-phasize the side effects of prolonged use of corticosteroids such as skin atrophy
- In severe cases, systemic corticosteroids may be indicated; prednisone can be given at 1 mg/kg, tapering slowly over a period of 1 to 3 weeks
- Oozing, vesicular lesions can be treated with wet dressings and drying solutions, such as Burow's solution (Domeboro®—available over the counter)
- Sedating night time oral antihistamines can be used to improve patients' sleep and decrease the amount of time they scratch during the night
  - Hydroxyzine (Atarax®, Vistaril®): 10 to 50 mg prn sleep (adults); hydroxyzine 0.3 mg/kg/day of 10 mg/5 ml suspen-sion (children)

- Diphenhydramine (Benadryl®): 25 to 50 mg prn sleep (adults); 0.3 mg/kg/day of 10 mg/5 ml suspension (children)
- Treat any secondary infections (*Staphylococcus aureus* most common)
  - Dicloxacillin: 500 mg bid for 10 days (adults); 12.5 to 25 mg/kg/day in children <40 kg
  - Cephalexin (Keflex®): 500 mg bid for 10 days (adults); 25 to 50 mg/kg/day in children
  - *Penicillin-allergic*: erythromycin 500 mg bid for 10 days (adults); 40 mg/kg/day for 10 days (children)

MANAGEMENT/FOLLOW-UP

- Patients who are treated with topical or oral corticosteroids should be followed up by a primary care physician or a dermatologist in 2 weeks to assess progress
- Patients who require patch testing should be evaluated by a physician trained to perform the tests

ICD-9 Code

692.9

CHAPTER 24

CORNS

- Painful lesions that occur on the feet or the hands, usually over bony prominences
- Lesions have usually been present for months or years
- Patients may relate a history of wearing tight-fitting and/or high-heeled shoes with repeated rubbing or pressure over a specific bony prominence

- Well-demarcated, painful, hyperkeratotic lesion that is usually present over a bony prominence, especially on the foot (Fig. 24-1)
- Most common site for corns is over the metatarsal heads, although the sides of the arches, the heels, and the dorsum of the foot can be involved as well

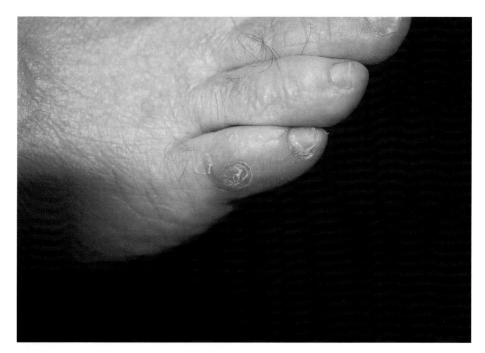

FIGURE 24-1 *Corn.*

- Soft corns appear different from hard corns, in that they are usually found between the fourth and fifth toes and appear macerated

- Diagnosis is made by history and clinical examination

- Verrucae vulgaris (warts): skin-colored lesions that vary in size and shape and can appear on any cutaneous surface; paring the lesion may reveal "black dots" representing thrombosed capillaries
- Callus: lesions that usually are present on the hands or feet and represent a response to chronic rubbing rather than focal pressure; appears as an ill-defined area of waxy, yellow thickening over which the skin markings may become indistinct
- Prurigo nodularis: keratotic flesh-colored to erythematous papules or nodules that occur secondary to chronic picking or scratching of the skin

- The treatment of corns is nonemergent
- The primary goals of treatment are to attempt to alleviate the mechanical problem and to provide symptomatic relief
- Symptomatic relief can be achieved through careful and regular paring of the skin lesion with either a blade, a pumice stone, or another abrasive device
- Salicylic acid preparations that are available over the counter can be used as a keratolytic agent and should be applied once to twice daily as needed; patients should be instructed to apply the acid only on the affected areas of skin, and they should be told that it may cause some irritation; examples include Compound W®, Dr. Scholl's, and DuoFilm®

- Patients can follow up with either a primary care physician, podiatrist, or dermatologist if they have lesions refractory to the above-mentioned treatments

ICD-9 Code

700

CHAPTER 25

DERMATOMYOSITIS

HISTORY

- Insidious development of muscle weakness
  - Severity of muscle weakness can range from nonexistent (dermatositis sine mysositis) to severe
  - Symmetric proximal muscle weakness of the shoulder and pelvic girdles is most commonly seen
    - The muscle weakness may be so profound as to be totally incapacitating
  - Dysphagia from esophageal dysfunction may occur
- Characteristic skin eruption preceding the myositis by weeks to years
  - Cutaneous eruption exacerbated by sunlight
- Associated with underlying neoplasm in some cases, including ovarian carcinoma, thymoma, and multiple myeloma
- Chronic fluctuating course is usual, although rapid progression in malignancy-associated and childhood cases is seen

PHYSICAL EXAMINATION

- Muscle examination
  - Symmetric proximal muscle weakness of the shoulder and pelvic girdles most commonly observed with muscle testing
  - Gait may be abnormal
- Skin examination is characterized by:
  - Heliotrope rash—edematous, violaceous periorbital eruption pathognomonic
  - Gottron's papules—red to violaceous, flat-topped, sometimes telangiectatic papules on the dorsal knuckles (Fig. 25-1)
  - Poikilodermatous eruption or the combination of hypopigmented and hyperpigmented skin with telangiectasia with atrophy
  - Raynaud's phenomenon
  - Thickness and roughness of the cuticles with erythema or telangiectasia at the base of the finger nails
  - Sausage-like fingers
  - Scalp involvement with red scaly plaques, sometimes with alopecia
  - Calcinosis cutis

DIAGNOSIS

- The diagnosis is primarily clinical, with confirmation by laboratory tests, including:
  - Elevated serum muscle enzymes (creatine kinase, aldolase, and lactate dehydrogenase)
  - Electromyographic abnormalities
  - Abnormal muscle biopsy histopathologic findings
  - Antinuclear antibodies in most patients, especially to Jo-1
  - Elevated erythrocyte sedimentation rate
  - Myoglobulinuria or creatinuria
  - A skin biopsy specimen demonstrating interface dermatitis

DIFFERENTIAL DIAGNOSIS

- Other collagen vascular diseases, especially lupus erythematosus; lupus does not commonly demonstrate Gottron's sign, muscle weakness, and a heliotrope rash

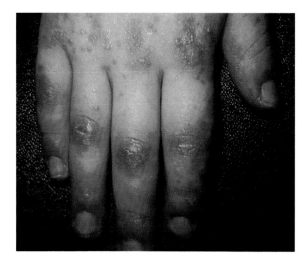

FIGURE 25-1 *Dermatomyositis.*

- Dermatomyositis-like mimics may be caused by drugs, including hydroxyurea, penicillamine, niflumic acid/diclofenac, tryptophan, and practolol

---

TREATMENT

- Under most circumstances treatment is non-emergent, but muscle disease may be so profound and of so rapid an onset that the patient may require admission for supportive care and intravenous corticosteroid treatment
- Local treatment for skin disease alone
  - Hats, protective clothing, and broad-spectrum sunscreens
  - Consider recommending moisturizers (e.g., Moisturel®, Lubriderm®, Eucerin®, Vaseline®, Cetaphil®) for relief of pruritus
  - Topical antipruritic agents such as high-potency corticosteroid agents (e.g., fluocinonide, halobetasol, clobetasol) for 4 or more weeks or tacrolimus 0.1% ointment for as long as needed
  - Antihistaminic agents have limited effect
- For myositis, systemic therapy is required
  - Systemic corticosteroids
    - Prednisone 1 to 1.5 mg/kg/day in divided doses for adults and 1 to 2 mg/kg/day for children
    - Most patients require 1 to 3 months of full-dose therapy before tapering

and will need more than 1 year of continuous therapy
  - Other agents play a secondary role and include:
    - Hydroxychloroquine 200 mg po bid/day
    - Quinacrine 100 mg/day
    - Chloroquine 250 mg/day
    - Azathioprine 1 to 2 mg/kg/day
    - Cyclophosphamide 1 to 2 mg/kg/day
    - Methotrexate 10 to 25 mg/week
    - Chlorambucil 2 to 6 mg/day
    - Cyclosporin 5 mg/kg/day
    - High-dose intravenous gamma-globulin therapy
  - Extracorporeal photochemotherapy has some demonstrated value

---

MANAGEMENT/FOLLOW-UP

- Close follow-up is required with multiple physicians including the patient's primary care physician, a rheumatologist, a dermatologist, and other physicians needed for the management of such patients
- Adults need careful evaluation for malignancy

ICD-9 Code
710.3

CHAPTER 26

DIAPER DERMATITIS

HISTORY

- Parents of the infant notice red, sometimes tender, areas in the perineal region that may spread to inguinal folds
- The infant may appear to be uncomfortable with manipulation in the diaper area
- Diaper dermatitis is more common in infants who use cloth diapers and in atopic children
- Diaper dermatitis is caused by chronic skin exposure to feces and the chronic occlusive nature of diapers
- There may be a superinfection with *Candida,* which causes an alarming red rash

PHYSICAL EXAMINATION

- Erythematous patches in the anogenital areas first appear, and with time patients develop scaling, papules, and erosions (Fig. 26-1)
- If patients become superinfected with *Candida,* one sees beefy red patches or plaques with pustules that develop in the erythematous areas and in the areas around the patches or plaques

DIAGNOSIS

- The diagnosis is based almost exclusively on the physical exam
- Examination of a KOH preparation of scale or pustule contents may reveal pseudohyphae or yeast forms

DIFFERENTIAL DIAGNOSIS

- Tinea infections: relatively uncommon in children, rarely involve the scrotum, and demonstrate central clearing
- Seborrheic dermatitis: may be seen in infants in intertriginous zones but is usually less well-demarcated; a KOH preparation examination is negative; infants may have cradle cap
- Inverse psoriasis: psoriasis is quite uncommon in infants and children, and patients will almost always have psoriatic lesions elsewhere on the body, including axillary and supraclavicular involvement

TREATMENT

- Mild topical corticosteroid agents such as hydrocortisone 1% to 2.5% ointment bid or desonide 0.05% (DesOwen®) ointment qid for 1 to 2 weeks may help to decrease the inflammation and irritation
- Long-term use of skin protectants such as Desitin® or A&D ointment® should be recommended as prophylaxis
- If there is any concern about candidal infection, consider prescribing nystatin powder, econazole (Spectazole®) cream, ketoconazole (Nizoral®) cream, or clotrimazole (Lotrimin®) cream bid for 1 to 2 weeks
- One should encourage appropriate cleansing of the diaper area and frequent diaper changes

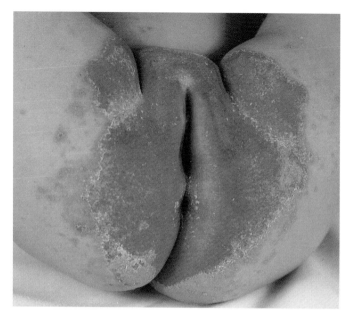

FIGURE 26-1 *Diaper dermatitis.*

- The patient may follow up with the primary care physician or dermatologist

- The cure for diaper dermatitis is successful toilet training

ICD-9-CM Code

694.0

CHAPTER 27

DISSEMINATED GONOCOCCAL INFECTION

- This condition is most frequently seen in young, sexually active patients and occurs worldwide
- Disseminated gonococcal infection is more common in women, occurring around the time of menses or in pregnancy
- Patients complain of fever, chills, arthralgias, and other systemic symptoms
  - Arthralgias are most common in the hands
- The primary infection is acquired through sexual activity and may involve infection of the genitourinary tract, anorectal area, or oropharynx, but disseminated disease occurs in 1% to 3% of patients infected with gonorrhea
  - A recent history of unprotected sexual exposure is sometimes obtained from patients

PHYSICAL EXAMINATION

- Patients are ill-appearing, with fever, arthritis, and tenosynovitis, and may present with petechial, papular, or pustular skin lesions on the hands or feet (Fig. 27-1)

- Early in dissemination, one can see petechiae or pink papules that are few in number with most of the lesions acrally distributed on the extremities and around joints
- Later (within 1 to 2 days), these lesions may evolve into hemorrhagic vesicles and pustules (Fig. 27-2)

DIAGNOSIS

- Gram's stain from the male urethra or female cervix and culture from the mucosal surface are the keys to diagnosis
- Caused by spread of *Neisseria gonorrhoeae,* a gram-negative diplococcus, into the bloodstream
- An immunofluorescence study of skin biopsy specimens shows gonococcus in 60% of specimens
- Blood culture may grow *N. gonorrhoeae*

DIFFERENTIAL DIAGNOSIS

- Bacteremias, including meningococcus and Rocky Mountain spotted fever, pustular psoriasis, Reiter's syndrome, and leukocytoclastic vasculitis

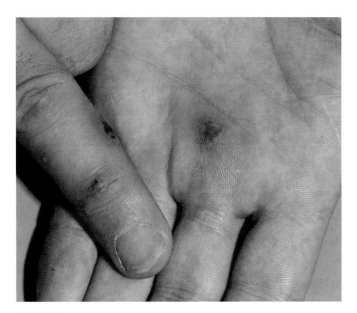

FIGURE 27-1 *Disseminated gonococcal infection.*

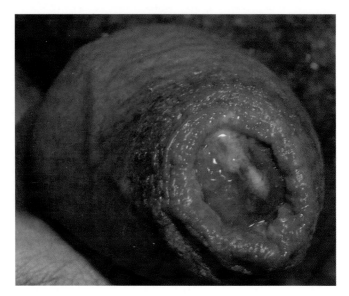

FIGURE 27-2 *Purulent urethral discharge.*

DISSEMINATED GONOCOCCAL INFECTION

- Treatment is an emergency
- Treatment of choice is hospitalization and ceftriaxone 1 g IM or IV every 24 hours or cefotaxime 1 g IV every 8 hours
- Treatment should continue for 24 hours after improvement occurs
  - At that time, begin oral therapy with cefixime 200 mg by mouth twice per day or ciprofloxacin 500 mg by mouth twice per day for 1 week
  - Ciprofloxacin is contraindicated in children and adolescents <17 years old and in pregnant and lactating women
- Patients should also be treated for presumed infection with *Chlamydia trachomatis*
- Joint effusions may need to be removed by aspiration, and all patients should be evaluated for evidence of endocarditis or meningitis

- Once the patient is treated, no specific follow-up is needed unless there are complications
- Safe sex practices should be discussed with all of these patients.

ICD-9-CM Code

098.89

CPT Code

11100   Biopsy

DISSEMINATED INTRAVASCULAR COAGULATION (DIC)

HISTORY

- Symptoms of bleeding from multiple sites or thrombosis with characteristic skin eruption in the setting of obstetric catastrophe, metastatic malignancy, massive trauma, sepsis, hepatic failure, or toxic reactions to venemous snake bites, or transfusion reactions

PHYSICAL EXAMINATION

- Widespread petechiae, ecchymoses, and hemorrhagic bullae, as well as ischemic necrosis of the skin (Fig. 28-1)
- Bleeding may be so severe that profuse bleeding is noted from all puncture sites including intravenous access lines
- Peripheral gangrene may be seen in late stages

DIAGNOSIS

- The diagnosis is a clinical diagnosis with supporting laboratory findings including: profound thrombocytopenia, fragmented red blood cells on smear, prolonged prothrombin time and activated partial thromboplastin time, reduced fibrinogen level, and elevated fibrin degradation products

DIFFERENTIAL DIAGNOSIS

- Warfarin necrosis: presents as limited or widespread ecchymoses within a few days of onset of warfarin therapy, but patients lack the severe signs and symptoms of disseminated intravascular coagulation
- Systemic vasculitides such as polyarteritis nodosa and nodular vasculitis: these generally present with large purpuric papules and nodules with ulceration, but not widespread purpura and bleeding
- Idiopathic (or autoimmune) thrombocytopenic purpura: occurs in both children (acute form) and adults (chronic form) and presents with petechiae and ecchymoses, gastrointestinal bleeding, menorrhagia, epistaxis, bleeding gums, and possibly intracranial hemorrhage with the presence of antiplatelet antibodies
- Thrombotic thrombocytopenic purpura: presents with petechiae and ecchymoses in association with thrombocytopenia, fever, microangiopathic hemolytic anemia, renal disease, and central nervous system symptoms
- Drug-induced thrombocytopenia: may cause purpura in the distribution of trauma but rarely becomes so severe as to cause the bleeding from every puncture and orifice seen in disseminated intravascular coagulation

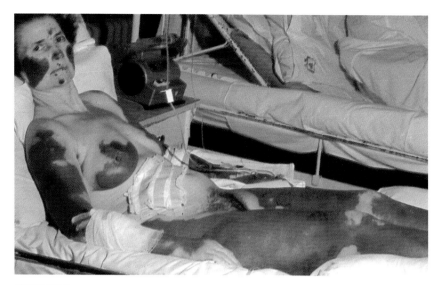

FIGURE 28-1 *Purpura fulminans in disseminated intravascular coagulation following surgery.*

- Waldenstrom's hyperglobulinemic purpura: this monoclonal IgM disease may produce lower extremity petechiae, but not widespread purpura and bleeding
- Thrombocytopenia: may cause purpura, but usually will not cause palpable purpura
- Meningococcemia: patients present with tiny petechiae to large ecchymoses, in conjunction with fever, headache, vomiting, and acute mental status changes
- Pigmented purpuric dermatoses: these conditions may present with purpura that is usually of chronic duration, limited to the distal lower extremities

TREATMENT

- Patients require intensive management to prevent death; this condition has a high mortality rate

- Control of the underlying disease if one can be identified is the single most important component to treatment
- Vitamin K replacement may be required
- Fresh frozen plasma replacement may be needed emergently in patients with active bleeding
- Platelet transfusions may be needed emergently for thrombocytopenia
- Heparin may be required emergently for patients with active thrombosis

MANAGEMENT/FOLLOW-UP

- Intensive care unit management

ICD-9-CM code

286.6

CHAPTER 29

DRUG ERUPTION (DRUG RASH)

HISTORY

- Onset of a characteristic cutaneous eruption temporally related to the initiation of a systemic agent
- Depending on the drug reaction mechanism, the patient may have taken the same medication previously without incident
- Most drug reactions involving the skin occur within 1 to 3 weeks of initiation, but this time interval can be longer for hypersensitivity syndromes
- In IgE-dependent drug reactions (e.g., to penicillin) reaction occurs in minutes after drug exposure
- The most common agents that cause drug eruptions include amoxicillin, trimethoprim/sulfamethoxazole, ampicillin, blood products, semisynthetic penicillins, cephalosporins, erythromycin, hydralazine, penicillin G, cyanocobalamin-B_{12}
- HIV-infected patients are 5 to 20 times more likely than the rest of the population to develop drug reactions

PHYSICAL EXAMINATION

- Several general categories of cutaneous drug eruption exist, as described below
  - *Exanthem* (*morbilliform*) is the most common; diffuse, pruritic, erythematous macules and papules first appear on the trunk and then generalize (Fig. 29-1)
  - *Urticaria* (*hives*) and/or *angioedema* appear as erythematous, pruritic, edematous wheals
    - Few lesions to hundreds can occur
    - Respiratory symptoms including bronchospasm and laryngeal edema may occur with associated sequelae of hypotension and death
    - Urticaria may be a component of the serum sickness reaction; 7 to 21 days after administration of the offending drug, urticaria, along with fever, myalgias, arthralgias, lymphadenopathy, and arthritis, develops; Serum sickness is self-limited, lasting 4 to 5 days

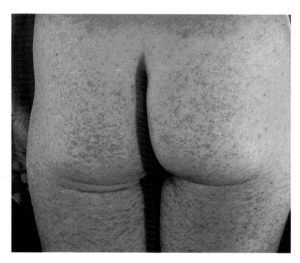

FIGURE 29-1 *Drug eruptions.*

- ○ *Photosensitive eruption* (may be *photoallergic* or *phototoxic* response) with patchy to confluent erythema, macules, papules, or vesicles in sun-exposed areas such as the arms and face
  - Agents particularly likely to cause such reactions include sulfa medications, fluoroquinolones, thiazides, tetracyclines, phenothiazines, tricyclic antidepressants, nalidixic acid, antimalarials, furosemide, griseofulvin, piroxicam, and ibuprofen
- ○ *Eczematous eruption* may occur with erythematous, scaly patches and plaques
  - Penicillins, sulfonamides, beta blockers, thiazides, aminophylline
- ○ *Acneiform eruptions* occur on the face, upper chest, and back in a pattern with monomorphous acneiform papules, pustules, and nodules without comedones
  - Agents particularly likely to cause such reactions include corticosteroids, androgenic steroids, oral contraceptives, androgens, phenytoin, halogens, lithium, phenobarbital, haloperidol, ethambutol, and isoniazid

- ○ *Pustular eruptions* are uncommon patterns that occur after an intense erythema
  - Streptomycin, piperazine, pyrimethamine, phenylbutazone, phenytoin, and amoxicillin with clavulanic acid
- ○ Hyperpigmentation (skin darkening) can occur in different patterns with specific drugs
  - Zidovudine may produce both nail and skin hyperpigmentation
  - Amiodarone may give a slate-blue coloration to the skin
  - Minocycline may also produce a gray-brown or gray-blue pigmentation
  - Heavy metals such as silver, gold, or bismuth may produce pigmentation
  - Phenytoin as well as oral contraceptives can produce a melasma-like pigmentation of the face
  - Clofazamine may give a red coloration to the skin
  - Nicotinic acid may produce a brown pigmentation
  - Antimalarials may produce a slate-gray or yellow pigmentation

- *Lupus erythematosus eruption* may rarely occur with a photosensitive eruption and related systemic findings
  - Agents particularly likely to cause such reactions include procainamide, phenytoin, minocycline, hydralazine, penicillamine, methyldopa, thiouracil, and carbamazepine
- *Fixed drug eruption* occurs as a single or several round erythematous patches or plaques that may contain central vesiculation
  - Each time an individual ingests the same medication, the eruption recurs in the same location
  - Agents particularly likely to cause such reactions include sulfa drugs, aspirin, ibuprofen, oxyphenylbutazone, tetracycline, phenolphthalein, and barbiturates
- *Erythema nodosum* presents as tender, deep, red nodules, usually on the anterior surface of the lower extremities
  - This may last weeks to years, and can result in depression of the skin
  - Agents particularly likely to cause such reactions include oral contraceptive agents, sulfonamides, halogens, tetracyclines, and penicillin
- *Vesiculobullous eruptions* produce a clinical pattern indistinguishable from pemphigus or bullous pemphigoid with the appearance of widespread erosions or bullae
  - Pemphigus-like reactions are most commonly due to drugs such as penicillamine and captopril
  - Bullous pemphigoid-like reactions are most commonly due to sulfa and thiol drugs, especially furosemide
  - Other drugs implicated in a variety of vesiculobullous eruptions include nonsteroidal antiinflammatory agents, griseofulvin, thiazide diuretics, barbiturates, mellaril, dipyridamole, chemotherapeutic agents, amoxapine, nalidixic acid, penicillamine, captopril, puva, penicillin, and sulfonamides
- *Anticoagulant necrosis* may be due to either coumadin or heparin, 3 to 5 days after the initiation of therapy; pain precedes the development of erythema on the thighs, breasts, and buttocks
  - This erythema rapidly becomes blue to black, sometimes with overlying blisters
  - Tissue necrosis may occur, even down to the subcutaneous tissues
- *Antiepileptic hypersensitivity reaction* occurs 2 to 6 weeks after the initiation of an aromatic amine-antiepileptic drug (phenytoin, carbamazepine, phenobarbital)
  - The skin eruption is variable, from a morbilliform erythematous eruption to toxic epidermal necrolysis
  - Facial edema, fever, lymphadenopathy, and leukocytosis are part of the reaction pattern and may be associated hepatitis, nephritis, and pneumonitis
- *Erythema multiforme/Stevens-Johnson syndrome/toxic epidermal necrolysis* (see separate chapters)

DIAGNOSIS

- Clinical history
- A skin biopsy is occasionally helpful

- Drug eruptions can mimic many disorders, and each type of drug eruption has innumerable mimics

- The treatment of drug eruption may be emergent or nonemergent
- Withdrawal of offending agent
- Symptomatic treatment

- Subsequent management is highly dependent upon the severity of the condition, and may range from follow-up with a primary care physician or dermatologist, to intensive care unit admission for supportive care

ICD-9 Code

693.0

DYSHIDROTIC DERMATITIS

HISTORY

- Patients complain of an eruption of itchy blisters on the fingers, palms, and soles that usually lasts for several weeks
- Patients often complain of having had similar eruptions in the past

PHYSICAL EXAMINATION

- Small, deep-seated vesicles located on the fingers, palms, and/or soles (Figs. 30-1 to 30-3)
- Larger bullae may occasionally develop

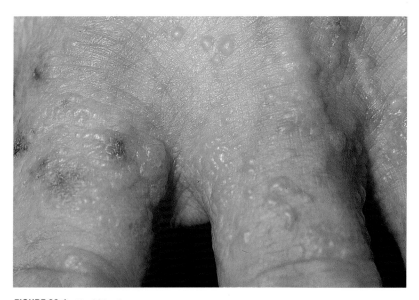

FIGURE 30-1 *Dyshidrotic eczema.*

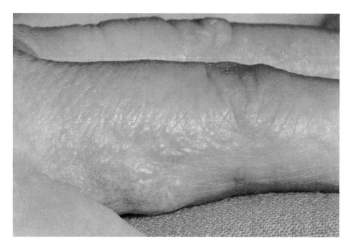

FIGURE 30-2 *Dyshidrotic eczematous dermatitis.*

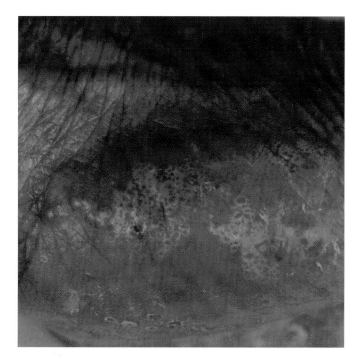

FIGURE 30-3 *Vesicular hand eczema.*

- Lichenification (thickened skin with accentuation of skin markings) and fissuring may be present with chronic lesions (from scratching and rubbing); ruptured vesicles may present as erosions and crusts
- Secondary infection may be present

- The diagnosis is usually made by history and physical examination
- A KOH preparation can be performed to exclude dermatophyte infection as a mimic
- A bacterial culture can be performed in the appropriate clinical setting to confirm secondary infection

DIFFERENTIAL DIAGNOSIS

- Atopic dermatitis: this may occur on the feet or hands; however, it tends to involve not only the palms and/or soles, as well as lateral aspects of the fingers and/or toes, but also other parts of the hands and feet
- Bullous tinea pedis: highly inflammatory large vesicles or vesiculopustules, often with interdigital web space scaling
  - This diagnosis can be confirmed by a positive KOH preparation
- Contact dermatitis (allergic or irritant)
- Palmoplantar pustulosis: a variant of psoriasis that presents with brightly erythematous plaques and pustules on the palms and soles
- Dermatophytid reaction: a vesicular eruption, usually on the palms, that is a reaction to a tinea infection elsewhere on the body, often on the feet
- Scabies: this pruritic infestation presents as interdigital and wrist scaling with tiny vesicles, associated with pruritus and lesions elsewhere on the body
  - Careful examination will often demonstrate tiny linear burrows

TREATMENT

- The treatment of dyshidrotic dermatitis is nonemergent
- Education regarding the need to use topical moisturizers frequently (e.g., Moisturel®, Lubriderm®, Eucerin®, Vaseline®, Cetaphil®) and to keep rubbing to a minimum is vital
- Large bullae can be punctured to allow the contents to drain, but they should not be unroofed
- Localized lesions can be treated with topical corticosteroids: a mid-potency to super-high-potency topical corticosteroid may be applied to the lesions bid for 2 weeks; should not be applied to the face, axillae, or groin
  - Mid-potency: prednicarbate (Dermatop®) 0.1% ointment or cream; triamcinolone acetonide (Aristocort®) 0.1% ointment or cream
  - High-potency: fluocinonide (Lidex®) 0.05% ointment or cream; clobetasol propionate (Temovate®) 0.05% ointment or cream; halobetasol propionate (Ultravate®) 0.05% ointment or cream, betamethasone dipropionate 0.05% in optimized ointment (Diprolene®)
  - Occlusion helps to facilitate penetration of the medication as well as prevent the patient from scratching or rubbing the area
  - Emphasize that the main side effect of prolonged use of a topical corticosteroid is skin atrophy
    - The use of topical tacrolimus (Protopic) 0.1% ointment has no atrophogenicity, and it may be used over the long term as a medium-potency corticosteroid equivalent

- White cotton gloves and cotton socks can be applied over the hands and feet, respectively, after application of a topical corticosteroid
- Sedating night time oral antihistamines can be used to improve patients' sleep and decrease the amount of time they scratch during the night
  - Hydroxyzine (Atarax®, Vistaril®) 10 to 50 mg prn sleep; syrup 10 mg/5 ml
  - Diphenhydramine (Benadryl®) 25 to 50 mg prn sleep
- Treat any secondary infections (*Staphylococcus aureus* most common cause)
  - Dicloxacillin: 500 mg bid for 10 days (adults); 12.5 to 25 mg/kg/day (children <40 kg)
  - Cephalexin (Keflex®): 500 mg bid for 10 days (adults); 25 to 50 mg/kg/day (children)
  - *Penicillin-allergic*: erythromycin 500 mg bid for 10 days (adults); 40 mg/kg/day for 10 days (children)
- Severe cases of dyshidrotic dermatitis may require systemic corticosteroids (0.5 to 1 mg/kg/day of prednisone for 1 to 2 weeks)

- Severe disease and disease that is nonresponsive to conventional therapy may require more complex forms of therapy, such as ultraviolet (UV) light therapy or oral immunosuppressive agents

MANAGEMENT/FOLLOW-UP

- Patients who are treated with topical corticosteroids should be followed up by a primary care physician or a dermatologist in 2 weeks to assess progress
- Patients who require more advanced forms of treatment, such as UV therapy or combination therapy, should be seen by a primary care physician or a dermatologist within a week for therapy

ICD-9 Code

705.81

ECTHYMA

HISTORY

- Immunocompromised and/or malnourished individual with history of trauma to the lower extremities (shins or dorsal feet)
  - Ecthyma may also seen in the elderly and children
  - Intravenous drug abusers are especially at risk
- Trauma followed by vesicle formation, which evolves into characteristic cutaneous ulceration

PHYSICAL EXAMINATION

- The most common locations are the shin and dorsal feet
- A vesicle evolves to a larger vesicopustule, which over the course of days enlarges and ulcerates and is covered by a thick yellow-gray crust (Fig. 31-1)
- The ulcer is saucer-shaped, with a raw base and elevated, indurated, violaceous edges

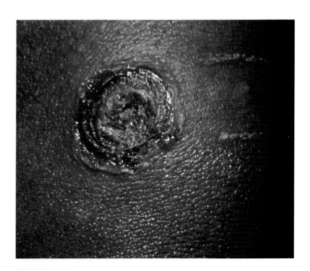

FIGURE 31-1   *Ecthyma.*

ECTHYMA

- This diagnosis is a clinical examination
- Skin bacterial culture (group A *Streptococcus, Staphylococcus aureus*)

DIFFERENTIAL DIAGNOSIS

- Must be distinguished from pseudomonal ecthyma, which usually occurs in patients who are neutropenic or who have *Pseudomonas aeruginosa* bacteremia

TREATMENT

- Penicillinase-resistant: semisynthetic penicillin or erythromycin orally for 7 to 10 days
- Cleanse locally at least bid with an antibacterial soap followed by topical application of mupirocin (Bactroban®)

MANAGEMENT/FOLLOW-UP

- Patients should be followed by their primary care physician or dermatologist within several days of evaluation
- If ecthyma is due to group A streptococcus, post-streptococcal glomerulonephritis may rarely occur
- Scarring usually occurs in deeper ulcers and autoinnoculation may occur

ICD-9-CM Code

686.8

CHAPTER 32

ECZEMA HERPETICUM

HISTORY

- Acute eruption, over a period of a few days to a week, of vesicles and erosions in areas of preexisting skin disorders, such as atopic dermatitis
- May have fever, malaise, and/or lymphadenopathy
- History of a preexisting skin disorder, such as atopic dermatitis or Darier's disease

PHYSICAL EXAMINATION

- Begins as small vesicles that enlarge, umbilicate, and become pustular and crusted; by the time the patient presents, may see large confluent areas of erosions, weeping, crust, and purulent hemorrhagic exudates (Figs. 32-1 and 32-2)
- Often presents on areas of preexisting skin disorders but can involve normal skin as well

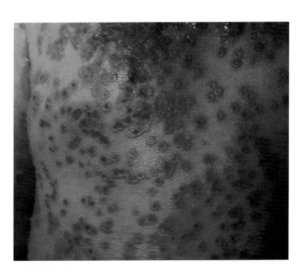

FIGURE 32-1 *Eczema herpeticum.*

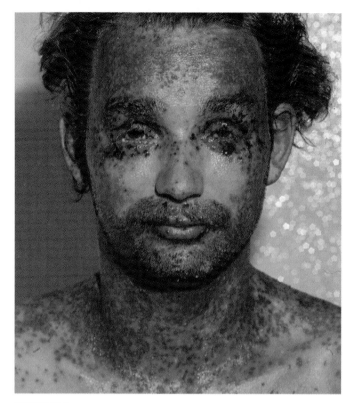

FIGURE 32-2 *Eczema herpeticum in areas of atopic dermatitis.*

- Superimposed secondary bacterial infection is often seen
- Patient may be ill-appearing and febrile

DIAGNOSIS

- The cause of eczema herpeticum is usually a herpes simplex virus-1 (HSV-1) superinfection of atopic dermatitis; but HSV-2 has been reported to cause it as well
- A Tzanck preparation can be useful for rapid diagnosis
  - Using a #15 blade, an intact blister is opened along one side
  - The base of the lesion is then gently scraped, and the contents are placed onto a glass slide and allowed to air dry
  - The material is then stained with Giemsa or Sedi-Stain, and the slide is viewed under a light microscope, looking for multinucleated giant cells
- Other approaches that can be confirmatory for diagnosis include obtaining a sample of blister fluid for polymerase chain reaction (PCR) testing or viral culture

DIFFERENTIAL DIAGNOSIS

- Bullous impetigo: vesicles and bullae filled with clear to yellow fluid; arises on normal-appearing skin and is usually seen in children and young adults
- Varicella: viral infection caused by the varicella-zoster virus; lesions are extremely pruritic and begin on the face and spread inferiorly; lesions appear in successive crops, with papules, vesicles, pustules, and crusts present simultaneously
- Disseminated zoster: viral infection caused by the varicella-zoster virus; patients are often immunosuppressed and ill-appearing; lesions appear as widespread necrotic papules and pustules
- Autoimmune blistering diseases: e.g., bullous pemphigoid, pemphigus vulgaris, epidermolysis bullosa acquista; intact vesicles and bullae and/or erosions arising on any cutaneous surface; usually not pustular and not localized to areas of preexisting dermatitis

TREATMENT

- The treatment of eczema herpeticum is emergent
- Oral therapy should be initiated for most cases
  - Acyclovir: 200 mg po 5x/day (adults) or acyclovir suspension (200 mg/5 ml) 5 mg/kg per dose qid (children) for 7 days for mild cases and IV 1.5 g/m^2/day for severe cases
  - Valacyclovir: 500 mg po bid for 7 days (adults)
  - Famciclovir: 250 mg po bid for 7 days (adults)

- Severe and widespread disease may require intravenous acyclovir, especially in immunocompromised patients
- Secondary impetiginization with *Staphylococcus aureus* should be treated with appropriate coverage
  - Dicloxacillin: 500 mg bid for 10 days (adults); 12.5 to 25 mg/kg/day in children <40 kg
  - Cephalexin: 500 mg bid for 10 days (adults); 25 to 50 mg/kg/day in children
  - *Penicillin-allergic*: erythromycin 500 mg bid for 10 days (adults); 40 mg/kg/day for 10 days (children)

- Patients should follow up with either a primary care physician or a dermatologist within a week

ICD-9-CM Code

054.0

CHAPTER 33

EPIDERMAL INCLUSION CYST

HISTORY

- A solitary lesion that usually occurs on face, neck, scalp, and upper trunk and has been present for months to years
- The lesions may occasionally become inflamed, with increased erythema, tenderness, and foul-smelling drainage

PHYSICAL EXAMINATION

- A solitary, freely moveable, dermal to subcutaneous nodule that may show a characteristic central punctum (Figs. 33-1 to 33-3)
- The lesions are usually located on the face, neck, scalp, and upper trunk

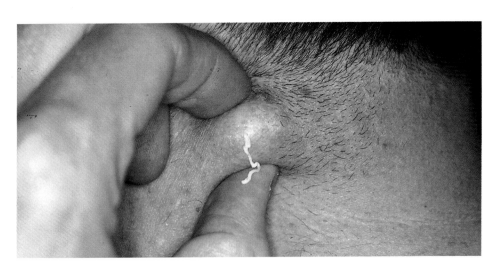

FIGURE 33-1 *Epidermoid cyst.*

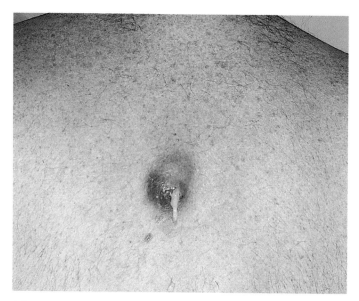

FIGURE 33-2 *Epidermoid cyst.*

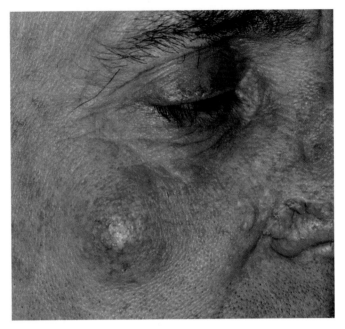

FIGURE 33-3 *Epidermoid cyst.*

- May be inflamed, with fluctuance, striking erythema, and tenderness, and have foul-smelling discharge

DIAGNOSIS

- Diagnosis usually based on history and clinical findings

DIFFERENTIAL DIAGNOSIS

- Lipoma: benign subcutaneous tumor that usually occurs on neck, trunk, and extremities; usually deeper than an epidermal inclusion cyst and does not become inflamed or have associated foul-smelling drainage

- Lymphadenopathy may also clinically resemble epidermal inclusion cysts, but the location and setting should help to differentiate between the two

TREATMENT

- Unless they are inflamed and tender, the treatment of epidermal inclusions cysts is nonemergent
- Definitive treatment involves removal of the entire lesion by surgical excision
- Incision and drainage may be helpful for very tender, inflamed, fluctuant cysts
- Most of the inflammation present in inflamed cysts is due to sterile foreign body response

- To decrease the inflammation, one can inject with triamcinolone acetonide (Kenalog®) 3 to 10 mg/ml to treat lesions; the amount injected will depend on the size of the lesion
- Many physicians treat patients with anti-staphylococcal antibiotics such as
  - Dicloxacillin: 500 mg bid for 10 days (adults); 12.5 to 25 mg/kg/day (children <40 kg)
  - Cephalexin (Keflex®): 500 mg bid for 10 days (adults); 25 to 50 mg/kg/day (children)
- *Penicillin-allergic*: erythromycin 500 mg bid for 10 days (adults); 40 mg/kg/day for 10 days (children)

MANAGEMENT/FOLLOW-UP

- Patients who request excision should be seen by a primary care physician or a dermatologist for excision of the lesion

ICD-9-CM Code

706.2

CPT Codes

10060   Incision and drainage
11900   Intralesional injection

CHAPTER 34

ERUPTIVE XANTHOMA

HISTORY

- Patients report the sudden appearance of crops of lesions most commonly located on extensor surfaces, thighs, and buttocks
- They may report itching lesions, but the lesions are usually asymptomatic
- May have a history of poorly controlled or undiagnosed diabetes mellitus or severe pancreatitis
- Patients may report a history of increased triglycerides

PHYSICAL EXAMINATION

- Small yellow and red papules measuring 2 to 4 mm in diameter located over elbows, knees, buttocks, and thighs (Figs. 34-1 and 34-2)
- The surface may be excoriated surfaces

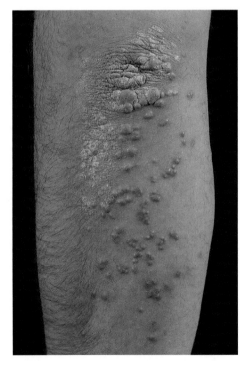

FIGURE 34-1 *Papular eruptive xanthomas.*

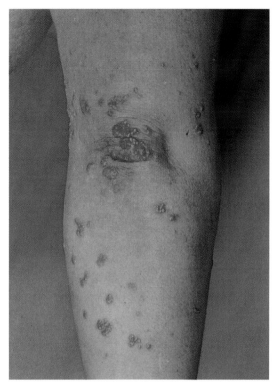

FIGURE 34-2 *Eruptive skin xanthomas.*

DIAGNOSIS

- The clinical exam is often diagnostic
- A skin biopsy can be performed to confirm clinical suspicion
- Patients need to have their underlying lipid abnormality and causative condition evaluated and treated

DIFFERENTIAL DIAGNOSIS

- Molluscum contagiosum: dome-shaped papules with a central keratotic plug that may be located on any cutaneous surface; often appears in clusters
- Verrucae vulgaris (warts): skin-colored lesions that vary in size and shape and can appear on any cutaneous surface
  - One may see "black dots" on surface; usually, lesions do not appear in clusters, as do the lesions of eruptive xanthoma

TREATMENT

- Treatment of eruptive xanthomas is non-emergent; however, a lipid profile including triglycerides should be obtained
- If clinical exam indicates, may need to rule out diabetes mellitus or pancreatitis
- Management of the skin lesions is aimed at correcting the associated hypertriglyceridemia via dietary manipulation, medications, or treatment of the underlying cause; eruptive xanthomas usually respond to such measures

MANAGEMENT/FOLLOW UP

- Patients should be seen by their primary care physician for further evaluation and management of underlying causes

ICD-9 Code

272.2

ERYTHEMA MULTIFORME AND STEVENS-JOHNSON SYNDROME

HISTORY

- Most commonly affects adolescents and young adults; characteristic cutaneous eruption with or without constitutional symptoms including fever, malaise, rhinitis, pharyngitis, cough, and arthralgias
- Outbreaks are most commonly idiopathic, but other precipitants are known
- Infections can precipitate erythema multiforme
  - A recent history of herpes simplex virus outbreak can precipitate both initial or recurrent episodes of erythema multiforme
  - Other associated infections include *Mycoplasma* infections, *Yersinia* infections, tuberculosis, histoplasmosis, coccidiomycosis, influenza, orf, ECHO infection, coxsackievirus infection, and mononucleosis
- Medications can precipitate erythema multiforme
  - Those particularly likely include sulfonamides, anticonvulsants and nonsteroidal antiinflammatory agents
  - Drug-induced erythema multiforme occurs 7 to 10 days after the drug is first given

- Other miscellaneous causes may include pregnancy, external beam radiation, and cancer
- Mucous membrane involvement can cause severe oral pain, anogenital pain, and photophobia
  - Patients may refuse to drink or void because of pain

PHYSICAL EXAMINATION

- Symmetric, small pink to red itchy or painful macules on the palms of the hands and extensor surfaces of the extremities evolving in hours into papules that persist for days (Fig. 35-1)
  - These papules may enlarge and develop dusky centers (target or iris lesions)
  - Some of these target lesions develop into small to large bullae
  - They may develop into polycyclic or geographic shapes
  - Isomorphism, the appearance of lesions at areas of cutaneous trauma, may be seen
- In more severe cases (Stevens-Johnson syndrome), skin and mucous membrane lesions rapidly enlarge or coalesce into large erythematous areas with epidermal necrosis and crusting

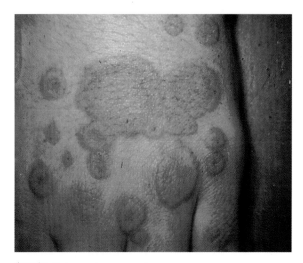

FIGURE 35-1   *Erythema multiforme.*

- Oral involvement may be minor, such as lip swelling, or severe in Stevens-Johnson syndrome, such as painful mucosal bullae, erosions, and crusting
- Anogenital involvement with erythema and bullae formation may occur
- Conjunctivitis in Stevens-Johnson syndrome may evolve to uveitis, panophthalmitis, ulceration, pseudomembrane formation, corneal perforation, and scarring

DIAGNOSIS

- Clinical examination
- Biopsy may be required to differentiate from vasculitis or immunobullous disorder

DIFFERENTIAL DIAGNOSIS

- Bullous pemphigoid can present with widespread tense vesicles, erosions, and mouth erosions, but target lesions are lacking
- Pemphigus can present with widespread erosions and mouth erosions, but target lesions are lacking
- Toxic epidermal necrolysis: this condition generally begins as large sheets of painful erythema, rather than as individual papules or plaques that become targetoid and vesicular
- Urticaria: urticaria-like papules and plaques may be present early in erythema multiforme, but the erythema multiforme rapidly progresses into targetoid lesions and bullae
- Urticarial vasculitis: urticaria-like papules and plaques may be present early in erythema multiforme, and purpura within these lesions may be the earliest sign of the development of a target lesion
  - However, true target lesions do not develop in urticarial vasculitis
- Viral exanthem: early erythema multiforme lesions appear to be nonspecific macules and papules and may have a diffuse distribution reminiscent of a viral exanthem

- Within a short time, evolution of individual lesions into erythema multiforme becomes evident

TREATMENT

- If a precipitating cause can be identified, it should be removed or treated
- Treatment may be emergent depending on the severity of the disease
  - Depending on the sites of involvement, consultation with ophthalmology, gynecology, urology, or dermatology may be required to develop a realistic treatment plan
- Systemic support
  - Fluid support with IV fluids may be required because of poor oral intake
  - Patients may require urinary catheterization if they refuse to micturate because of urethral involvement and pain
  - Systemic corticosteroids such as prednisone 1 to 2 mg/kg/day for 7 days may be indicated for mild disease
    - Corticosteroids are controversial in severe disease with large portions of body surface areas covered by erosions
- Topical support
  - Bland emollients (Vaseline® or Aquaphor®) or silver sulfadiazine cream (Silvadene®) may be helpful to apply to lips, genitalia, and skin erosions
  - Painful mouth lesions may benefit from Magic Mouthwash or similar anesthetic agents
- Hospitalization or burn unit transfer may be required for severe cases skin and mucous membrane involvement

- Milder courses of erythema multiforme often resolve in 1 to several weeks
  - Systemic symptoms are rare, with complete recovery expected and no adverse sequelae except some postinflammatory skin color changes
  - Mucous membrane involvement, if present, is localized to the oral and anogenital mucosae
  - If patients present with recurrent erythema multiforme, further recurrences are common and systemic antiviral therapy (acyclovir, valacyclovir, or famciclovir) may be beneficial
- Severe cases are more likely to be associated with drug intake
  - In severe cases, burn unit treatment is necessary
  - Pneumonia, sepsis, and renal failure have resulted in death in severe cases
  - If eye involvement is present, ophthalmologic consultation is mandatory to avoid complications of uveitis, panophthalmitis, ulceration, pseudomembrane formation, corneal perforation, and scarring
    - Blindness can occur if untreated
  - Multisystem involvement of mucosal surfaces may occur characterized by gastrointestinal bleeding, hepatitis, diarrhea, cystitis, nephritis, arthritis, pneumonitis, or otitis media
  - Esophageal strictures, anal strictures, vaginal stenosis, and urethral meatus stenosis have been documented

ICD-9 Code

695.1

CHAPTER 36

ERYTHEMA NODOSUM

HISTORY

- More common in women than men, and most common in the third to fourth decades of life
- Patients present with a history of painful subcutaneous nodules, often on the shins
- Most patients have idiopathic disease, but some may have identifiable precipitants
  - Examples of etiologic factors include streptococcal infections in children, sarcoidosis, inflammatory bowel disease (ulcerative colitis), tuberculosis, pregnancy, Behçet's syndrome, lymphoma, toxoplasmosis, adenocarcinoma, psittacosis, cat scratch disease, lymphogranuloma venereum, *Chlamydia* infection, deep and superficial fungal infections, viral and bacterial infections, mycobacterial infections, and acne conglobata
  - Drug exposures may also precipitate disease; and common drugs implicated include oral contraceptives, halides, sulfonamides, penicillins, gold, thiazides, and phenytoin
- Some patients have preceding upper respiratory infection or influenza-like symptoms 1 to 2 weeks prior to cutaneous eruption
  - Symptoms may include coryza, fatigue, headache, malaise, diarrhea, anorexia, and abdominal pain
- Occasionally patients may have a fever to 39°C associated with myalgias and arthralgias, which accompany the onset of cutaneous eruption

- Lofgren's syndrome consists of a febrile illness with erythema nodosum and evidence of sarcoidosis with bilateral enlargement of the hilar glands

PHYSICAL EXAMINATION

- Tender red nodules and plaques that become more purplish in color and flatter after 1 to 2 weeks (Fig. 36-1)
- Pretibial distribution bilaterally is common, although lesions can be found on virtually any body surface (e.g., thighs, buttocks, arms, face, and neck)
- Usually no ulcerated lesions are present
- Lymphadenopathy may be present

DIAGNOSIS

- The diagnosis may be made upon clinical findings alone
  - A definitive diagnosis requires a skin biopsy to a septal panniculitis pattern of inflammation
- Evaluation may also require in some patients a chest x-ray, complete blood count, and other tests to identify precipitating disorders such as sarcoidosis, tuberculosis, and other concurrent conditions

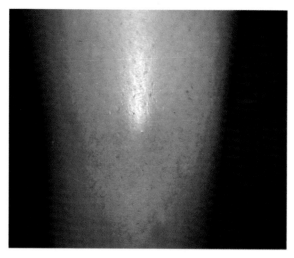

FIGURE 36-1 *Erythema nodosum.*

- Pancreatic panniculitis: patients with acute pancreatitis may develop erythema nodosum-like lesions, but patients may have a history of abdominal pain and other factors that would help identify pancreatitis
- Nodular vasculitis: generally presents with purpura, in addition to tender papules or nodules
- Erythema nodosum leprosum: seen in patients undergoing treatment for leprosy (Hansen's disease)
- Polyarteritis nodosa: generally presents with purpura, in addition to tender papules or nodules

TREATMENT

- In most patients, bed rest and leg elevation are helpful measures
- Systemic nonsteroidal antiinflammatory agents such as indomethacin
- Potassium iodine (400 to 900 mg/day) tapered over 2 to 8 weeks after resolution of skin eruption
- Systemic corticosteroids such as prednisone 1 mg/kg/day tapered over a 2-week period may give rapid relief

MANAGEMENT/FOLLOW-UP

- Patients should follow up with their primary care physician or dermatologist within 1 week
- The eruption persists for 3 to 6 weeks
- Recurrences are not uncommon
- The associated arthropathy may persist beyond the resolution of the cutaneous eruption

ICD-9-CM Code

695.2

CHAPTER 37

ERYTHRASMA

- Asymptomatic red scaling of the toe-web spaces, groin, axillae, or submammary skin
- Risk factors include diabetes mellitus, obesity, increasing age, and residence in tropical climates
- May be present for months to years

- If present in one or more toe-web spaces, there is erythema, scaling, fissuring, and maceration (Figs. 37-1 and 37-2)

- In the groin, axillae, or inframammary skin, there are well-marginated irregularly shaped red to brown patches
- By shining a Wood's lamp on the area, one can demonstrate coral-red fluorescence, whereas tinea infections lack such fluorescence
- If desired for confirmation, a Gram stain of the scale demonstrates gram-positive rods (*Corynebacterium minutissimum*)

- The diagnosis is a clinical one, confirmed onlyu if necessary by Wood's lamp examination or laboratory measures

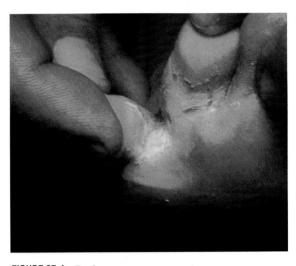

FIGURE 37-1 *Erythrasma.*

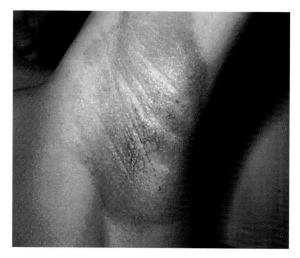

FIGURE 37-2 *Erythrasma.*

- Intertriginous dermatitis
- Inverse psoriasis
- Seborrheic dermatitis
- Tinea cruris

- Topical erythromycin 2% solution bid for 2 weeks
- Econazole 1% cream (Spectazole®) or similar azole antifungal agent bid for 2 weeks
- Systemic erythromycin 500 mg bid for 2 weeks for resistant cases

- The disease may relapse, often within 6 to 12 months
- Antibacterial soaps used in bathing may decrease the risk of recurrence

ICD-9-CM Code

039.0

CHAPTER 38

EXFOLIATIVE ERYTHRODERMA

HISTORY

- The patient complains of rapidly developing generalized redness and scaling over most if not the entire body surface
- Patients may also complain of alopecia and thickened nails
- There may or may not be a prior history of a preexisting dermatologic condition such as psoriasis or atopic dermatitis
- Patients often report a history of fever, chills, and malaise

PHYSICAL EXAMINATION

- Confluent and generalized bright red erythema and scale over a significant portion of the skin, with or without skin thickening (Fig. 38-1)
- Palms and soles are usually involved with thickening, erythema, scale, and fissuring
- Hair may be thin in areas and the nails may be thickened or absent
- +/– Lymphadenopathy, fever, tachycardia

DIAGNOSIS

- Exfoliative erythroderma may occur as an idiopathic entity, as a part of a systemic disease, or secondary to the ingestion of certain drugs
- The cause of erythroderma is often very difficult to ascertain without a history of a preexisting dermatosis or exposure to certain drugs, and in many cases, the cause remains undetermined
- The history and physical examination may help to narrow the likely causes, but a skin biopsy is often required to confirm the diagnosis

DIFFERENTIAL DIAGNOSIS

Generalized Conditions

- Psoriasis: psoriatic erythrodermas are often seen in patients with a prior history of psoriasis, and an examination suggesting psoriasis will often demonstrate nail pits, silvery scale, and occasionally pustules

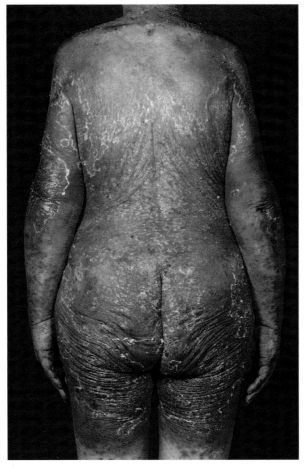

A.

FIGURE 38-1 *Psoriatic erythroderma.*

- Pityriasis rubra pilaris: presents with a rapidly progressive erythematous eruption with follicular papules, "islands" of normal skin amid striking erythema, and extreme thickening of the palm and sole skin
- Atopic dermatitis: patients usually have a history of atopic disease (atopic dermatitis, allergic rhinitis, and/or asthma), severe pruritus, and inadequate treatment for progressive atopic dermatitis
- Cutaneous T-cell lymphoma (Sézary's syndrome): this malignant condition may present with a slowly progressive onset of total body erythema and scale, associated with lymphadenopathy, large numbers of atypical lymphocytes visible on a peripheral blood smear
- Contact dermatitis: rarely would a contact dermatitis with small or large vesicles produce an exfoliative erythroderma, since direct skin contact is required for the eruption to occur
- Toxic epidermal necrolysis: early in toxic epidermal necrolysis, broad areas of painful erythema occur, rapidly followed by sloughing

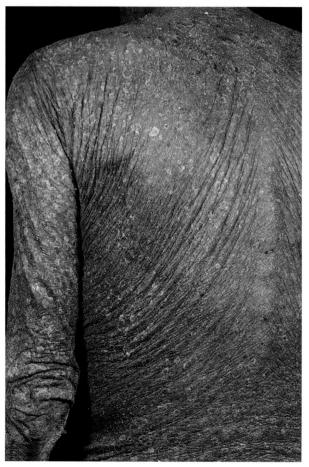

B.

- Staphylococcal scalded skin syndrome: this
  condition occurs most often in children;
  patients are feverish, with very rapid onset
  of brightly erythematous, tender skin
- Idiopathic disease: at least 25% of patients,
  despite adequate evaluation, prove to have
  idiopathic disease
- Medications: must be considered as a cause
  of exfoliative erythroderma, and any drug
  initiated within the month prior to the onset
  of the eruption should be considered a
  possible cause
  - Examples of agents responsible include
    antibiotics, antiseizure medications,
    antihypertensive agents, allopurinol, and
    other agents

- Initial management of a patient with exfoliative erythroderma will vary depending on
  their hemodynamic stability, general
  appearance, whether or not they are febrile,
  and whether or not a known cause has been
  established
  - Unstable/febrile patient
    - Patients who are not stable and are
      ill-appearing should be admitted and
      stabilized

EXFOLIATIVE ERYTHRODERMA

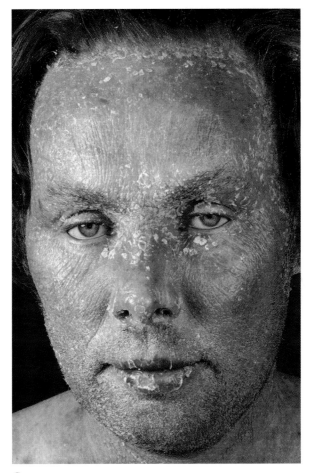

C.

- Blood cultures should be drawn if sepsis is a concern, and cultures from the skin should be performed if a secondary infection is suspected
- Prophylactic antibiotics should be initiated if sepsis or skin infection is suspected
- Once the patient is stabilized, a search for the cause of the erythro-derma should be undertaken and treatment can begin
○ Stable patient
  - Patients who are not ill-appearing, are hemodynamically stable, and are afebrile may be closely evaluated and monitored on an outpatient basis

• Optimal therapy of patients with exfoliative erythroderma depends on establishment of its cause
  ○ Drug-induced reactions: the suspected offending agent should be withdrawn, which often leads to a rapid improve-ment of the erythroderma
  ○ Systemic causes: in these patients, the erythroderma often resists therapy until the underlying condition is treated; thus appropriate treatment should be initiated
  ○ Idiopathic causes: these patients, as well as patients in the above two categories who require supplemental treatment, should be treated as for any subacute dermatitis

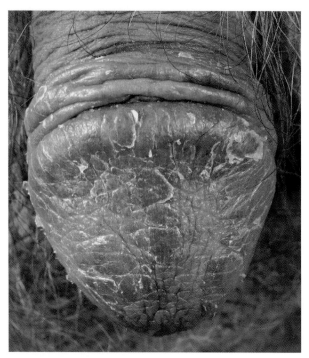

D.

- Topical therapy
  - Generous use of emollients (e.g., Vaseline® or Aquaphor®) should be encouraged on a daily basis
  - Harsh soaps should be replaced with no soaps or mild agents such as Cetaphil®, Aquanil®, or Dove®
  - Water baths or whirlpool therapy to debride the skin surface followed by application of emollients should be encouraged
  - Topical corticosteroids can be used to decrease the inflammation in the skin and provide symptomatic relief; application of warm, wet towels for 10 to 15 minutes prior to application of the topical steroids may help to enhance penetration of the topical agent
    - A mid-potency topical corticosteroid such as triamcinolone acetonide (Aristocort®) 0.1% cream or ointment may be applied to the trunk and extremities bid for 2 or more weeks and should be prescribed by the pound
    - A low-potency topical corticosteroid such as hydrocortisone 2.5% cream or ointment and desonide (DesOwen®) 0.05% cream or ointment should be prescribed for use on the face and neck
    - Emphasize that prolonged use of corticosteroids may cause skin atrophy

- Systemic therapy
  - Systemic corticosteroids should be used with caution until a cause is established
    - These agents may cause a severe rebound phenomenon in patients with psoriasis
  - Systemic retinoids such as acitretin (Soriatane®) may be indicated for treatment of an underlying skin condition
    - Initiation of retinoid therapy is never appropriate for the emergency department setting
  - Other immunosuppressive agents, such as methotrexate or azathioprine (Imuran®), have been of benefit in these patients
    - Initiation of immunosuppressive agents therapy is never appropriate for the emergency department setting
  - Sedating night time oral antihistamines can be used to improve patients' sleep and decrease the amount of time they scratch during the night
    - Hydroxyzine (Atarax®): 10 to 50 mg prn
    - Diphenhydramine (Benadryl®): 25 to 50 mg prn

- Any patient with an exfoliative erythroderma who is being treated on an outpatient basis should follow up with either a primary care physician or a dermatologist within a few days for further evaluation of possible causes of the condition, as well as for continued therapy

ICD-9-CM Code

695.9

FIFTH'S DISEASE (ERYTHEMA INFECTIOSUM)

HISTORY

- Child presenting with low-grade fever, headache, coryza, pharyngitis, and malaise followed in approximately 2 days by characteristic eruption
- Patients may have nausea and diarrhea, and 10% of children develop arthritis or arthralgias
- Outbreaks occur most commonly in the late winter and early spring within schools or families
- The eruption lasts for 5 to 9 days but may recur for weeks to months with triggers such as sunlight, bathing, and temperature changes
- Pruritus may be severe

- When the disease occurs in adults, there may be an acute onset of a self-limited arthropathy affecting the small joints of the hands, knees, wrists, ankles, and feet
  - In adults, fever, adenopathy, and mild arthritis without a rash is characteristic

PHYSICAL EXAMINATION

- Rosy, blanchable, confluent erythema on the cheeks (slapped cheek appearance), sparing the skin around the mouth (Fig. 39-1)

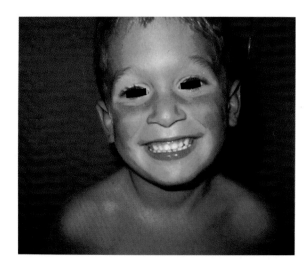

FIGURE 39-1 *Fifth's disease.*

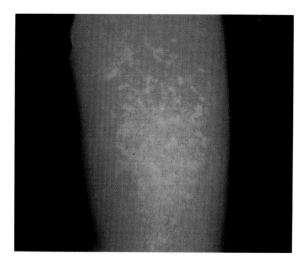

FIGURE 39-2 *Fifth's disease.*

- As this eruption, a distal-spreading maculopapular erythema develops on the extensor extremities and buttocks that becomes lace-like (reticular) from its characteristic central clearing (Fig. 39-2)

DIAGNOSIS

- Clinical examination is usually all that is required
- Serum laboratory confirmation detecting parvovirus B19 can be performed by the Centers for Disease Control and Prevention (CDC)

DIFFERENTIAL DIAGNOSIS

- Other viral exanthems are too numerous to mention and may differ only in subtle ways from roseola; a few include:
  ◦ Enterovirus
  ◦ Rubella
  ◦ Adenovirus
  ◦ Coxsackievirus
  ◦ Rotavirus
  ◦ Measles
- Scarlet fever: associated with streptococcal disease, and the constellation of oropharyngeal findings and positive streptococcal testing

- Drug reactions: patients should have a history of a new drug having been administered within 1 to 3 weeks prior to the onset of the eruption; constitutional symptoms are uncommon with drug eruptions
  ◦ Although morbilliform drug reactions can appear quite varied, the typical "slapped cheek" and reticulate eruption of the extremities would be most unusual in a drug eruption

TREATMENT

- Symptomatic treatment

MANAGEMENT/FOLLOW-UP

- The disease usually runs a self-limited course
- The infection may lead to transient aplastic crisis in patients with chronic hemolytic anemias
- In immunocompromised patients, chronic parvovirus B19 infection may lead to prolonged anemia
- Intrauterine infection of parvovirus B19 may result in hydrops fetalis

ICD-9-CM Code

057.0

FOLLICULITIS

HISTORY

- Lesions are present for days to months over hair-bearing regions of the skin
- Patients may have had a prior history of follicultitis or may have had chaffing in the affected area
- Patients frequently have itching and/or pain

DIAGNOSIS

- The diagnosis usually made by history and physical examination
- If there is uncertainty in the diagnosis, a Gram stain and culture can be performed to identify the organism
- A KOH preparation can also be performed to rule out a fungal etiology

PHYSICAL EXAMINATION

- Patients have erythematous papules or pustules confined to the opening of hair follicles (Figs. 40-1 to 40-3)
- Lesions are often surrounded by an erythematous halo
- Lesions usually located on the hair-bearing areas of the skin, with common sites including the beard area, posterior neck, chest, abdomen, back, and upper thighs
- Lesions may be excoriated or may have ruptured, leading to superficial erosions and crusting
- Lighter or darker macules may be present at sites of previous lesions (postinflammatory pigment change)

DIFFERENTIAL DIAGNOSIS

- Eosinophilic folliculitis: an chronic, extremely itchy follicular eruption, occasionally associated with peripheral eosinophilia, that occurs in patients with the acquired immunodeficiency syndrome
  - In the right clinical setting it cannot always be easily clinically differentiated from other forms of folliculitis, but a skin biopsy shows characteristic histologic differences
- Keratosis pilaris: chronic, tiny, follicularly based papules with central keratin plugs that are usually located on the upper, outer arms and upper thighs

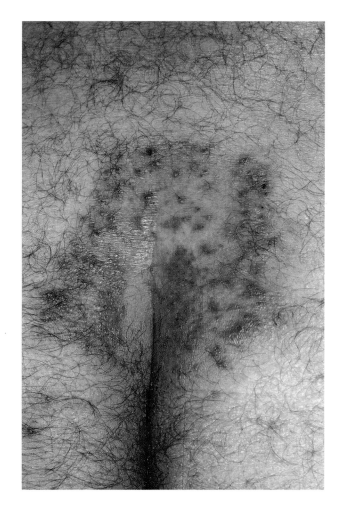

FIGURE 40-1 *Infectious folliculitis.*

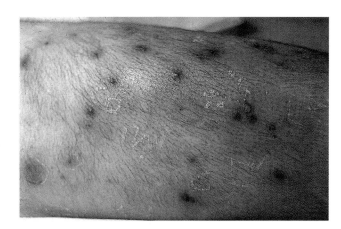

FIGURE 40-2 *Folliculitis of stump skin.*

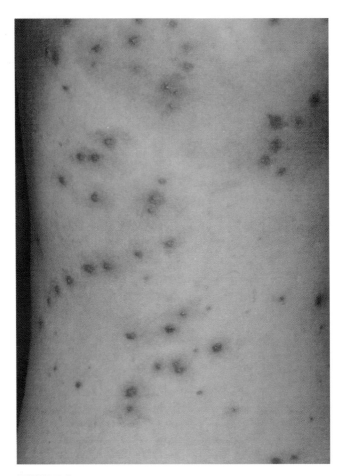

FIGURE 40-3 Pseudomonas aeruginosa: *"hot tub folliculitis."*

- This condition is often found in atopic patients, and the diagnosis is a clinical one
- Perforating folliculitis: a chronic, mildly itchy dermatosis that involves the hair-bearing regions of the arms, forearms, thighs, and buttocks; lesions are discrete, erythematous follicular papules with a central keratin plug that often heals with a scar
  - The diagnosis is confirmed by a biopsy
- Hidradenitis suppurativa: a chronic, suppurative, scarring disease of the apocrine glands associated with draining sinus tracts and ulcerations
  - Occurs in sites with large numbers of apocrine glands including the axillae, inframammary areas, groin, and perirectal area
- Transient and persistent acantholytic dermatosis (Grover's disease): an itchy eruption consisting of papules and papulovesicles, usually located on the central trunk; patient presents with abrupt onset of crops of lesions, often correlated with heavy exercise, excessive sun exposure, or fever

TREATMENT

- The treatment of infectious folliculitis is nonemergent
- By far the most common organism that causes folliculitis is *Staphylococcus aureus*; all other forms of folliculitis are rare
  - *Staphylococcus aureus* can be treated systemically
    - Dicloxacillin: 500 mg bid for 10 days (adults); 12.5 to 25 mg/kg/day (children <40 kg), or
    - Cephalexin (Keflex®): 500 mg bid for 10 days (adults); 25 to 50 mg/kg/day (children)
    - *Penicillin-allergic*: erythromycin ethyl-succinate 500 mg bid for 10 days (adults); 40 mg/kg/day for 10 days (children)
  - *Staphylococcus aureus* can be treated topically with 2% mupirocin ointment (Bactroban®) bid to the involved skin

- In patients with recurrent disease, consider intranasal administration to decrease *S. aureus* colonization
- *Pseudomonas aeruginosa* folliculitis: also known as "hot tub" folliculitis, this condition commonly occurs following exposure to a communal hot tub
  - This condition often resolves spontaneously, but symptomatic lesions can be treated with oral ciprofloxacin (Cipro®) 500 mg bid
- Gram-negative folliculitis: often associated with systemic antibiotic therapy
  - Discontinue oral antibiotic use and consider topical and/or systemic therapies
  - Wash with topical benzoyl peroxide, such as Benzac AC® 5% wash or Brevoxyl® 4% creamy wash
  - Treat systemically with either oral ampicillin 250 mg qid or trimethoprim-sulfamethoxazole double strength (Septra DS®) bid
- Fungal folliculitis: *Pityrosporum ovale* folliculitis or candidal folliculitis can be treated with itraconazole (Sporanox®) 100 mg po bid for 10 to 14 days or fluconazole (Diflucan®) 100 mg po bid for 10 to 14 days
- Herpetic folliculitis
  - Oral therapy can be initiated for more severe cases
    - Acyclovir (Zovirax®): 400 mg po 5x/day for 7 days
    - Valacyclovir (Valtrex®): 500 mg po bid for 7 days
    - Famciclovir (Famvir®): 250 mg po bid for 7 days

MANAGEMENT/FOLLOW-UP

- Patients treated may be seen within 2 to 4 weeks by a primary care physician or a dermatologist to assess progress and determine whether further therapy will be required

ICD-9 Code
704.8

CHAPTER 41

GRANULOMA ANNULARE

HISTORY

- Patients report the gradual appearance, over months to years, of lesions often arranged in circles over the dorsum of the hands, feet, elbows, or knees
- Lesions are usually asymptomatic

PHYSICAL EXAMINATION

- Firm, flesh-colored to erythematous papules and plaques often arranged in a circle or semicircle

- Usually located on the dorsum of hands or feet or over the elbows or knees (Figs. 41-1 to 41-3)
- In subcutaneous granuloma annulare, tender, deeper, isolated nodules most commonly located over the shins are seen

DIAGNOSIS

- The diagnosis is often made by clinical exam
- A skin biopsy can be performed to verify the diagnosis

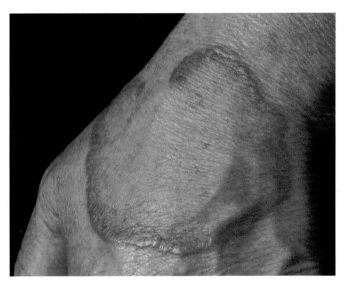

FIGURE 41-1 *Granuloma annulare.*

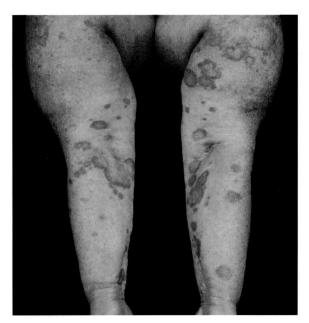

FIGURE 41-2   *Generalized granuloma annulare.*

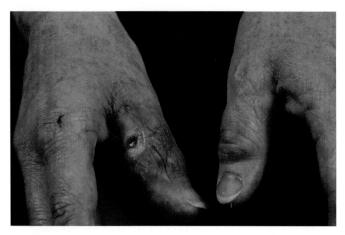

FIGURE 41-3 *Nodular granuloma annulare.*

- Dermatophyte infection: one sees scaly erythematous plaques affecting the skin of the body that can be diagnosed by examination of KOH preparation or fungal culture
- Sarcoidosis: presents with brown to violaceous papules and plaques that may appear on any cutaneous surface
  - Sarcoidosis may only be distinguishable from granuloma annulare by skin biopsy examination
- Necrobiosis lipoidica diabetacorum: presents with yellow to orange atrophic plaques that have indurated borders, often located on the shins
  - Telangectasia may be visible in central portion of the lesion

- Treatment of granuloma annulare is nonemergent
- Approximately 50% of patients improve spontaneously in 2 years
- Topical therapy
  - Topical corticosteroids: a mid-potency to super high-potency topical corticosteroid may be applied to the borders of the lesions bid for 2 weeks; should not be applied to the face, axillae, or groin
    - Mid-potency: prednicarbate (Dermatop®) 0.1% ointment or cream; triamcinolone acetonide (Aristocort®) 0.1% ointment or cream

- High-potency: fluocinonide (Lidex®) 0.05% ointment or cream; clobetasol propionate (Temovate®) 0.05% ointment or cream; halobetasol propionate (Ultravate®) 0.05% ointment or cream, betamethasone diproprionate 0.05% in optimized ointment (Diprolene®)
  - Emphasize side effects of prolonged use of corticosteroids, such as skin atrophy
- Intralesional corticosteroids
  - Can inject with triamcinolone acetonide (Kenalog®) 2.5 to 5.0 mg/ml to borders of the lesion
  - Inject along border using about 0.1 ml with each injection

- Patients should be seen within 3 to 4 weeks by either a primary care physician or a dermatologist if they underwent treatment for their lesions
- Patients who do not wish to have their lesions treated can follow up as needed

ICD-9-CM Code

695.89

CPT Code

11900 Intralesional injection ≤7 sites

HAND-FOOT-AND-MOUTH DISEASE

HISTORY

- Children under 10 years of age are most commonly affected
- Patients have a sore mouth and may refuse to eat
- Other symptoms may include fever, sore throat, cough, headache, malaise, diarrhea, anorexia, abdominal pain, and occasional arthralgias
- Highly contagious
- Summer and fall in temperate climates

PHYSICAL EXAMINATION

- Both oral and cutaneous lesions may be present (Figs. 42-1 and 42-2)
- Small, erythematous 2- to 8-mm macules and/or papules on the oropharynx (hard palate, buccal mucosa, tongue, and gingiva)
  - These form small, 1- to 3-mm gray ovoid vesicles with a peripheral zone of erythema
  - They ulcerate quickly, leaving shallow yellow to gray ulcerations

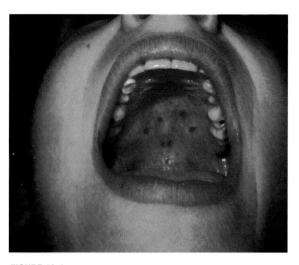

FIGURE 42-1   *Hand-foot-and-mouth disease.*

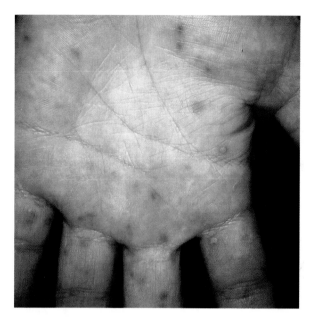

FIGURE 42-2 *Hand-foot-and-mouth disease.*

- Oral lesions usually number between 5 and 10
- Cutaneous lesions, which may vary in number from a few to over 100, may appear with or shortly after the oral lesions
  - They begin as red macules and papules then become round to ovoid vesicles that ulcerate These heal without scarring in 7 to 10 days
  - The dorsum and sides of fingers and toes are the most commonly affected cutaneous locations

DIAGNOSIS

- Clinical presentation or oral and distal extremity lesions sufficient for diagnosis
- When the diagnosis is in question, enzyme-linked immunosorbent assay detection of virus-specific IgM is useful
- Polymerase chain reaction and viral culture from multiple sites can be performed

DIFFERENTIAL DIAGNOSIS

- Aphthous stomatitis (canker sores): may cause lesions in the mouth that look similar to vesicles but lesions of the palms and soles are lacking
- Drug eruption: mucositis may be the result of a drug exposure, but vesicles on palms and soles would be highly unusual
- Erythema multiforme: can cause oral vesiculation and ulceration, but typical targetoid lesions elsewhere are not similar to the ovoid palm and sole vesicles of hand-foot-and-mouth disease
- Herpangina: produces scattered tiny vesicles with petechiae, along with fever and pharyngitis
- Herpes simplex: produces painful grouped vesicles, often on the lips; hand and foot involvement is lacking
- Rubella: petechiae are found on the posterior oral mucosa
- Varicella-zoster virus: unilateral painful grouped vesicles are seen

- Supportive care
- Antipyretics and antitussives
- Topical analgesics
  - Benzocaine (Lanacane®) or lidocaine (Xylocaine®) ointment for especially painful lesions
- Acyclovir has been used anecdotally, although the mechanism of action is unknown

- Severely affected patients should follow up with their primary care physician within days
- This is a self-limited disease, with resolution occurring over the course of 1 week
- Oral lesions resolve in 5 to 19 days without treatment
- Infection during the first trimester of pregnancy may result in spontaneous abortion

ICD-9-CM Code

074.3

CHAPTER 43

HERPES GESTATIONIS [PEMPHIGOID GESTATIONIS]

HISTORY

- Female, usually in fourth to seventh month of pregnancy, with extremely pruritic papulovesicular eruption
- May occur in the immediate postpartum period initially or as an exacerbation of previous eruption
- May be exacerbated by estrogen-containing medications

PHYSICAL EXAMINATION

- Variable morphology of lesions is seen (Figs. 43-1 and 43-2)
- One may observe erythematous and edematous urticarial papules and plaques to larger bullae
- This condition primarily involves the abdomen but may also involve the face, chest, back, palms, and soles

DIAGNOSIS

- Clinical examination with appropriate histopathologic findings of biopsy specimens

- Diagnostic confirmation is obtained by direct immunofluorescence study of perilesional skin or indirect immunofluorescence study of the patient's serum

DIFFERENTIAL DIAGNOSIS

- Polymorphous eruption of pregnancy (pruritic urticarial papules and plaques of pregnancy [PUPPP]): this nonvesicular condition presents during pregnancy with papules and excoriations on the abdomen, and generalization of lesions subsequently occurs
- Dermatitis herpetiformis: this autoimmune condition is highly pruritic and displays tiny vesicles, but vesicles are so pruritic that they are usually removed by scratching and none are visible
- Bullous pemphigoid: generally occurs in older adults, but the morphology of individual lesions is quite similar

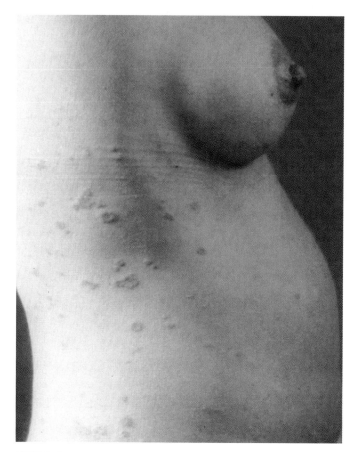

FIGURE 43-1 *Herpes gestationis.*

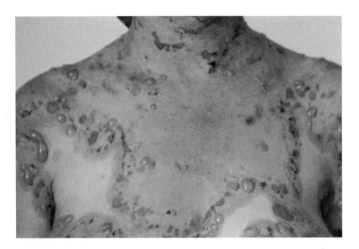

FIGURE 43-2 *Herpes gestationis.*

- Treatment is used to suppress blister formation and decrease pruritus
- Prednisone 20 to 40 mg daily in divided doses may be needed, with higher doses for disease flares (e.g., after parturition)
- Milder cases can be managed by bid application of potent topical corticosteroids
  - Fluocinonide (Lidex®) 0.05% ointment or cream; clobetasol propionate (Temovate®) 0.05% ointment or cream; halobetasol propionate (Ultravate®) 0.05% ointment or cream, betamethasone diproprionate 0.05% in optimized ointment (Diprolene®)
- Severe cases, after parturition, require immunosuppressive agents in addition to systemic prednisone

MANAGEMENT/FOLLOW-UP

- All patients require follow-up evaluation by their primary care physician and/or dermatologist

- The disease may flare during the first few postpartum menstrual periods and may or may not recur in later pregnancies
- The fetal prognosis is uncertain, since some studies demonstrate risk for fetal death and prematurity, whereas other studies show no significant fetal risk
- Infants born to mothers who received prednisone should be examined for adrenal insufficiency
- Infants born to mothers with herpes gestationis may develop vesicles and bullae, but these are transient and require no therapy

ICD-9-CM Code
646.8

HERPES SIMPLEX VIRUS

Primary herpetic infection

- The patient complains of painful ulcers, most commonly in the mouth or genital area, that have been present for a few days to a week
  - Lesions can be found on any skin surface from scalp to toes
- The lesions are occasionally accompanied by fever, headache, myalgia, malaise, and/or lymphadenopathy

Recurrent herpetic infection

- The patient complains of groups of painful blisters, pustules, or erosions present on any cutaneous surface
- Commonly affected areas include the skin of the perioral area, lumbosacral area, and external genitalia
- Patients may report a prodrome of tingling, itching, or burning that precedes the eruption by 1 to 2 days
- Patients may report a history of such lesions in the past

Neonatal herpes simplex virus infection

- Neonates may be infected during delivery, either on the skin or mucosa, and present with blisters, erosions, pustules, or ulcers
- Mothers of infected neonates may or may not relate a personal history of prior herpes simplex virus infections
- Lesions may occur in a local or widespread (disseminated) pattern

Immunosuppressed patients

- Patients may present with chronic lesions on any cutaneous or mucocutaneous surface, including the esophagus and anorectal area; they may also have widespread visceral involvement
- Lesions may be present for days, months, or years
- Disseminated disease is more common in immunosuppressed individuals, and these patients present complaining of flu-like symptoms and generalized lesions

Primary herpetic infection

- Multiple, painful erosions are found on any skin or mucous membrane (Figs. 44-1 and 44-2)
- The mouth, genitalia, and lumbosacral areas are most commonly affected
- The skin or mucosa is erythematous and edematous and has small to large grouped vesicles with central umbilication
- As lesions mature, vesicles may coalesce, become vesiculopustules, and become erosions
- The patient may appear ill and present with fever and/or dehydration
- Lymphadenopathy may be present

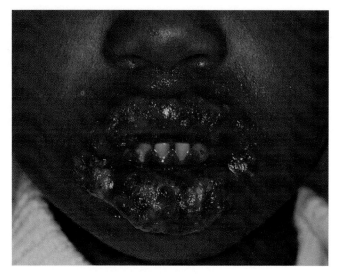

FIGURE 44-1 *Primary herpetic gingivostomatitis in a child.*

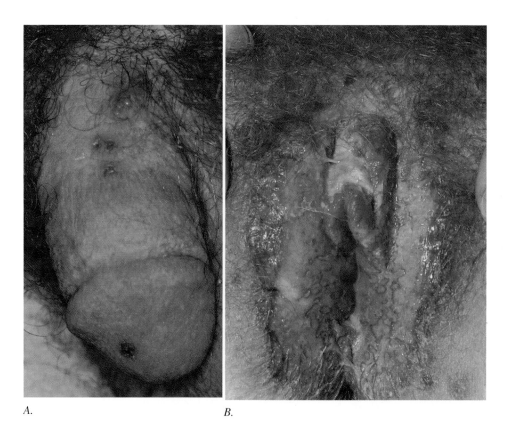

A.   *B.*

FIGURE 44-2 A. *Primary genital herpes simplex.* B. *Primary herpetic vulvitis.*

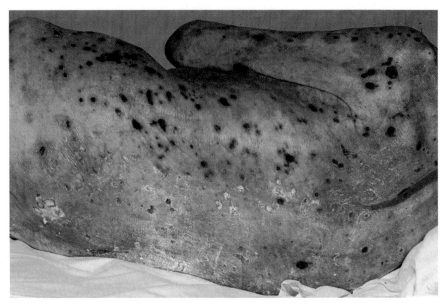

A.

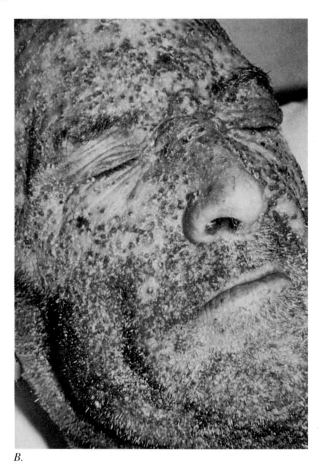

B.

FIGURE 44-3 *Disseminated herpes simplex infection.*

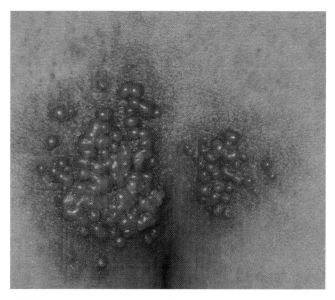

FIGURE 44-4   *Recurrent lumbosacral herpes simplex.*

Recurrent herpetic infection

- Groups of umbilicated vesicles, vesico-lopustules, or erosions on an erythematous base may be present on any mucocutaneous surface (Figs. 44-3 and 44-4)
- Oral mucosal herpetic lesions are almost always associated with primary herpetic infection, whereas genital mucosal ulcers may be found in primary and recurrent infection
- Systemic findings are not usually present in immunocompetent hosts

Neonatal and immunosuppressed patients

- Localized disease: presentation is similar to that in immunocompetent patients
- Disseminated disease: presents with non-grouped vesicles and pustules that often rupture and leave "punched-out" erosions

- The diagnosis can generally be made by history and physical examination
- A Tzanck preparation can be performed to confirm that a herpetic infection is present, but it cannot distinguish between herpes simplex virus and varicella-zoster virus infections
  - Using a #15 scalpel blade, unroof the skin of an intact blister
  - Using a sterile cotton-tipped applicator or the scalpel blade, either obtain the fluid from the blister or scrape the base of the blister and apply directly to a dry glass slide
  - Allow the specimen to air dry on the slide, and then place a drop of either Wright's or Giemsa stain on the slide

- The appearance of multinucleated giant cells or large viropathic cells indicates a positive finding
- Interpretation of a Tzanck smear can be quite difficult; an experienced individual should interpret the slide, and other tests can be performed to confirm infection
- The diagnosis of herpes simplex can only be made tentatively in the acute setting, and definitive diagnosis requires other laboratory approaches
  - Polymerase chain reaction studies for herpes simplex virus and varicella-zoster virus infections can be performed on vesicle fluid or biopsy specimens and is the most sensitive and reliable approach
  - A viral culture can be performed using appropriate viral media
    - Optimally, an intact blister should be opened and the vesicular fluid obtained for culture
    - Herpes simplex virus I is usually associated with oral-labial infection and herpes simplex virus II with genital infection, but this is not always the case

DIFFERENTIAL DIAGNOSIS

Local disease

- Herpes zoster (shingles) may be clinically indistinguishable from herpes simplex virus infections and can only be distinguished by polymerase chain reaction or viral culture confirmation
  - Populations of patients with herpes simplex tend to be younger, and more commonly herpes simplex involves the perioral area, lumbosacral area, and external genitalia
- Hand-foot-and-mouth disease: this viral disease in children is associated with vesicles and papules on the hands, the feet, and occasionally the buttocks area, along with constitutional symptoms
- Erythema multiforme: this reaction pattern produces oral ulcerations and mucosal erosions associated with constitutional symptoms and a typical targetoid skin rash

- Chronic oral aphthosis: one sees painful, recurrent, intraoral erosions that remain localized to mucosal surfaces of the skin
- Chancroid: a tender erythematous papule first appears that evolves into a pustule, erosion, and then an ulcer with sharp, undermined borders and a friable gray-yellow base of granulation on the external genitalia
- Traumatic ulceration: this may occur in any location including the genitalia, and unusual, angular shapes suggesting external causes are found
- Lymphogranuloma venereum: this infection involves a painless, nonindurated superficial ulcer in association with painful regional lymphedenopathy
- Granuloma inguinale: presents with one or more painless nodules in the genital areas
- Crohn's disease: this inflammatory bowel disease may present ulcers that are usually linear and resemble lacerations
- Squamous cell or basal cell carcinoma: these cancers may occur in the anogenital area or anywhere on the body, but they have a chronic, slowly enlarging course lasting months to years
- Behçet's disease: recurrent oral and genital ulceration associated with eye disease, arthritis, vasculitis, and other skin lesions

Disseminated disease

- Varicella (chickenpox): this viral infection is caused by the varicella-zoster virus
  - Lesions are extremely pruritic, begin on the face, and spread inferiorly
  - Lesions appear in successive crops, with papules, vesicles, pustules, and crusts present simultaneously
- Disseminated zoster: this viral infection is caused by the varicella-zoster virus; patients are often immunosuppressed and ill-appearing; lesions appear as widespread necrotic papules and pustules
- Eczema herpeticum: this widespread herpes simplex virus infection occurs in the setting of preexisting atopic dermatitis

- Bullous impetigo: vesicles and bullae filled with clear to yellow fluid arise on normal-appearing skin and are usually seen in children and young adults

TREATMENT

- Treatment of herpes simplex virus is non-emergent unless there is ophthalmologic involvement
  - However, prompt treatment is recommended to decrease the duration of symptoms and viral shedding
- Skin to skin contact should be avoided during the outbreak of cutaneous herpes simplex infection
- Patients should be made aware that asymptomatic viral shedding does occur; therefore it is possible to transmit the infection during periods of clinical remission
- Antiviral therapy
  - Antiviral therapy should be considered for the groups of patients described below.

Primary herpetic infection

- Immunocompetent patients with mild to moderate disease whose lesions have been present for 48 hours or less
- Immunocompetent patients with severe disease
- Immunosuppressed individuals, pregnant women, and neonates

Recurrent herpetic infection

- Any patient with confirmed herpes simplex virus is susceptible to recurrent infections and should be considered for prophylactic therapy
- In general, patients with six or more episodes a year are encouraged to use daily suppressive antiviral therapy
- Antiviral therapy has been shown to decrease the duration of symptoms and viral shedding if used early in disease

- Intravenous acyclovir should be strongly considered in immunosuppressed individuals, neonates with severe or disseminated disease, or those with ophthalmologic involvement

Primary herpetic infection

Acyclovir   400 mg orally tid for 7 to 10 days or 200 mg orally 5x/day for 7 to 10 days or
Famciclovir   250 mg orally tid for 7 to 10 days or
Valacyclovir   500 mg to 1 gm orally bid for 7 to 10 days

Episodic recurrent infection

Acyclovir   400 mg orally tid for 5 days or 200 mg orally 5x/day for 5 days or
Famciclovir   125 mg orally bid for 5 days or
Valacyclovir   500 mg orally bid for 5 days

Suppressive therapy

Acyclovir   400 mg orally bid or
Famciclovir   250 mg orally bid or
Valacyclovir   500 mg bid

MANAGEMENT/FOLLOW-UP

- Patients with primary infection should be educated regarding the signs and symptoms of recurrent infection so that they may seek prompt treatment
- Patients with recurrent infection should be given the option of daily suppressive therapy
- Immunosuppressed patients or neonates who are treated as outpatients should be followed up by a primary care physician or a dermatologist within a few days to assess progress

ICD-9 Code

054.9

HERPES ZOSTER (SHINGLES)

HISTORY

- The patient complains of pain or paresthesia in a localized area that precedes a skin rash by 3 to 5 days
- The rash is primarily localized to one side of the body
- The lesions are occasionally accompanied by fever, headache, myalgia, malaise, and/or lymphadenopathy

- Immunosuppressed individuals often present with more widespread lesions or disseminated disease, and they are more likely to have recurrent episodes

PHYSICAL EXAMINATION

- Grouped and confluent vesicles, pustules, or crusted papules in a dermatomal and unilateral distribution (on one side of the midline; Figs. 45-1 to 45-3)

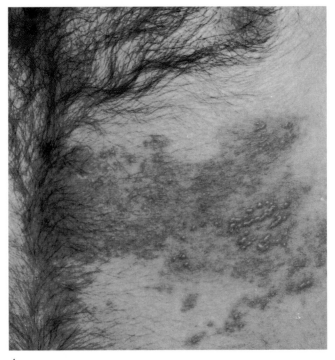

A

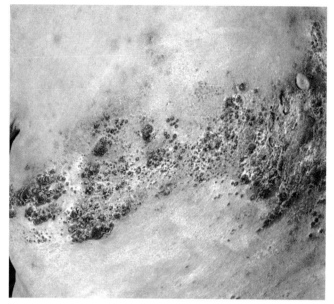

B.

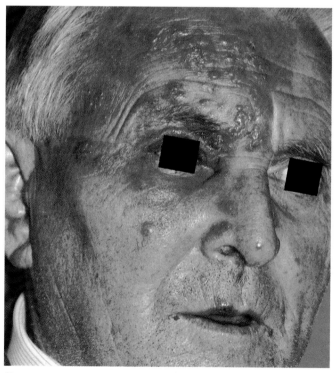

C.

FIGURE 45-1 *Herpes zoster.*

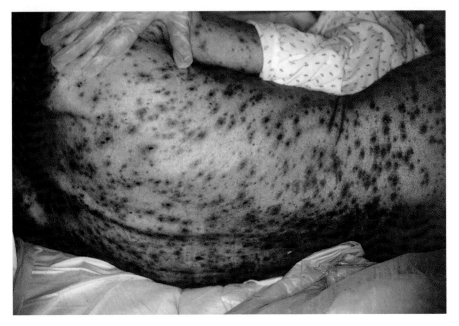

FIGURE 45-2 *Patient with disseminated herpes zoster.*

- A few lesions may be found outside of the primary affected dermatome, and an immunocompetent individual may occasionally present with more than one dermatome involved
- Most common sites involved include thoracic, trigeminal, lumbosacral, and cervical dermatomes
- Depending on the dermatome involved, mucosal lesions may occur as well
- In trigeminal disease (usually cranial nerve V_1 distribution), involvement of the nasociliary branch occurs in one-third of the cases
  - These patients present with lesions on the sides and tip of the nose
  - Such lesions could be a harbinger to ophthalmologic involvement
- Immunosuppressed individuals often have more than one dermatome involved and are more likely to present with disseminated disease

DIAGNOSIS

- Diagnosis can be made by history and physical exam
- A Tzanck preparation can be performed to confirm that a herpetic infection is present, but it cannot distinguish between herpes simplex virus and varicella-zoster virus infections
  - Using a #15 scalpel blade, unroof the skin of an intact blister
  - Using a sterile cotton-tipped applicator or the scalpel blade, either obtain the fluid from the blister or scrape the base of the blister and apply directly to a dry glass slide
  - Allow the specimen to air dry on the slide, and then place a drop of either Wright's or Giemsa stain on the slide

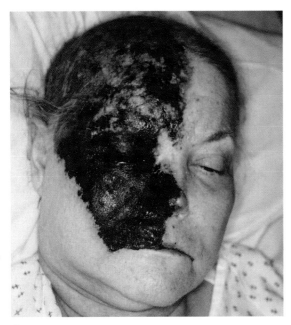

A.

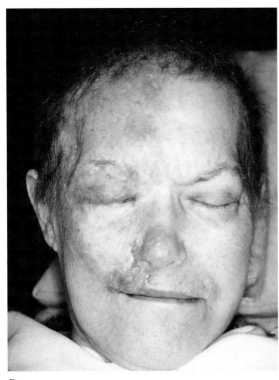

B.

FIGURE 45-3 *Acute, necrotic herpes zoster.*

- The appearance of multinucleated giant cells or large viropathic cells indicates a positive finding
  - Interpretation of a Tzanck smear can be quite difficult; an experienced individual should interpret the slide, and other tests can be performed to confirm infection
- The diagnosis of herpes simplex can only be made tentatively in the acute setting, and definitive diagnosis requires other laboratory approaches
  - Polymerase chain reaction studies for herpes simplex virus and varicella zoster virus infections can be performed on vesicle fluid or biopsy specimens and is the most sensitive and reliable approach
  - A viral culture can be performed using appropriate viral media
    - Optimally, an intact blister should be opened and the vesicular fluid obtained for culture
    - The yield from viral culture is generally quite low

DIFFERENTIAL DIAGNOSIS

Local Disease

- Herpes simplex virus infections may be clinically indistinguishable from herpes zoster infections and can only be distinguished by polymerase chain reaction or viral culture confirmation
  - Populations of patients with herpes zoster tend to be older, and more commonly herpes simplex involves the perioral area, lumbosacral area, and external genitalia
- Hand-foot-and-mouth disease: this viral disease in children is associated with vesicles and papules on the hands, the feet, and occasionally the buttocks area, along with constitutional symptoms
- Erythema multiforme: oral ulcerations and mucosal erosions associated with constitutional symptoms and a typical targetoid skin rash

- Chronic oral aphthosis: painful, recurrent, intraoral erosions that remain localized to mucosal surfaces of the skin
- Behçet's disease: recurrent oral and genital ulceration associated with eye disease, arthritis, vasculitis, and other skin lesions
- Aphthous ulcerations: rarely, patients may present with persistent forms of aphthae due to systemic problems, such as iron deficiency, vitamin B_{12} deficiency, HIV infection, or gluten-sensitive enteropathy
- Major acute systemic conditions: patients with chest zoster may mimic patients with myocardial infarction, and patients with abdominal involvement may mimic patients with abdominal emergencies such as bowel perforation, appendicitis, cholecystitis, etc.

Disseminated Disease

- Varicella: this viral infection is caused by the varicella-zoster virus
  - Lesions are extremely pruritic and begin on the face and spread inferiorly; lesions appear in successive crops, and with papules, vesicles, pustules, and crusts are present simultaneously
- Disseminated herpes simplex virus: this viral infection is caused by the herpes simplex virus; patients are often immunosuppressed and ill-appearing
  - Lesions appear as widespread necrotic papules and pustules and may be clinically indistinguishable from disseminated zoster
- Eczema herpeticum: widespread herpes simplex virus infection occurring in the setting of preexisting atopic dermatitis
- Bullous impetigo: vesicles and bullae filled with clear to yellow fluid that arise on normal-appearing skin and are usually seen in children and young adults

TREATMENT

- Treatment of zoster is nonemergent unless there is ophthalmologic involvement

- However, prompt treatment is recommended to decrease the duration of symptoms and viral shedding
- Education regarding the condition should be given to the patient:
  - Lesions of zoster are contagious several days before the exanthem appears until the last crop of vesicles have crusted over
  - Transmission of zoster does not occur through contact with an individual with zoster; it requires previous infection with varicella, with subsequent reactivation of the virus that has been latent in the sensory ganglia
  - Exposure to a person with zoster can cause varicella (chickenpox) in another patient who has not had varicella previously, but such exposure cannot cause zoster in another individual; any contact with individuals who have not yet had primary varicella should be avoided
  - Infected patients should avoid contact with pregnant females or immunosuppressed individuals
- Antiviral therapy
  - Antiviral therapy should be considered for the following groups of patients:
    - Immunocompetent patients with mild to moderate disease whose lesions have been present for 48 hours or less
    - Immunocompetent patients with severe disease
    - Immunosuppressed individuals, pregnant women, and neonates
  - Antiviral therapy has been shown to decrease the duration of symptoms and viral shedding if used early in disease
  - Intravenous acyclovir should be strongly considered in immunosuppressed individuals; oral antiviral therapy may be administered as follows:
    - Acyclovir   800 mg orally 5x/day for 7 to 10 days or

- Famciclovir   500 mg orally tid for 7 to 10 days or
- Valacyclovir   1 g orally tid for 7 to 10 days
- Topical therapy
  - The use of topical antiviral agents has not been proved useful in the setting of zoster infection
  - Topical antibiotic agents, such as 2% mupirocin (Bactroban®) cream or ointment, can be prescribed for bid use if secondary infection is suspected
  - Topical 1% silver sulfadiazine cream (Silvadene® cream) can be used twice daily for its antiinflammatory properties (do not use in sulfa-allergic patients)
- Pain management: the pain of herpes zoster may be severe and may require opiate analgesia such as acetaminophen with codeine (Tylenol #3®) or oxycodone
- Postherpetic neuralgia (PHN)
  - PHN is pain localized to an area of previous zoster infection that persists after the rash has subsided
  - PHN may last for months to years
  - PHN may respond to analgesics, but other popular treatments include tricyclic antidepressants, capsaicin cream, topical anesthetics, and nerve blocks

MANAGEMENT/FOLLOW-UP

- Immunosuppressed individuals should be educated regarding the signs and symptoms of recurrent infection so that they may seek prompt treatment
- Immunosuppressed patients who are treated as outpatients should be followed up by a primary care physician or a dermatologist within a few days to assess progress
- Other patients can follow up as needed

ICD-9-CM Code
053.9

CHAPTER 46

HIDRADENITIS SUPPURATIVA

- Painful and tender lesions related to abscess formation in the axillae, inframammary areas, and/or anogenital areas

- Lesions usually present for months to years, and the patient often presents with marked scarring from previous lesions
- Patient may also have a history of recurrent nodular acne vulgaris

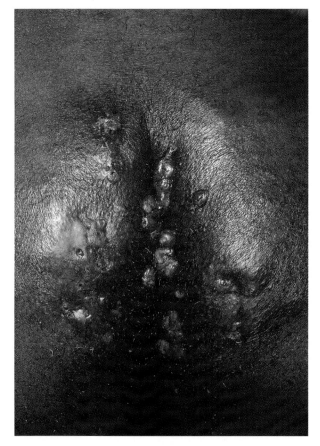

FIGURE 46-1 *Hidradenitis suppurativa.*

- Erythematous, tender nodules and/or abscesses that may have purulent drainage are found in the axillae, inframammary areas, and/or anogenital areas (Figs. 46-1 to 46-3)
- Sinus tracts may be evident, as may severe scarring
- Scarring is usually hypertrophic or keloidal in nature
- Chronic hidradenitis usually has associated open comedones ("blackheads")

DIAGNOSIS

- The diagnosis is usually made by history and physical exam

DIFFERENTIAL DIAGNOSIS

- Psuedofolliculitis barbae and acne keloidalis nuchae: multiple papules, pustules, and keloids occurring on the beard area and posterior scalp areas, respectively; commonly seen in African-American males
- Abscess, furuncle, or carbuncle: very painful, tender papules and pustules presenting on any cutaneous region, particularly hair-bearing sites; usually arises over a period of a few days and is associated with foul-smelling discharge; usually not associated with scarring or sinus tracts

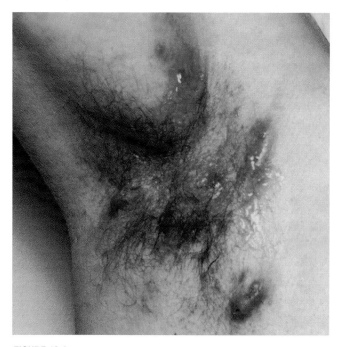

FIGURE 46-2 *Stage I hidradenitis suppurativa.*

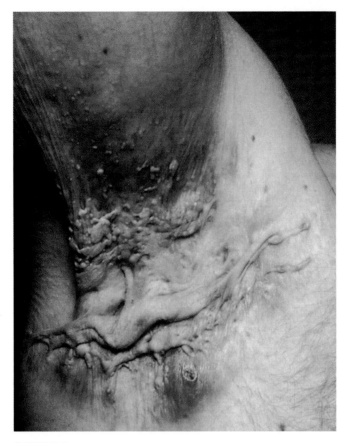

FIGURE 46-3 *End-stage hidradenitis suppurativa.*

- Ruptured epidermal inclusion cyst: an erythematous, tender plaque associated with foul-smelling drainage; patient often reports a history of a chronic cyst that recently became inflamed and tender
- Other dermatoses that produce fistulas and sinuses should also be included in the differential diagnosis, such as actinomycosis, tularemia, tuberculosis, and cat-scratch disease; in the inguinal area, granuloma inguinale, lymphogranuloma venereum, and cutaneous inflammatory bowel disease should also be considered

- Treatment of hidradenitis supparativa is nonemergent

Medical management
- Antimicrobial therapy appropriate for staphylococcus coverage can provide short-term relief
  - Dicloxacillin: 500 mg bid for 10 days (adults); 12.5 to 25 mg/kg/day (children <40 kg)

- ○ Cephalexin (Keflex®): 500 mg bid for 10 days (adults); 25 to 50 mg/kg/day (children)
- ○ *Penicillin-allergic*: erythromycin 500 mg bid for 10 days (adults); 40 mg/kg/day for 10 days (children)
- Intralesional corticosteroids
  - ○ Can inject with triamcinolone acetonide (Kenalog®) 3 to 10 mg/ml to treat lesions; the amount injected will depend on the size of the lesion
  - ○ Firm, fibrotic lesions may be very difficult/impossible to inject
- Application of heat to the lesions often promotes drainage as well; warm wet towel compresses can be applied 2 to 3 times daily for 10 minutes each time
- Other systemic therapy
  - ○ Isotretinoin (Accutane®) or dapsone may be of benefit in patients refractory to other forms of therapy but should not be dispensed in an emergency department setting because of the need for strict laboratory monitoring and close outpatient management

Surgical management
- Incision and drainage of acute abscesses can be performed for immediate relief of lesions; often combined with antibiotic therapy and/or intralesional corticosteroids
- Chronic, fibrotic nodules and sinus tracts may be excised to remove scar tissue

MANAGEMENT/FOLLOW-UP

- Hidradentitis supparativa is a chronic condition that will require long-term management by either a primary care physician or a dermatologist
- Patients should follow up within 1 month for further therapy

ICD-9-CM Code

705.83

CPT Code

11900   Intralesional injection ≤7 sites
10060   Incision and drainage

CHAPTER 47

HYPERSENSITIVITY VASCULITIS (LEUKOCYTOCLASTIC VASCULITIS)

HISTORY

- Patients may have a history of an associated condition such as:
  - A recent drug exposure approximately 1 week prior to onset of vascultitis
  - An infection including streptococcal, staphylococcal, and rickettsial bacterial infections; hepatitis A, B, or C viral infections
  - Inflammatory bowel disease including ulcerative colitis and Crohn's disease may be related
  - Autoimmune disorder such as systemic lupus erythematosus, dermatomyositis, Sjögren's syndrome, or rheumatoid arthritis
  - Malignancy can induce vascultitis as a paraneoplastic event
  - Cryoglobulinemia can induce vascultitis
  - Antiphospholipid antibody syndrome can induce vascultitis
- Most commonly patients present with idiopathic disease

- History of either characteristic cutaneous eruption or visceral symptoms, which may include:
  - Fever, malaise
  - Gastrointestinal symptoms: abdominal pain, gastrointestinal bleeding, intussusception
  - Musculoskeletal: arthralgias, arthritis
  - Renal: glomerulonephritis
- The crops of lesions may have a burning or pruritic feeling
- In children generally 4 to 8 years old, Henoch-Schönlein purpura presents with a cutaneous purpuric eruption, arthralgias, abdominal pain, and renal disease
  - Most children have a preceding upper respiratory tract infection

PHYSICAL EXAMINATION

- Palpable purpuric papules and plaques are more prominent in gravity-dependent sites (Fig. 47-1)

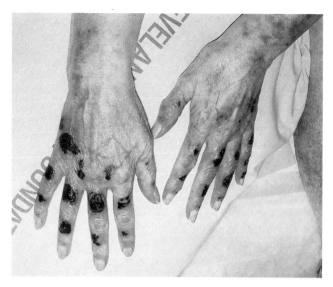

FIGURE 47-1 *Digital purpura (leukocytoclastic angiitis).*

- There may be an associated edema of the extremities
- Urticarial plaques, livedo reticularis, vesicles and ulcers may be seen
- Examine for evidence of disease in the following systems: cardiopulmonary, renal, musculoskeletal, and gastrointestinal

DIAGNOSIS

- Diagnosis usually requires obtaining a skin biopsy specimen for histopathologic confirmation of vasculitis
- A search to identify the underlying process and sequelae of vasculitis; should consist at the minimum of a complete blood count with differential, erythrocyte sedimentation rate (ESR), urinalysis, blood chemistry panel, and antinuclear antibody determination
  - Other tests that may be beneficial in individuals may include stool guaiac, chest x-ray, direct immunofluorescence testing of skin biopsy specimen, complement tests, HIV antibody tests, and cryoglobulins and hepatitis screen
  - A wide variety of other organ-specific laboratory and radiologic tests may be indicated

DIFFERENTIAL DIAGNOSIS

- Thrombocytopenia: this may cause purpura, but not usually palpable
- Septic emboli: patients are usually febrile, have malaise, and have relatively few distal purpuric papules
- Meningococcemia: patients present with tiny petechiae to large ecchymoses, in conjunction with fever, headache, vomiting, and acute mental status changes
- Disseminated intravascular coagulation: this appears with widespread petechiae, ecchymoses, and hemorrhagic bullae, as well asischemic necrosis of the skin and profuse bleeding
- Pigmented purpuric dermatoses: these conditions may present with purpura that is usually of chronic duration, limited to the distal lower extremities
- Other systemic vasculitides such as polyarteritis nodosa and nodular vasculitis: these less common conditions generally present with larger purpuric papules and nodules, often with large ulcerations

- Treatment is directed towards the underlying process
  - Potentially offending drugs in drug-hypersensitivity vasculitis should be withdrawn
  - Any evident infection should be treated
- If there is any evidence of internal organ involvement, such as glomerulonephritis in Henoch-Schönlein purpura, emergent intervention may be required with the assistance of appropriate specialists
- For many patients, nonsteroidal antiinflammatory drugs such as aspirin and indomethacin may decrease the severity of the condition
- Colchicine and dapsone have some ability to decrease the onset of new lesions in idiopathic disease

- Other reported treatments have included pentoxyfylline, systemic corticosteroids, methotrexate, azathioprine, cyclophosphamide, cyclosporin, and plasmapheresis

MANAGEMENT/FOLLOW-UP

- In most patients, palpable purpura lasts for 1 to 4 weeks, resolving with transient hyperpigmentation and possibly atrophic scarring
- Henoch-Schönlein Purpura resolves in the majority of patients in 6 to 16 weeks, although 5-10% of patients will have recurrent or persistent disease

ICD-9-CM Code

287.0

IMPETIGO

- Crusted, scaly lesions or blisters present for days to weeks over any cutaneous surface
- Lesions may arise on areas of underlying dermatoses, such as atopic dermatitis, or on areas of minor breaks in the skin, such as arthropod bites

- Nonbullous impetigo: superficial small vesicles or pustules, erosions, and/or honey-colored crusted papules located most commonly on the face and extremities (Figs. 48-1 to 48-3)

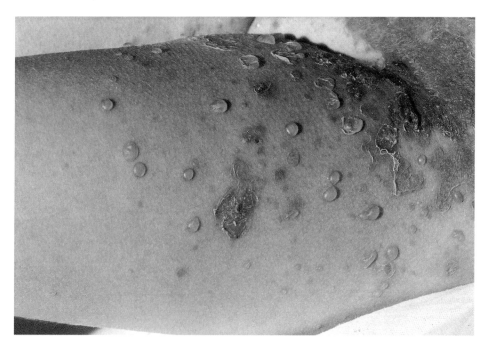

FIGURE 48-1 *Bullous impetigo:* S. aureus.

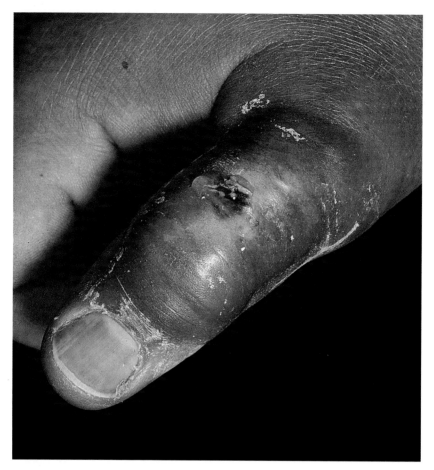

FIGURE 48-2 *Bullous impetigo:* S. aureus.

- Bullous impetigo: vesicles or bullae containing clear to yellow fluid, usually located on the trunk, extremities, face, or intertriginous areas
- Patient may have clinical findings of preexisting dermatoses, such as atopic dermatitis
- May occur in any age group, although children and young adults are most commonly affected

DIAGNOSIS

- Diagnosis is usually made by history and clinical examination
- The organisms most likely to cause impetigo are *Staphylococcus aureus* and *Streptococcus pyogenes*; a Gram stain can be performed and will reveal gram-positive cocci in clusters or chains, respectively

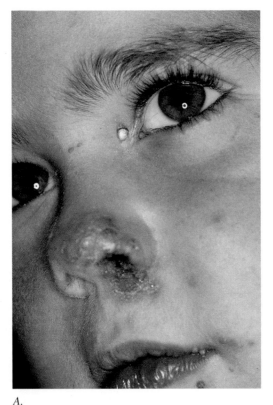

A.

FIGURE 48-3 *Impetigo:* S. aureus.

- Herpes simplex virus (HSV) and herpes zoster: HSV and herpes zoster lesions occur as grouped vesicles or erosions on an erythematous base; in primary HSV infection, patients usually appear ill and may have constitutional symptoms such as fever and malaise; recurrent oral lesions occur in groups and almost always involve only the vermilion of the lip rather than intraoral areas
- Perioral dermatitis: erythematous papules and pustules on an erythematous background that most commonly occurs around the mouth, although the periorbital area may be involved as well; there is often sparing directly around the lips
- Seborrheic dermatitis: yellow to red, greasy and scaly papules and plaques usually located on the scalp, eyebrows, glabellar areas, ears, and nasolabial folds, as well as hair-bearing sites on the face and chest
- Allergic contact dermatitis: an allergen elicits an inflammatory reaction on the skin, causing well-demarcated plaques of erythema with superimposed vesicles if the reaction is acute; plaques of lichenification (thickened skin with accentuation of skin lines) occur if the process is chronic

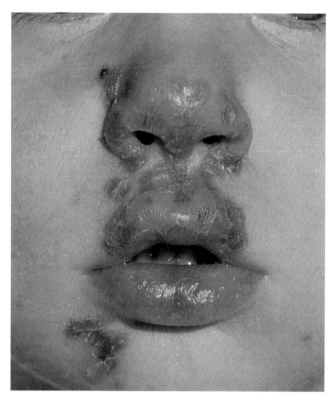

B.

- The treatment of impetigo is nonemergent, but prompt treatment is recommended to prevent deeper tissue infections
- Topical therapy
  - 2% Muciprocin ointment (Bactroban®) is highly effective against the gram-positive organisms that commonly cause impetigo; apply the ointment 2 to 3x/day for 7 to 10 days to affected areas
  - Approximately 20% of individuals are nasal carriers of *Staphylococcus aureus*; thus muciprocin should be applied to the distal nares 2 to 3x/day for 7 to 10 days as well
- Systemic therapy
  - Dicloxacillin: 500 mg bid for 10 days (adults); 12.5 to 25 mg/kg/day (children <40 kg)
  - Cephalexin: 500 mg bid for 10 days (adults); 25 to 50 mg/kg/day (children)
  - *Penicillin-allergic*: erythromycin 500 mg bid for 10 days (adults); 40 mg/kg/day for 10 days (children)

MANAGEMENT/FOLLOW-UP

- Patients should be encouraged to follow up with a primary care physician or dermatologist if the lesions do not resolve after a course of topical or systemic antibiotics

ICD-9 Code

684

CHAPTER 49

INGROWN NAIL

- Patient presents complaining of pain, tenderness, swelling, and redness of the lateral nail fold of a finger or toe
- Patient may have had similar episodes in the past

PHYSICAL EXAMINATION

- The most frequent cause of ingrown nails is improper trimming of a nail, resulting in a spicule of nail that protrudes into the lateral nail fold (Fig. 49-1)
- Most commonly, patients present for infection secondary to the ingrown nail, with a lateral nail fold that is erythematous, edematous, and tender and may have pustular drainage

DIAGNOSIS

- Diagnosis of an ingrown nail is made by history and physical examination

DIFFERENTIAL DIAGNOSIS

- Paronychia: infection of the nail fold usually caused by a break in the skin; etiology is bacterial, fungal, or candidal and may be exacerbated by frequent exposure of the digits to water

TREATMENT

- The treatment of ingrown nail infection is nonemergent, but prompt treatment should be provided to prevent further complications
- Oral antibiotics appropriate for *Staphylococcus* coverage should be administered to patients with signs and symptoms of an ingrown nail infection
  - ◦ Dicloxacillin: 500 mg bid for 10 days (adults); 12.5 to 25 mg/kg/day (children <40 kg)
  - ◦ Cephalexin: 500 mg bid for 10 days (adults); 25 to 50 mg/kg/day (children)
  - ◦ *Penicillin-allergic*: erythromycin 500 mg bid for 10 days (adults); 40 mg/kg/day for 10 days (children)

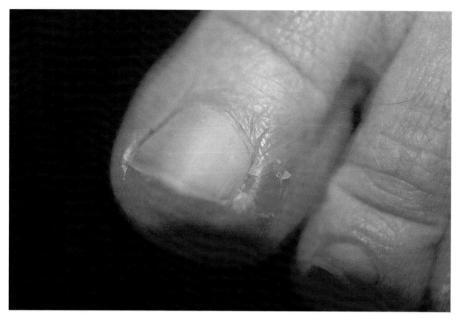

FIGURE 49-1 *Ingrown nail.*

- To prevent further nail spicule formation, the nail should be trimmed straight across and slightly distal to the hyponychium; tight-fitting shoes should also be avoided

MANAGEMENT/FOLLOW-UP

- Patients should be told that if their symptoms do not improve within a week of oral antibiotic therapy, they should follow up with either a primary care physician or a dermatologist

ICD-9-CM Code

703.0

CPT Code

10060   Drainage of infected nail area, simple or single

CHAPTER 50

KAWASAKI'S DISEASE

HISTORY

- If this syndrome is suspected, the history and physical examination should focus on elucidation of the criteria for diagnosis
- Patients require five of the six principle criteria to diagnose Kawasaki's disease definitively
  - Infants or children present with 5 days or more of a spiking fever up to 40°C
  - Acute nonsuppurative cervical lymphadenopathy
  - Changes in peripheral extremities, including edema and erythema, progressing to desquamation
  - Bilateral conjunctival injection
  - Oral mucosal disease, including oropharyngeal erythema, erythematous to fissured lips, and "strawberry" tongue
  - Scarlatiniform eruption
- Other findings may include arthralgias and arthritis; urethritis and sterile pyuria, aseptic meningitis, diarrhea, vomiting, abdominal pain, and perineal erythema
- Abnormal cardiac findings may include myocarditis, pericardial effusions, congestive heart failure, coronary artery aneurisms, or aortic or mitral valve regurgitation secondary to valvulitis

PHYSICAL EXAMINATION

- Almost all patients develop cherry red lips, which are dry and cracked or fissured (Fig. 50-1)

- Almost all patients develop erythema and edema of the distal hands and feet within a few days of the onset of illness (Figs. 50-2 to 50-4)
  - These areas desquamate in the subacute phase of the illness, 10 to 18 days after starting
- Truncal and proximal extremities with a variable exanthem
  - This eruption may be morbilliform, macular, papular, or urticarial
  - It is indistinguishable from viral exanthem or drug eruption
- Diffuse macular or plaque-like erythema of the perineum, which may be tender (Fig. 50-5)
- 90% of patients have nonexudative bilateral conjunctival injection (more bulbar than palpebral) that is noncrusting
  - More than 80% of these patients develop anterior uveitis
- Unilateral cervical lymphadenopathy is often present
- "Strawberry" tongue is present in half of patients, with erythematous, hypertrophied papillae
- Generalized desquamation in some patients during the subacute phase of the illness
- On cardiac exam, patients may demonstrate tachycardia, gallop rhythms, pericardial friction rub, dysrhythmias, aortic/mitral regurgitation, findings of congestive heart failure, and/or peripheral arterial aneurysms
- Electrocardiographic (ECG) abnormalities such as prolonged PR interval, left ventricular hypertrophy, abnormal Q waves, and nonspecific ST-T changes

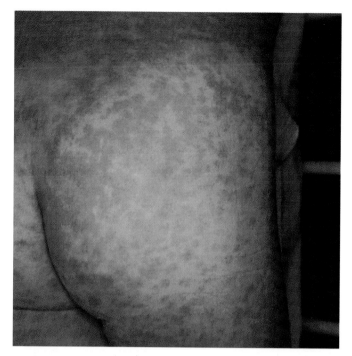

FIGURE 50-1 *Kawasaki's disease.*

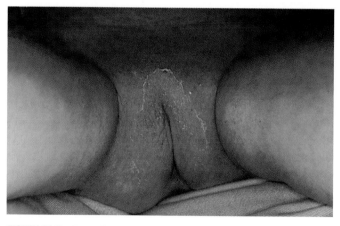

FIGURE 50-2 *Generalized morbilliform eruption in the early stages of Kawasaki's disease.*

- Clinical presentation and fulfilling criteria
- ECG abnormalities; echocardiography for demonstration of coronary artery changes

- There are very few conditions that present with the constellation of features of Kawasaki's disease

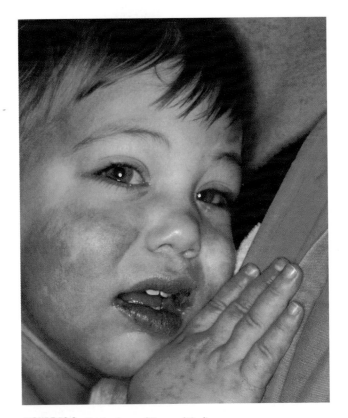

FIGURE 50-3   *Early phase of Kawasaki's disease.*

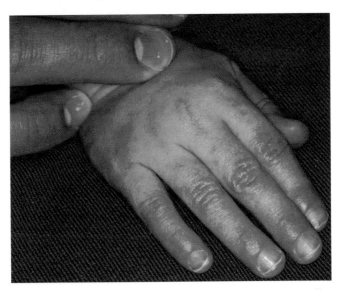

FIGURE 50-4   *Desquamation starting at the fingertips in infant with Kawasaki's disease.*

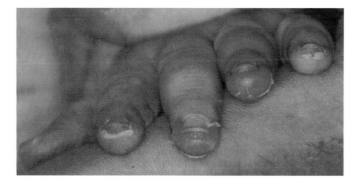

FIGURE 50-5 *Generalized erythema and early desquamation in perineal area of a young girl with Kawasaki's disease.*

- Juvenile rheumatoid arthritis: this condition may display fever, arthritis, and a diffuse salmon-colored eruption, but it lacks other aspects of the criteria listed above
- Drug eruption: widespread drug eruptions may cause erythema and mucositis but should not cause marked fever and cervical lymphadenopathy
- Viral exanthem: these exanthems can display exanthems and enanthems, but it would be atypical to see the prolonged duration of fever, cervical lymphadenopathy, and other features

TREATMENT

- Treatment of Kawasaki's disease is emergent
- Combination of ASA with high dose IVIG for reduction of myocardial and coronary artery inflammation and prevention of coronary artery thrombosis
  - Aspirin 80 to 100 mg/kg/day to achieve serum salicylate level of 20 to 25 mg/dl
    - Dose is reduced after defervescence (2 weeks) to 3 to 5 mg/kg/day, and discontinued at 6 to 8 weeks if no coronary abnormalities are noted
    - Aspirin is continued indefinitely for patients with coronary artery aneurysms
  - Dipyridamole 4 mg/kg/day to inhibit platelet aggregation further in certain cases
  - IVIG, a single dose of 2 g/kg

- Cardiology evaluation
  - Echocardiography for detection and progression of coronary artery changes
  - Anticoagulant therapy or use of thrombolytics in cases of cardiac ischemia/thrombosis
  - Angioplasty and coronary artery bypass grafting have been required

MANAGEMENT/FOLLOW-UP

- After resolution of the acute illness, most children return to their prior state of health; fatality rate is 2%
- Cardiovascular morbidity is the major complication
  - Between one-half and two-thirds of children with arterial aneurysms demonstrate regression on angiography within 6 to 24 months
  - Coronary artery aneurysms may occur in 25% patients not treated with IVIG
  - Children with large (greater than 8 mm) aneurysms are at risk for stenosis or obstruction
- All children with Kawasaki's disease, regardless of the presence of aneurysm, should have long-term cardiology follow-up to guard against the development later in life of myocardial dysfunction, late-onset valvular regurgitation, or premature coronary artery disease

ICD-9 Code

446.1

KELOID SCAR

HISTORY

- Development of a thickened scar usually following injury to the skin (e.g., surgical scar, trauma, acne, body piercing, etc); may develop spontaneously, without preceding injury
- Itching and/or pain may be associated with the lesion
- Common sites include the earlobe, shoulders, upper back, and chest; spontaneous lesions often occur on the presternal area

PHYSICAL EXAMINATION

- Flesh-colored to deep red papules, nodules, or tumors that extend in a "claw-like" fashion beyond the original site of injury (Figs. 51-1 and 51-2)
- Usually the lesions are firm, with a smooth surface, and are occasionally painful
- Spontaneous presternal lesions often have a "bowtie" shape (Fig. 51-3)

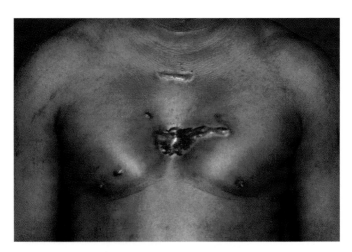

FIGURE 51-1 *Hypertrophic keloidal scars.*

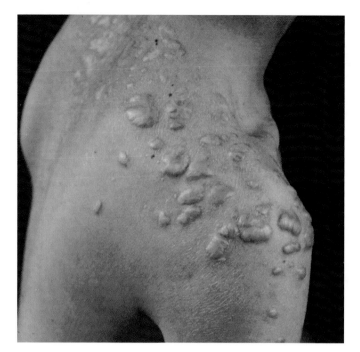

FIGURE 51-2 *Keloidal scarring.*

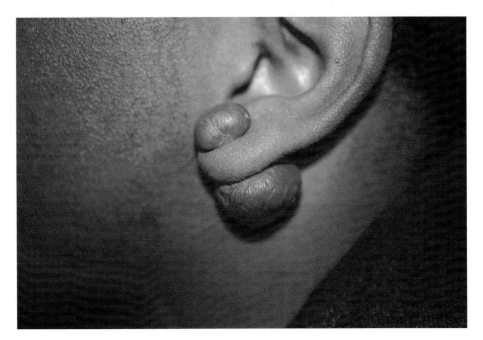

FIGURE 51-3 *Two keloids in the presternal region.*

- Diagnosis made by history and clinical exam

DIFFERENTIAL DIAGNOSIS

- Hypertrophic scar: also follows skin injury; however, the scar is confined to approximately the original site of injury
- Dermatofibroma: these lesions are either dome-shaped or depressed below the plane of normal surrounding skin; lateral compression of the lesion from both sides produces a characteristic "dimpling" or depression of the lesion
- Sarcoidosis: brown to violaceous papules and plaques that may appear on any cutaneous surface of the skin; may or may not be associated with systemic sarcoidosis
- Kaposi's sarcoma: blood vessel tumor often seen in immunosuppressed patients; purple nodules and tumors located on any cutaneous or mucosal surface

TREATMENT

- Treatment of keloids is nonemergent
- Patient should be made aware that any invasive measure may induce additional scar formation
- Intralesional corticosteroids
  - Can inject with triamcinolone acetonide (Kenalog®) 10 to 40 mg/ml to treat lesions; the amount injected will depend on the size of the lesion

- Firm, fibrotic lesions may be very difficult/impossible to inject
  - Intralesional corticosteroids may help to reduce pruritus and/or pain associated with these lesions, as well as reduce the thickness and firmness of the lesions
  - Patients generally require a series of injections every 4 to 6 weeks for several months to obtain maximum benefit
- Surgical excision
  - Lesions that are surgically excised have the potential to recur larger than the original lesion
  - This treatment is often combined with other therapies, such as intralesional corticosteroids, to attain maximum benefit
  - Earlobe lesions are often excised, with subsequent use of "pressure earrings" to prevent the lesions from recurring
- Patients prone to keloids or hypertrophic scars should avoid invasive cosmetic procedures, such as ear piercing

MANAGEMENT/FOLLOW-UP

- Patients who have been treated with intralesional corticosteroids should be seen by either a primary care physician or a dermatologist within 4 to 6 weeks

ICD-9-CM Code

701.4

CPT Code

11900   Intralesional injection ≤7 sites

KERATOACANTHOMA

- Patients report a very rapidly growing tumor, commonly located on the face or arms, appearing over a period of weeks
- Untreated, the patient may have the lesion for months to years
- Patient may report pain and/or bleeding within the lesion

- One finds a skin-colored to red dome-shaped nodule that occasionally has a central keratotic plug (Figs. 52-1 to 52-3)
- Usually there is a single, isolated, lesion on sun-exposed areas of the body
- Clinically and histologically mimics squamous cell carcinoma

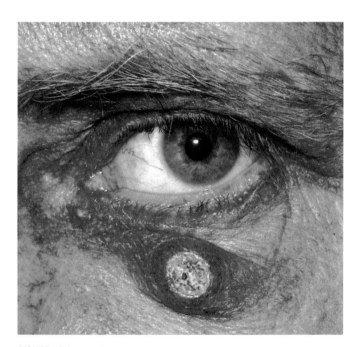

FIGURE 52-1   *Keratoacanthoma.*

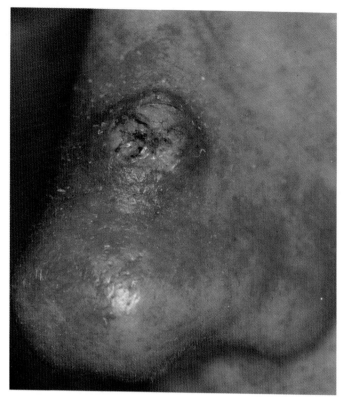

FIGURE 52-2 *Keratoacanthoma.*

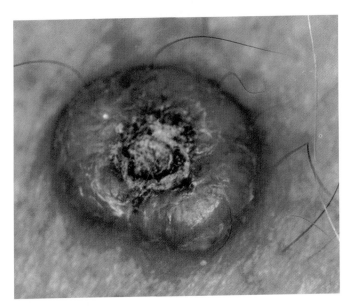

FIGURE 52-3 *Keratoacanthoma.*

DIAGNOSIS

- Clinical findings should be confirmed by a procedure designed to remove the lesion, such as an excision

DIFFERENTIAL DIAGNOSIS

- Squamous cell carcinoma: a slowly evolving malignant skin tumor that occurs on Sun-exposed areas of skin
- Verrucae vulgaris (warts): skin-colored lesions that vary in size and shape and can appear on any cutaneous surface; may see "black dots" on surface
- Basal cell carcinoma: a slowly evolving malignant skin tumor that occurs on sun-exposed areas of the skin; presents as either a pearly, erythematous papule with telangiectasia or a scaly, erythematous plaque
- Prurigo nodularis: keratotic flesh-colored to erythematous papule or nodule that occurs secondary to chronic picking or scratching of the skin

TREATMENT

- The treatment of keratoacanthomas is nonemergent
- Nevertheless, keratoacanthomas cannot be readily distinguished from squamous cell carcinomas clinically or histologically; thus prompt treatment is recommended
- Surgical excision is recommended for the treatment of keratoacanthomas

MANAGEMENT/FOLLOW-UP

- Patients who are suspected of having a keratoacanthoma should be referred within the next week to either their primary care physician or a dermatologist for further management

ICD-9-CM Codes

173.1   Skin of lip
173.1   Eyelid, including canthus
173.2   Skin of ear and external auditory canal
173.3   Skin of other and unspecified parts of face
173.4   Scalp and skin of neck
173.5   Skin of trunk, except scrotum
173.6   Skin of upper limb, including shoulder
173.7   Skin of lower limb, including hip
173.8   Other specified sites of skin
173.9   Skin, site unspecified

CHAPTER 53

LICHEN NITIDUS

HISTORY

- Patients report the gradual appearance of groups of tiny asymptomatic papules on any cutaneous surface
- Occasionally patients may report itching associated with the lesions

PHYSICAL EXAMINATION

- Flesh-colored to slightly pink pinpoint, discrete, dome-shaped papules; occasionally they have a "glistening" surface (Fig. 53-1)
- Most frequent sites of predilection include flexural surfaces of arms and wrists, lower abdomen, breast, and external genitalia (Fig. 53-2)
- Lesions are often grouped

DIAGNOSIS

- The diagnosis is often made by clinical exam
- A skin biopsy may be performed to confirm clinical suspicion

DIFFERENTIAL DIAGNOSIS

- Molluscum contagiosum: dome-shaped papules with a central keratotic plug that may be located on any cutaneous surface; often are symmetrically distributed in occluded areas because of their viral etiology; appear in clusters
- Verrucae vulgaris (warts): skin-colored lesions that vary in size and shape and can appear on any cutaneous surface; may see "black dots" on surface; usually, lesions are larger than those of lichen nitidus
- Keratosis pilaris: follicularly based papules that most commonly occur on the shoulders, upper arms, and upper thighs; often seen in the setting of atopic dermatitis
- Lichen planus: flat-topped violaceous polygonal papules that are sharply defined and located on any cutaneous surface; often has white lines on surface known as Wickham's striae

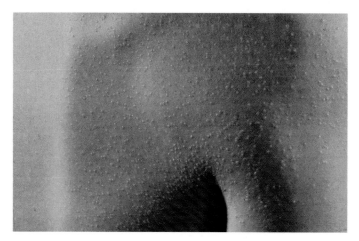

FIGURE 53-1 *Lichen nitidus.*

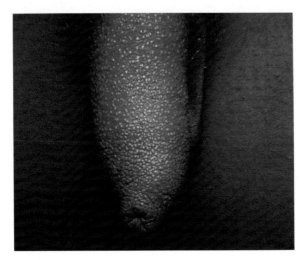

FIGURE 53-2 *Lichen nitidus on the penis.*

- Treatment of lichen nitidus is nonemergent
- The disease is usually asymptomatic and self-limiting, so no treatment is needed in most cases; those patients with symptomatic lesions or with cosmetic concerns can be offered treatment
- Local treatment
  - Topical corticosteroids: a mid- to high-potency topical corticosteroid may be applied to the lesions bid for 2 weeks; should not be applied to the face, axillae, or groin
    - Mid-potency: prednicarbate (Dermatop®) 0.1% ointment or cream; triamcinolone acetonide (Aristocort®) 0.1% ointment or cream
    - High-potency: fluocinonide (Lidex®) 0.05% ointment or cream; clobetasol propionate (Temovate®) 0.05% ointment or cream; halobetasol propionate (Ultravate®) 0.05% ointment or cream, betamethasone dipropionate 0.05% in optimized ointment (Diprolene®)
  - Emphasize side effects of prolonged use of corticosteroids, such as skin atrophy
  - Tacrolimus (Protopic®) 0.1% ointment can be used for prolonged periods without risk of atrophy
- Systemic therapy
  - Oral prednisone can be used in patients with more extensive disease; a 4- to 6-week taper is generally used, with the dose depending on age and weight; generally 1 mg/kg/day can be used as the starting dose

- Patients who are treated with topical corticosteroids should be followed up by a primary care physician or a dermatologist in 2 weeks to assess progress
- Patients treated with systemic steroids should be seen within a week of completing therapy

ICD-9-CM Code

697.1

LICHEN PLANUS

HISTORY

- Patient complains of violaceous papules on the skin and/or mucosal erosions arising over days to weeks
- Lesions may be asymptomatic, but itching or pain may be severe
- Obtain a drug history to assess the possibility of a lichenoid drug eruption

PHYSICAL EXAMINATION

- Flat-topped violaceous polygonal papules that are sharply defined and located on any cutaneous surface (Figs. 54-1 and 54-2)
- Surface of lesions have white lines known as Wickham's striae
- Oral mucosa: lesions on oral mucosa most commonly present in a net-like pattern of white hyperkeratosis; usually on buccal mucosa but may occur on gingiva, tongue, or lips (Fig. 54-3)
- Genitalia: patient may get papular, annular, or erosive lesions on the penis, scrotum, or vulva
- Koebner phenomenon: may develop lichen planus at sites of trauma, often in a linear distribution

DIAGNOSIS

- Diagnosis is often made by clinical exam
- A skin biopsy can be performed to confirm clinical suspicion

DIFFERENTIAL DIAGNOSIS

- Lichenoid drug eruption: many drugs can cause a generalized eruption that closely resembles lichen planus, both clinically and histologically; examples include angiotensin-converting enzyme inhibitors, tetracycline, antimalarials, pencillamine, thiazides, gold, furosemide, propranolol, and methyldopa
- Guttate psoriasis: bright red, scaly papules that can be seen in the setting of psoriasis vulgaris, classically after a streptococcal pharyngitis; psoriasis vulgaris is most commonly located on the scalp, ears, flexor surfaces, umbilicus, and gluteal cleft, but lesions of guttate psoriasis are often more generalized
- Pityriasis rosea: erythematous to pink scaly papules and plaques classically in a "Christmas tree" distribution over the trunk; begins with a "herald patch," which is slightly larger than the other lesions; self-limited eruption that spontaneously regresses in 6 to 12 weeks
- Lichenoid graft-versus-host disease: cutaneous finding of chronic graft-versus-host disease; presents with a lichen-planus–like reaction with flat-topped papules and confluent areas of dermal induration seen in patients with a history of bone marrow transplant
- Kaposi's sarcoma: blood vessel tumor often seen in immunosuppressed patients; purple nodules and tumors located on any cutaneous or mucosal surface

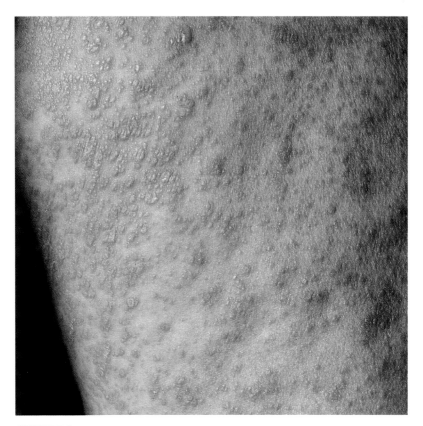

FIGURE 54-1 *Generalized lichen planus.*

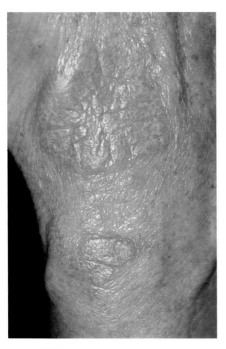

FIGURE 54-2 *Lichen planus.*

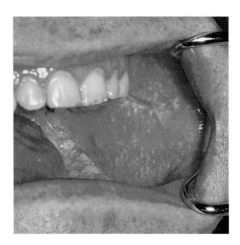

FIGURE 54-3 *Mucosal lichen planus.*

TREATMENT

- The treatment of lichen planus is nonemergent
- Local therapy
  - Topical corticosteroids: a mid- to super-high-potency topical corticosteroid may be applied to the lesions bid for 2 weeks; should not be applied to the face, axillae, or groin
    - Mid-potency: prednicarbate (Dermatop®) 0.1% ointment or cream; triamcinolone acetonide (Aristocort®) 0.1% ointment or cream
    - High-potency: fluocinonide (Lidex®) 0.05% ointment or cream; clobetasol propionate (Temovate®) 0.05% ointment or cream; halobetasol propionate (Ultravate®) 0.05% ointment or cream, betamethasone dipropionate 0.05% in optimized ointment (Diprolene®)
  - Emphasize side effects of prolonged use of corticosteroids, such as skin atrophy
  - Tacrolimus 0.1% (Protopic®) ointment bid may be useful for prolonged application to the skin without risk of atrophy

- ○ Intralesional corticosteroids
    - - Can inject with triamcinolone acetonide (Kenalog®) 2.5 to 5.0 mg/ml to treat small lesions, using about 0.1 ml with each injection
- • Systemic therapy
    - ○ Oral prednisone can be used in patients with symptomatic lichen planus, or in those with extensive disease who are bothered by cosmetic disfigurement; a 4- to 6-week taper is generally used, with the dose depending on age and weight; generally 1 mg/kg can be used as the starting dose
    - ○ Other treatment options include systemic retinoids (e.g., acitretin), immunosuppressive agents (methotrexate or azathioprine), and photochemotherapy
        - - These treatments are more complex, require frequent lab monitoring, are contraindicated in pregnancy, and should not be offered in the emergency department setting

MANAGEMENT/FOLLOW-UP

- • Patients who are treated with topical corticosteroids should be followed up by a primary care physician or a dermatologist in 4 weeks to assess progress

ICD-9 Code

697.0

CPT Code

11900   Intralesional injection ≤7 sites

CHAPTER 55

LICHEN SCLEROSIS

HISTORY

- Cutaneous lesions that may affect all areas of the skin, although there is a predilection for genital surfaces
- Usually disease has been present for months to years prior to detection
- The disease is often asymptomatic, but genital lesions may be painful and very itchy, with associated dysuria or dyspareunia
- The condition usually affects middle-aged women, but prepubertal females as well as adult males may be affected

PHYSICAL EXAMINATION

- Ivory or porcelain-white, semitransparent and atrophic papules and plaques usually located on genital surfaces (Figs. 55-1 and 55-2)
- As the disease evolves, papules become confluent and form depressions with fine "cigarette paper" wrinkling (Fig. 55-3)
- May form a "figure-of-eight" arrangement on the anogenital area of females
- Lesions may be located over any cutaneous surface
- In females, fusion of labia minora and majora may occur, and the vulva may become atrophic, with a decrease in vaginal introitus size; vulvar architecture becomes distorted, with a pale white or yellow appearance

- In uncircumcised males, the prepuce may become sclerotic and may not be retractable; also known as balanitis xerotica obliterans
- Squamous cell carcinoma may uncommonly develop in long-standing lesions of lichen sclerosis et atrophicus

DIAGNOSIS

- The diagnosis is usually made by clinical exam
- A skin biopsy should be performed to confirm clinical suspicion

DIFFERENTIAL DIAGNOSIS

- Morphea: indurated, violaceous to hyperpigmented plaques are located on any cutaneous surface, which may show some to profound atrophy
- Chronic cutaneous lupus: well-marginated, atrophic scaly plaques with erythematous borders
  - Lesions can cause scarring and may be located on any cutaneous surface, but anogenital areas are rarely involved
- Necrobiosis lipoidica diabetacorum: yellow to orange telangiectatic atrophic plaques with an indurated border are often located on the shins

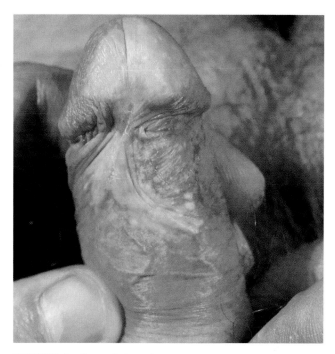

FIGURE 55-1 *Chronic lichen sclerosus.*

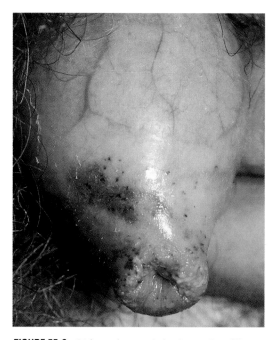

FIGURE 55-2 *Lichen sclerosus: balantis xerotica obliterans.*

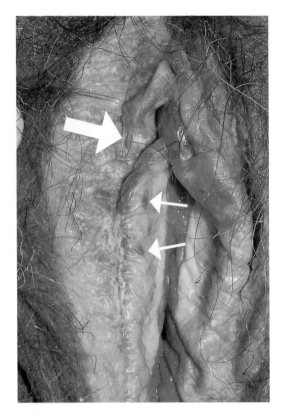

FIGURE 55-3 *Waxy or crinkled texture, purpura (small arrow), and erosions (large arrow) are diagnostic of lichen sclerosus.*

- Vitiligo: completely depigmented patches that differ from genital lichen sclerosis by completely lacking induration
- Squamous cell carcinoma: indurated lesions of the anogenital mucosa could represent squamous cell carcinoma, and skin biopsy readily distinguishes the conditions

TREATMENT

- The treatment of lichen sclerosis is nonemergent
- Symptomatic treatment can be offered to the patient, but no curative therapy exists
- Topical therapy
  - Topical corticosteroids
    - Clobetasol propionate (Temovate®) 0.05% ointment should be applied bid for 1 month
    - Emphasize that the side effect of prolonged use of corticosteroids is skin atrophy
  - One may also consider the use of tacrolimus (Protopic) 0.1% ointment bid for 1 or more months
    - This noncorticosteroidal agent is more likely to cause transient burning upon application, but does not cause atrophy

MANAGEMENT/FOLLOW-UP

- Patients who are treated with topical corticosteroids should be followed up by a primary care physician or a dermatologist in 4 weeks to assess progress
- The occurrence of squamous cell carcinoma in areas of lichen sclerosis et atrophicus, particularly of the genitalia, is possible, and patients should be evaluated once yearly for this reason

ICD-9-CM Code

701.0

CHAPTER 56

LICHEN SIMPLEX CHRONICUS

- Patients complain of pruritic skin lesion(s) that have been present for weeks to years over any cutaneous surface
- Pruritus is usually an associated feature, although patients may not relate a history of scratching or rubbing the area

PHYSICAL EXAMINATION

- A lichenified plaque is the primary skin lesion, in which there is thickened skin with accentuated skin markings (Figs. 56-1 and 56-2)
- Excoriations are often superimposed, and the lesion may be scaly as well
- The color is usually a dull red initially and later may become brown from postinflammatory hyperpigmentation
- Site is characteristically over areas that can be reached by the patient; common areas include the neck, ankles, vulva, scrotum, anal area, and scalp
  - The midback is often spared
- One or more lesions may be present

DIAGNOSIS

- The diagnosis is made by history and clinical findings, but occasionally a skin biopsy is performed to exclude other conditions from consideration

DIFFERENTIAL DIAGNOSIS

- Dermatophyte infection: scaly erythematous plaques affecting the skin of the body that can be diagnosed by KOH preparation examination
  - Majocchi's granuloma is a deep fungal infection that involves the hair follicles and is diagnosed by skin biopsy or culture
- Contact dermatitis (allergic or irritant): acute or chronic inflammatory reaction to agents that come into contact with the skin
  - Acute: well-demarcated plaques of erythema, edema, and vesicles, often with superimposed erosions and crusting
  - Chronic: erythematous and lichenified plaques with scale
  - Arranged in linear or bizarre patterns, indicating an exogenous etiology
- Mycosis fungoides: a cutaneous T-cell lymphoma that presents with erythematous scaly patches and plaques that may be located on any cutaneous surface
  - More than one plaque is usually present, and these lesions are often resistant to treatment
- Psoriasis: inflammatory skin disease characterized by thick, erythematous papules and plaques with silvery scale; pruritus is common
  - Sites of predilection include elbows, knees, scalp, ears, umbilicus, and gluteal cleft

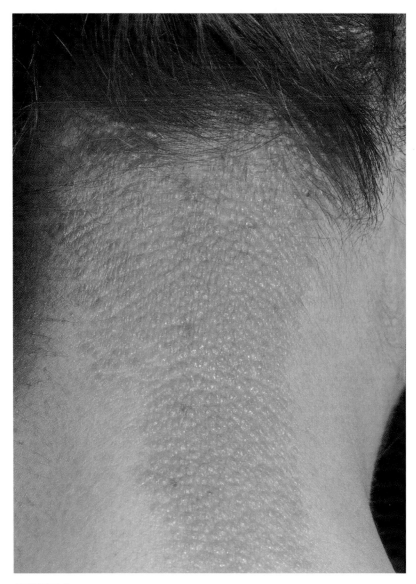

FIGURE 56-1 *Lichen simplex chronicus.*

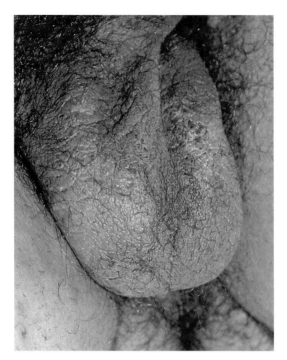

FIGURE 56-2 *Lichen simplex chronicus.*

TREATMENT

- The treatment of lichen simplex chronicus is nonemergent
- The etiology of this condition should be discussed with the patient; it should be explained that rubbing and/or scratching should be stopped
- Localized lesions can be treated with topical corticosteroids: a mid- to super-high-potency topical corticosteroid may be applied to the lesions bid for 2 weeks; should not be applied to the face, axillae, or groin
  - Mid-potency: prednicarbate (Dermatop®) 0.1% ointment or cream; triamcinolone acetonide (Aristocort®) 0.1% ointment or cream
  - High-potency: fluocinonide (Lidex®) 0.05% ointment or cream; clobetasol propionate (Temovate®) 0.05% ointment or cream; halobetasol propionate (Ultravate®) 0.05% ointment or cream, betamethasone dipropionate 0.05% in optimized ointment (Diprolene®)
  - Occlusion helps to facilitate penetration of the medication as well as prevent the patient from scratching or rubbing the area, and the topical agent flurandrenolide (Cordan®) tape can provide treatment and occlusion together
  - Emphasize the side effects of prolonged use of corticosteroids, such as skin atrophy
- Occlusive dressings can be applied over the topical corticosteroid, to facilitate penetration of the medication, as well as prevent the patient from scratching or rubbing the area
- Intralesional corticosteroids
  - One can inject with triamcinolone acetonide 2.5 to 5.0 mg/ml to treat small lesions, using about 0.1 ml with each injection
- Treat any secondary infections (*Staphylococcus aureus* most common)
  - Dicloxacillin: 500 mg bid for 10 days (adults); 12.5 to 25 mg/kg/day (children <40 kg)
  - Cephalexin (Keflex®): 500 mg bid for 10 days (adults); 25 to 50 mg/kg/day (children)
  - *Penicillin-allergic*: erythromycin 500 mg bid for 10 days (adults); 40 mg/kg/day for 10 days (children)

MANAGEMENT/FOLLOW-UP

- Patients who are treated with topical corticosteroids should be followed up by a primary care physician or a dermatologist in 4 weeks to assess progress

ICD-9-CM Code

698.3

CPT Code

11900   Intralesional injection ≤7 sites

CHAPTER 57

LUPUS

HISTORY

- Patients may complain of skin lesions or a rash that has been present for days, weeks, or months
- Patients often relate a history of new-onset skin photosensitivity or sun intolerance
- Constitutional symptoms may be present, including fatigue, fever, weight loss, and/or malaise
- Review of systems may reveal additional symptoms, most commonly including arthralgias and/or arthritis
- A family history of lupus may be present

PHYSICAL EXAMINATION

Physical examination may reveal one or more of the following clinical findings:
- Skin
  - Malar rash (the "butterfly" rash): confluent, fixed, symmetric erythema and macular or papular edema centered over the malar eminences and over the nose, with sparing of the nasolabial folds (Fig. 57-1)
  - Discoid lesions: erythematous plaques with a scarred, atrophic center with scales that extend into the openings of dilated hair follicles, most commonly located on the face, scalp, ears, and neck (Fig. 57-2 to 57-4)
  - Photosensitivity: skin rash or persistent "burn" resulting from sun sensitivity

  - Other rash: hyperkeratotic, nonscarring annular plaques located on photodistributed areas of the trunk including the neck, chest, and arms
- Mucous membranes: oral or nasopharyngeal ulceration
- Nails: nail fold telangiectasias may be present, which are dilated capillaries noted along the proximal nail folds
- Hair abnormalities may include:
  - Scarring alopecia: discoid lesions of lupus may cause a scarring hair loss, most commonly presenting with patchy areas of hair loss and plugged hair follicles
  - Nonscarring alopecia: a telogen effluvium may occur after a flare of lupus, resulting in a "shed" of about 70% of actively growing hairs
    - Complete regrowth is expected within 8 to 12 months
- Extracutaneous multisystem involvement
  - Arthritis
  - Renal disease
  - Pericarditis
  - Pleuritis
  - Neurologic disorders
  - Hepatosplenomegaly
  - Lymphadenopathy

DIAGNOSIS

- Diagnosis of systemic lupus erythematosus is based on the 1982 Revised Criteria for Classification of Systemic Lupus Erythematosus; 4 of 11 criteria are required to

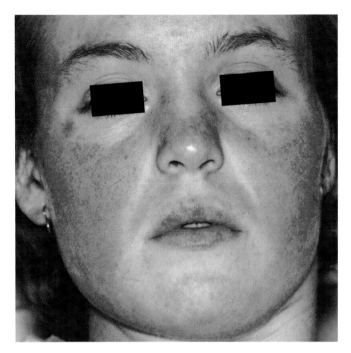

FIGURE 57-1 *Localized acute cutaneous lupus erythematosus (ACLE).*

make the diagnosis:

1. Malar rash
2. Discoid rash
3. Photosensitivity
4. Oral or nasopharyngeal ulcers, observed by a physician
5. Arthritis: nonerosive arthritis involving two or more peripheral joints, characterized by tenderness, swelling, or effusion
6. Serositis
   a. Pleuritis: convincing history of pleuritic pain or rub heard by physician or evidence of pleural effusion
      -or-
   b. Pericarditis: documented by electrocardiography (ECG) or rub or evidence of pericardial effusion
7. Renal disorder
   a. Persistent proteinuria: >0.5 g/day or >3+ if quantitation not performed
      -or-
   b. Cellular casts: may be red cell, hemoglobin, granular, tubular, or mixed

8. Neurologic disorder
   a. Seizures: in the absence of offending drugs or known metabolic derangements, e.g., uremia, ketoacidosis, or electrolyte imbalance
      -or-
   b. Psychosis: in the absence of offending drugs or known metabolic derangements, e.g., uremia, ketoacidosis, or electrolyte imbalance
9. Hematologic disorder
   a. Hemolytic anemia: with reticulocytosis
      -or-
   b. Leukopenia: <4000/μl total on two or more occasions
      -or-
   c. Lymphopenia: <1500/μl on two or more occasions
      -or-
   d. Thrombocytopenia: <100,000/μl in the absence of offending drugs

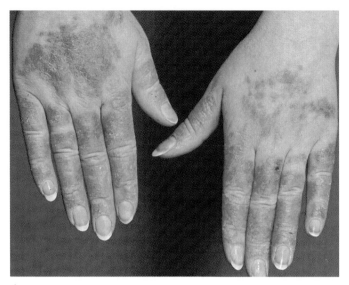

A.

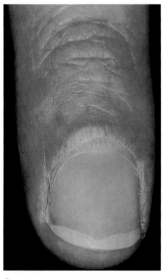

B.

FIGURE 57-2 *Generalized ACLE.*

10. Immunologic disorder
   a. Anti-DNA antibody: antibody to native DNA in abnormal titer
      -or-
   b. Anti-Sm antibody: antibody to Smith nuclear antigen
      -or-
   c. Positive finding of antiphospholipid antibodies based on
      i. Abnormal serum level of IgG or IgM anticardiolipin antibodies
      ii. Positive test result for lupus anticoagulant using a standard method, or

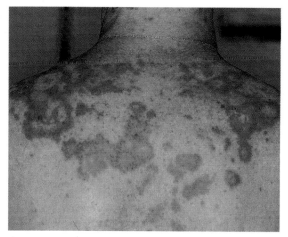

A.

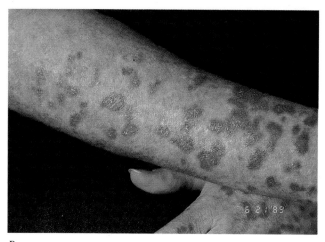

B.

FIGURE 57-3 *Subacute cutaneous lupus erythematosus (SCLE).*

iii. A false-positive serologic test for syphilis known to be positive for at least 6 months and confirmed by *Treponema pallidum* immobilization or fluorescent treponemal antibody absorption test

11. Antinuclear antibody (ANA): an abnormal titer of antinuclear antibody by immunofluorescence or an equivalent assay at any point in time and in the absence of drugs known to be associated with "drug-induced lupus" syndrome

- Chronic cutaneous lupus (CCL)
  - A patient who presents with discoid lesions of lupus but does not fulfill the criteria for systemic lupus erythematosus is said to have CCL
  - ANA is present in low titer in about 30% to 40% of patients with CCL; less than 5% of patients have high titers of ANA
  - About 5% of patients with CCL eventually develop systemic lupus erythematosus

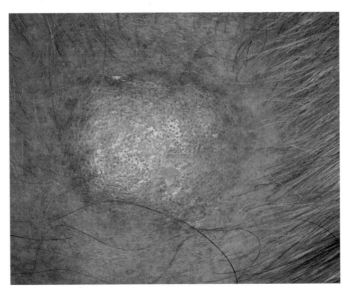

FIGURE 57-4 *Classic discoid lupus erythematosus (DLE).*

- Subacute cutaneous lupus (SCLE)
  - A patient who presents with annular, polycyclic plaques that are photodistributed and proved to be lesions of lupus via biopsy but who does not fulfill the criteria for systemic lupus erythematosus is said to have SCLE
  - 70% to 90% of patients with SCLE have autoantibodies to SS-A/Ro, and 30% to 50% of patients have autoantibodies to SS-B/La
  - Low titers of ANA are commonly found in patients with SCLE
  - About 15% to 20% of patients with SCLE eventually develop systemic lupus erythematosus

DIFFERENTIAL DIAGNOSIS

- Acne rosacea: this chronic acneiform condition occurs on the face, affecting the facial pilosebaceous units
  - Patients present with facial flushing, telangiectasias, and acneiform papules and pustules
  - Patients may have associated rhinophyma

- Dermatomyositis: this systemic disease is characterized by photosensitivity and proximal muscle weakness; creatine kinase and aldolase levels are frequently elevated in patients with dermatomyositis, and characteristic skin findings include violaceous periorbital discoloration, flat-topped papules over the metacarpophalangeal and interphalangeal joints of the hands, and nail fold telangiectasias
- Seborrheic dermatitis: a chronic dermatosis associated with redness and scaling on areas where sebaceous glands are prominent, such as the scalp ("dandruff"), face, and chest; lesions are yellowish red, greasy scaling macules and papules of various sizes
- Polymorphous light eruption: this group of photodermatoses is characterized by delayed reactions to ultraviolet radiation
  - Skin manifestations vary morphologically and may resemble cutaneous findings of lupus
  - The history, physical exam, and skin biopsy examination can help to differentiate the two conditions

- The treatment of cutaneous limited lupus is nonemergent; however, systemic lupus erythematosus should be treated promptly to prevent sequelae from renal destruction, or other internal manifestations
- All patients should be advised to avoid direct sun exposure and protect themselves using hats, protective clothing, and topical sunscreens with a minimum sun protection factor (SPF) of 30
- Localized lesions can be treated with topical corticosteroids: a mid- to high-potency topical corticosteroid may be applied to the borders of the lesions on the scalp, trunk, or extremities bid for 2 weeks; a low-potency topical corticosteroid may be applied to lesions on the face, groin, or axillae
  - Low-potency: hydrocortisone 2.5% ointment or cream; desonide (DesOwen®) 0.05% ointment or cream
  - Mid-potency: triamcinolone acetonide (Aristocort®) 0.1% ointment or cream
  - High-potency: fluocinonide (Lidex®) 0.05% ointment or cream; clobetasol propionate (Temovate®) 0.05% ointment or cream; halobetasol propionate (Ultravate®) 0.05% ointment or cream, betamethasone dipropionate 0.05% in optimized ointment (Diprolene®)
  - Emphasize that the side effect of prolonged use of corticosteroids is skin atrophy
  - Over the long term, the safest topical treatment is tacrolimus 0.1% (Protopic®) ointment bid, with no known risk of atrophy
- Intralesional corticosteroids
  - One can inject with triamcinolone acetonide (Kenalog®) 2.5 to 5.0 mg/ml to treat small lesions
  - Inject about 0.1 ml at several points along the border of the lesions

- Systemic therapy
  - Antimalarial agents: hydroxychloroquine (Plaquenil®) is commonly prescribed for photoaggravated conditions and if administered, should be done with appropriate laboratory screening, ophthalmologic monitoring, and follow-up
  - Other agents used in patients with refractory disease include oral retinoids including isotretinoin (Accutane®), dapsone, thalidomide (Thalidomid®), prednisone, cyclophosphamide (Cytoxan®), and other corticosteroid-sparing immunosuppressive agents

MANAGEMENT/FOLLOW-UP

- All patients with a diagnosis of lupus should establish ongoing care with either a primary care physician, a rheumatologist, or a dermatologist
- Any patient with evidence of acute internal disease such as pericarditis or glomerulonephritis needs emergent intervention in a hospital setting
- Patients who are treated with topical corticosteroids should be followed up by a primary care physician or a dermatologist within 2 weeks to assess progress
- Any patient requiring systemic therapy should first be evaluated on an outpatient basis to ensure appropriate follow-up and to obtain adequate screening lab work

ICD-9-CM Code

695.4   Chronic cutaneous lupus
710.0   Systemic lupus

CPT Code

11900   Intralesional injection ≤7 sites

CHAPTER 58

MALIGNANT MELANOMA

HISTORY

- A patient notices a dark brown or black spot changing in size, color, or developing symptoms, such as itching or bleeding
- Lesions are often noticed by a doctor, family member, or hairstylist, and the patient is unaware
- Risk factors: sun exposure, fair skin with red or blond hair, family history of melanoma, numerous atypical melanocytic nevi, and immunosuppression
- Four main types of invasive malignant melanoma are known:
  - Superficial spreading melanoma: represents 70% of all melanomas; usually does not arise within a preexisting nevus

  - Lentigo maligna melanoma: most often seen in elderly patients on sun-damaged skin, especially in head and neck area
    - Lentigo maligna is an in situ melanoma
    - Lentigo maligna melanoma displays dermal invasion
  - Nodular melanoma: second most common type of melanoma; usually seen on trunk, head, or neck areas
  - Acral lentiginous melanoma: affects palms, soles, and nail beds most commonly
- Most malignant melanomas, except for nodular melanoma, are believed to progress through a radial growth phase into a vertical growth phase
- If diagnosed in radial growth phase, has highest chance of cure

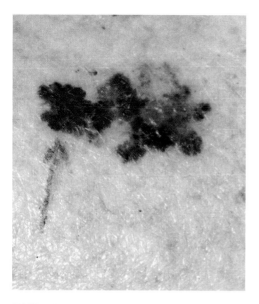

FIGURE 58-1 *Lentigo maligna.*

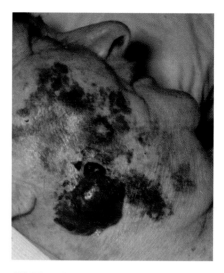

FIGURE 58-2 *Malignant melanoma.*

- Lesions should be grossly assessed for size, shades of color, color variegation, border irregularity, and symmetry
- Lentigo maligna: hyperpigmented macule or patch with irregular shape and pigmentation (Figs. 58-1 and 58-2)
  - With growth radially and no treatment, this lesion may begin to extend vertically and become a lentigo maligna melanoma (invasive melanoma) with a palpable component
- Superficial spreading melanoma: darkly pigmented macule or papule with an irregular surface and focal areas that are darker than the rest of the lesion (Fig. 58-3)
  - Often has significant border irregularity and multiple shades of brown, black, red, blue, or white

- Nodular melanoma: dark blue-black, brownish-red, or flesh-colored papule or nodule that may be pedunculated and often arises in normal-appearing skin
- Acral lentiginous melanoma: hyperpigmented, irregular macule beneath the nail plate, or on palms or soles
  - Hutchinson's sign may be noted, which is the finding of pigment extending from the subungual lesion onto the posterior nail fold

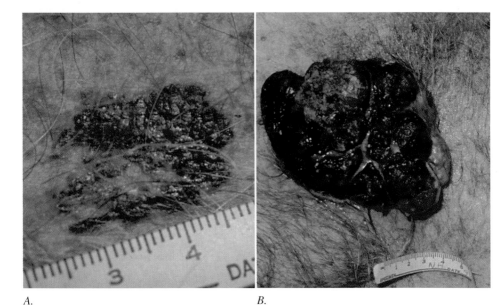

A.   B.

FIGURE 58-3 *Superficial spreading melanoma.*

- A skin biopsy should be considered as soon as is feasible to establish or exclude the diagnosis
- A thorough physical exam looking for any lymphadenopathy or evidence of metastasis should be performed
- Further evaluation is highly dependent on the definitive diagnosis, thickness, and presence or absence of evidence of metastasis

- Atypical nevus: appears to have many of the same visible and microscopic architectural features of melanomas, but the degree of atypia is mild compared with true melanoma
- Solar lentigo: these pigmented macules appear on sun-damaged skin and are usually regular in contour and color

- Pigmented basal cell carcinoma: often has tiny stipples of pigmentation at the border of an otherwise typical basal cell carcinoma
- Seborrheic keratosis: has a keratotic surface with superficial scale, but can at times mimic melanoma closely

- Malignant melanoma is staged according to the American Joint Commission on Cancer (AJCC) Staging System for melanoma
- Poor prognostic signs include advanced age, location on trunk, palms, or soles, tumor thickness, level of invasion, vertical growth phase, high number of mitoses, ulceration, brisk inflammatory response, and areas of regression
- Early recognition and surgical excision of the primary tumor are the only standards of treatment for cutaneous melanoma
- Once the lesion metastasizes, it does not respond well to chemotherapy, immuno-therapy, or radiotherapy
  - For distant metastases, numerous sys-temic chemotherapeutic treatments have been tried; however, none of these treat-ments are uniformly effective and all may be associated with significant toxicity

- Patients should be referred for a biopsy and definitive treatment as soon as possible
- Further evaluation and management de-pends on the stage of the melanoma

ICD-9-CM Codes

172.0   Skin of lip
172.1   Eyelid, including canthus
173.2   Skin of ear and external auditory canal
173.3   Skin of other and unspecified parts of face
172.4   Scalp and skin of neck
172.5   Skin of trunk, except scrotum
172.6   Skin of upper limb, including shoulder
172.7   Skin of lower limb, including hip
172.8   Other specified sites of skin
172.9   Skin, site unspecified

ACUTE MENINGOCOCCEMIA (Neisseria meningitidis INFECTION)

HISTORY

- Adolescent or child younger than 4 years
- Late winter to early spring
- May occur in epidemics
- Variable prodrome that may include cough, headache, nausea, vomiting, sore throat followed by sudden spiking fever, chills, myalgias and arthralgias, and in fulminant cases, stupor and hypotension within hours
- Symptoms of meningitis, which may include agitated or maniacal behavior
- Symptoms of meningococcal infection in other organ systems besides the central nervous system: pneumonia, endocarditis, pericarditis, arthritis, and osteomyelitis

PHYSICAL EXAMINATION

- Patient appears ill, with fever, tachycardia, tachypnea, and mild hypotension
- Pink maculopapular eruption begins on the extremities and generalizes; this becomes petechial, and lesions may become papular as the infection progresses; the petechiae appear "smudged," with pale, grayish, sometimes vesicular centers (Fig. 59-1)
- Large ecchymoses may develop
- Splenomegaly
- Splinter hemorrhages in nail beds may be present
- Conjunctivitis may be present

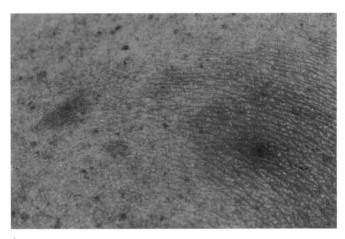

A.

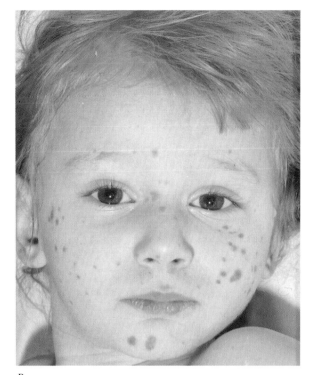

B.

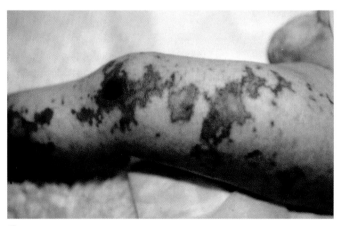

C.

FIGURE 59-1 Neisseria meningitidis: *Acute meningococcemia.*

- Clinical picture
- Cerebrospinal fluid smear, culture, and analysis
- Blood culture

DIFFERENTIAL DIAGNOSIS

- Acute bacteremias
- Endocarditis
- Hypersensitivity vasculitis
- Toxic shock syndrome
- Leptospirosis
- Rocky Mountain spotted fever
- Henoch-Schönlein purpura
- Gonococcemia
- Purpura fulminans
- Disseminated intravascular coagulation (DIC)
- Viral exanthem

TREATMENT

- For adults
  - Cefotaxime 2 g q4-6hr IV or
  - Ceftriaxone 2 g q12hr IV or
  - Chloramphenicol (1 g IV q6hr)
- Supportive measures for prevention of brain swelling (fluid monitoring, mannitol expanders, dexamethasone), for shock (fluid expanders, dopamine, etc.), and for DIC

- Meningococcemia may be acute and lethal or mild, or may be chronic and relapsing
- Meningococcal infection may result in pneumonia, endocarditis, pericarditis, arthritis, osteomyelitis, or meningitis. Multiple organ failure has been documented
- Acute respiratory distress syndrome, renal failure, or multiple organ failure may lead to death; these cases have been associated with adrenal hemorrhage (Waterhouse-Friderichsen syndrome)

- Immunization protection is available
- Prophylaxis for at-risk individuals (adults) with rifampin 600 mg orally bid for 2 days

ICD-9-CM Code

036.2

MOLLUSCUM CONTAGIOSUM

HISTORY

- A child or young adult presents with asymptomatic or pruritic papules
- Molluscum is more severe in immunocompromised patients
- Lesions may be present for months to years
- Individual lesions last for about 2 months with spontaneous resolution

PHYSICAL EXAMINATION

- Smooth, dome-shaped, flesh-colored to pink papules 3 to 6 mm in diameter, caused by a poxvirus (Fig. 60-1)
- A central dell or umbilication with a keratotic core is sometimes seen
- When lesions are resolving, one may see erythema around the papules

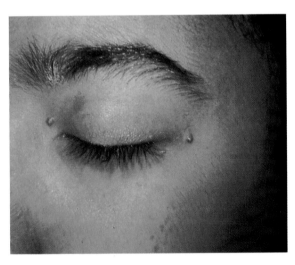

FIGURE 60-1   *Molluscum contagiosum.*

- Multiple lesions are usually grouped in one or two areas
  - Most patients have less than 20 lesions, but thousands may be present
  - The face and trunk are common sites in children
  - Genitals are a common locations in adults
- Lesions may be linearly arranged, as they can spread through skin trauma (Koebner phenomenon)
- In immunocompromised patients, lesions can be very numerous and grow extremely large
- Children with atopic dermatitis may develop widespread lesions

DIAGNOSIS

- The diagnosis is based on a clinical exam
- Giemsa staining of expressed keratotic core demonstrates round molluscum bodies (inclusion bodies—rarely necessary)

DIFFERENTIAL DIAGNOSIS

- Must be differentiated from cutaneous cryptococcal infection and *Histoplasma capsulatum* in immunocompromised patients—if there is any doubt about the diagnosis, a skin biopsy should be obtained
- Warts: these lesions are usually rough on the surface
- Keratoacanthoma: if molluscum presents as a single, large lesion, it may be difficult to distinguish from a squamous cell carcinoma

TREATMENT

- Treatment of molluscum contagiosum is nonemergent
- Treatment is not required in most cases since lesions are self-limited, resolving spontaneously in 6 to 9 months, but may last for years in immunocompromised patients
- If treatment is desired:
  - Gentle manual expression of the central core with a sterile needle or comedo extractor
  - Light curettage or Light electrocautery
  - Cryotherapy with liquid nitrogen in adults is effective
  - Topical cantharidin application can promote destruction
  - Topical imiquimod (Aldara®) may speed resolution

MANAGEMENT/FOLLOW-UP

- If patients are interested in therapy, they should visit their primary care physician or dermatologist

ICD-9-CM Code

078.0

CPT Code

17110   Destruction of molluscum

MORPHEA (LOCALIZED SCLERODERMA)

- Patients report the slow onset of localized skin thickening that may be located on any cutaneous surface
- The disease is usually asymptomatic
- If located over a joint, the patient may experience difficulty moving that joint

- Well-circumscribed violaceous and erythematous plaques that later become ivory-colored (Figs. 61-1 to 61-3)
- Chronic lesions may become hyperpigmented
- Upon palpation, lesions feel very indurated

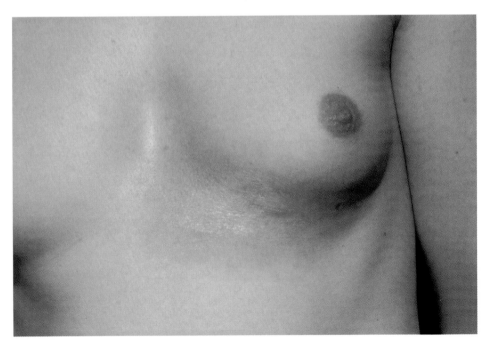

FIGURE 61-1   *Morphea.*

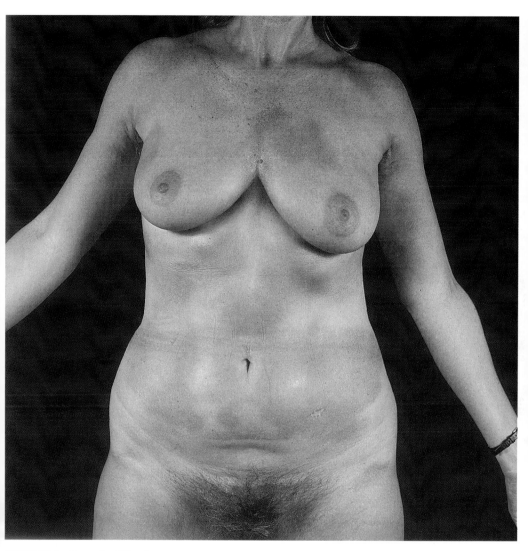

FIGURE 61-2   *Generalized Morphea.*

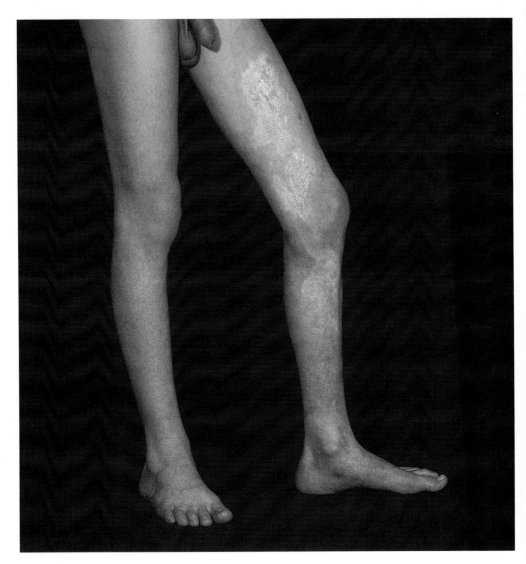

FIGURE 61-3 *Linear morphea.*

- Deeper involvement may be associated with atrophy of muscle and bones
- Joint involvement may lead to flexion contractures

DIAGNOSIS

- The diagnosis is usually made by clinical exam
- A skin biopsy should be performed to confirm clinical suspicion

DIFFERENTIAL DIAGNOSIS

- Progressive systemic sclerosis: this multisystem disorder with inflammatory, vascular, and sclerotic changes of the skin as well as internal organs presents with widespread disease and other findings
  - Patients often have Raynaud's phenomenon
  - The CREST syndrome presents with cutaneous calcinosis, Raynaud's phenomenon, esophageal dysmotility, sclerodactyly, and cutaneous telangiectasias
- Acrodermatitis chronica atrophicans: this late cutaneous finding of Lyme disease begins with violaceous erythema and edema on an extremity that later becomes an indurated atrophic plaque
- Nongenital lichen sclerosis et atrophicus: ivory-white atrophic plaques that may affect any genital or cutaneous surface
- Eosinophilic fasciitis: symmetric induration of the extremities often following an episode of unusual exertion; is associated with pain, edema, and peripheral eosinophilia

TREATMENT

- Treatment of morphea is nonemergent
- No proven effective treatments exist for morphea, but some success has been reported with the use of topical corticosteroids, topical calcipotriene, ultraviolet therapy, and immunosuppressive agents
- As first-line treatment, consider mid- to high-potency corticosteroid agents for 1 month
  - Mid-potency: prednicarbate (Dermatop®) 0.1% ointment or cream; triamcinolone acetonide (Aristocort®) 0.1% ointment or cream
  - High-potency: fluocinonide (Lidex®) 0.05% ointment or cream; clobetasol propionate (Temovate®) 0.05% ointment or cream; halobetasol propionate (Ultravate®) 0.05% ointment or cream, betamethasone dipropionate 0.05% in optimized ointment (Diprolene®)

MANAGEMENT/FOLLOW-UP

- Patients can follow up with a primary care physician or a dermatologist for symptomatic treatment of their lesions

ICD-9-CM Code

701.0

CHAPTER 62

NECROBIOSIS LIPOIDICA DIABETICORUM

HISTORY

- Patients report the appearance of lesions over months to years
- Many patients have a history of diabetes mellitus
- Lesions often located on the shins, but may be on any cutaneous surface
- Patients report asymptomatic lesions unless ulcers develop within the lesions

PHYSICAL EXAMINATION

- Well-demarcated shiny, nontender, atrophic plaques of yellow-orange color are often located on the shins (Fig. 62-1)
- Telangiectatic vessels may be visible within the lesions
- Older lesions may develop ulcers, especially following minor trauma

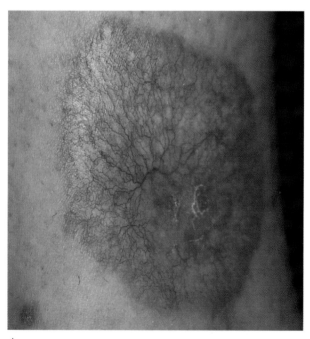

A.

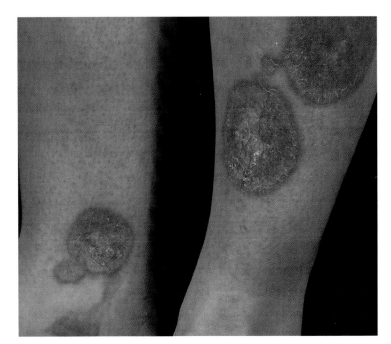

B.

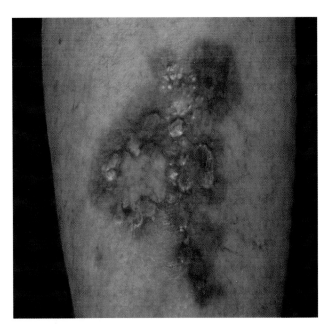

C.

FIGURE 62-1 *Necrobiosis lipoidica diabeticorum.*

- The diagnosis is usually made by clinical exam, but examination of a skin biopsy specimen can be performed to confirm clinical suspicion

- Granuloma annulare: presents with skin-colored papules and plaques, often arranged in an annulus
  - Most common locations include the dorsum of hands or feet, elbows, and knees
- Dermatophyte infection: scaly erythematous plaques without atrophy affecting any cutaneous surface that can be confirmed by examination of a KOH preparation
- Sarcoidosis: brown to violaceous papules and plaques appear on any cutaneous surface of the skin, and cutaneous disease may or may not be associated with systemic sarcoidosis
- Nongenital lichen sclerosis et atrophicus: ivory-white atrophic plaques that may affect any genital or cutaneous surface

- Treatment of necrobiosis lipoidica diabeticorum is nonemergent
- Patients often have associated diabetes mellitus or abnormal glucose tolerance tests; blood sugar, glycosylated hemoglobin, and/or glucose tolerance tests should be evaluated
- Topical therapy
  - Topical corticosteroids: a mid- to super-high-potency topical corticosteroid may be applied only to the borders of the lesions bid for 2 weeks; should not be applied to the face, axillae, or groin
    - Mid-potency: prednicarbate (Dermatop®) 0.1% ointment or cream; triamcinolone acetonide (Aristocort®) 0.1% ointment or cream
    - High-potency: fluocinonide (Lidex®) 0.05% ointment or cream; clobetasol propionate (Temovate®) 0.05% ointment or cream; halobetasol propionate (Ultravate®) 0.05% ointment or cream, betamethasone dipropionate 0.05% in optimized ointment (Diprolene®)

- ○ Although topical corticosteroids are indicated for use for a few weeks, emphasize the side effects of prolonged use of corticosteroids such as skin atrophy
  - ○ Consider the use of tacrolimus 0.1% (Protopic®) ointment bid, which can be used for prolonged periods with no risk of atrophy
- Intralesional corticosteroids
  - ○ Can inject with triamcinolone acetonide (Kenalog®) 2.5 to 5.0 mg/ml to borders of the lesion
  - ○ Inject along border using about 0.1 ml with each injection
- Ulcerated lesions require local wound care, including oral antibiotics if needed

- Patients should be seen within 3 to 4 weeks by either a primary care physician or a dermatologist if treatment for necrobiosis lipoidica diabeticorum is initiated
- Patients who do not wish to have their lesions treated can follow up as needed

ICD-9-CM Code

250.8

CPT Code

11900   Intralesional injection ≤7 sites

NEUROTIC EXCORIATIONS

HISTORY

- Lesions are present for weeks to months on any skin surface that the patient can reach
- Produced by habitual picking or manipulating of the skin with the fingernails
- Patient may relate history of stress or other preceding stimuli
- Patients often deny picking or scratching at the lesions
- There may be a history of neuropsychiatric disease

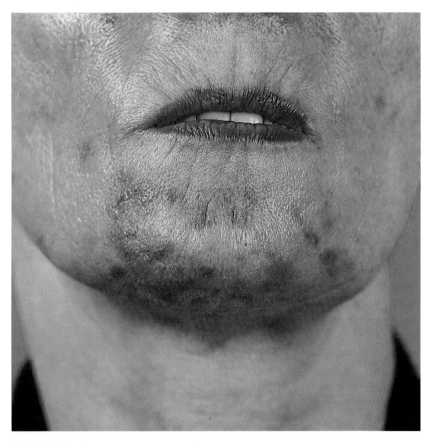

FIGURE 63-1 *Neurotic excoriations on the chin.*

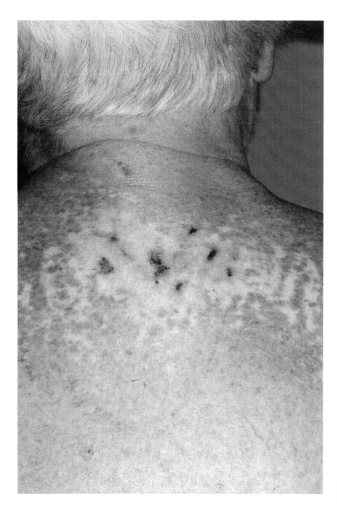

FIGURE 63-2 *Neurotic excoriations on the upper back.*

- New lesions appear as excoriations, whereas older lesions appear as scars
- No primary lesions such as papules or vesicles are seen
- Lesions most commonly appear on areas that the patient can reach, thus sparing the midback (Figs. 63-1 to 63-3)
- Lesions are usually linear in shape, although bizarre geometric shapes are common as well

- The diagnosis is primarily based on history and clinical findings
- If indicated a careful evaluation for systemic causes of pruritus is sometimes necessary

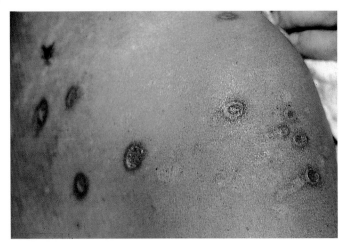

FIGURE 63-3 *Neurotic excoriations.*

- Scabies: this skin infestation of a mite causes intense, widespread itching that often interferes with sleep; classically, serpiginous intraepidermal burrows are noted on any cutaneous surface
  - Interdigital web spaces of hands are the most common sites, followed by wrists and ankles
  - The diagnosis is confirmed by scraping a burrow and demonstrating a mite or scybala (fecal material) under light microscopic examination
- Dermatitis herpetiformis: an autoimmune blistering disorder that causes intense itching at the sites of lesions; often, scratching results in excoriations, which may be present along with vesicles, papules, and/or urticarial lesions
  - Most commonly this presents on extensor surfaces

- Atopic dermatitis: poorly defined erythematous patches and plaques
  - Acute lesions appear edematous, whereas chronic lesions appear thickened, with the accentuation of skin markings (lichenified)
  - Often the disease is associated with hay fever and asthma
- Pruritus of systemic disease: many systemic diseases may cause pruritus, which results in excoriations on the skin including thyroid disorders, renal disease, obstructive biliary disease, polycythemia vera, HIV, hepatitis, diabetes, and malignancies (lymphoma, multiple myeloma)
  - Evaluation for systemic conditions should be guided by history and physical examination

- The treatment of neurotic excoriations is nonemergent
- The patient should be educated as to the cause of the lesions and should be informed that picking of lesions must be stopped
- Localized lesions can be treated with topical corticosteroids
  - A low-potency topical corticosteroid may be applied to lesions on the face, groin, or axillae bid for 2 weeks
    - Desonide (DesOwen®) 0.05% ointment, cream, or lotion; hydrocortisone 2.5% ointment or cream
  - Mid-potency: prednicarbate (Dermatop®) 0.1% ointment or cream; triamcinolone acetonide (Aristocort®) 0.1% ointment or cream
  - High-potency: fluocinonide (Lidex®) 0.05% ointment or cream; clobetasol propionate (Temovate®) 0.05% ointment or cream; halobetasol propionate (Ultravate®) 0.05% ointment or cream, betamethasone dipropionate 0.05% in optimized ointment (Diprolene®)
    - Although topical corticosteroids are indicated for use for a few weeks, emphasize the side effects of prolonged use of corticosteroids such as skin atrophy
- Topical antipruritic preparations such as menthol-camphor lotion (Sarna®) or benzocaine (Lanacane®) can be used for the long term and may be of some benefit
- If evidence of depression, obsessive-compulsive disorder, monosymptomatic hypochondriasis, or other neuropsychiatric disease is present, therapy may need to be directed toward amelioration of the neuropsychiatric disease

- Patients who are treated with topical corticosteroids should be followed up by a primary care physician or a dermatologist in 2 weeks to assess progress

ICD-9-CM Code

698.4

CHAPTER 64

NUMMULAR ECZEMA

HISTORY

- Round and scaly lesions on skin develop over weeks to months

- Patient often reports tendency toward atopic conditions (atopic dermatitis, asthma, and/or allergic rhinitis)
- Pruritus is often associated

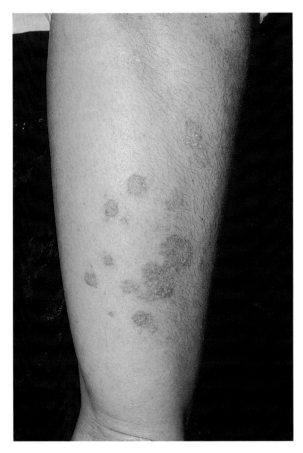

FIGURE 64-1 *Nummular eczema.*

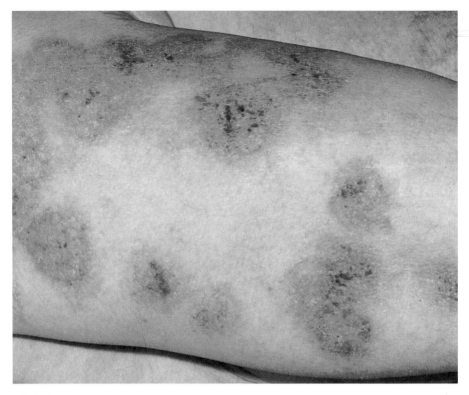

FIGURE 64-2 *Nummular eczematous dermatitis.*

- Scaly erythematous papules, often coalescing into plaques, that are commonly located on the lower extremities (Fig. 64-1)
- Well-demarcated lesions that often form coin-shaped plaques, thus the name "nummular" (Fig. 64-2)
- Any cutaneous surface may be affected

- The diagnosis is usually made based on clinical findings

- Dermatophyte infection: scaly erythematous plaques with central clearing affecting the skin of the body that can be diagnosed by examination of a KOH preparation
- Contact dermatitis (allergic or irritant): acute or chronic inflammatory reaction to agents that come into contact with the skin; arranged in linear or bizarre patterns, indicating an exogenous etiology
  - Acute: well-demarcated plaques of erythema, edema, and vesicles are often found with superimposed erosions and crusting
  - Chronic: erythematous and lichenified (thickened skin with accentuation of skin markings) plaques with scale
- Mycosis fungoides: this cutaneous T-cell lymphoma presents with scaly patches and plaques that may be located on any cutaneous surface
  - Lesions have usually been present longer than those of nummular eczema and are more resistant to treatment
- Psoriasis: this inflammatory skin disease is characterized by thick, erythematous papules and plaques with silvery scale
  - Pruritus is common, and sites of predilection include elbows, knees, scalp, ears, umbilicus, and gluteal cleft
- Pityriasis rosea: this condition presents with erythematous to pink scaly papules and plaques classically in a "Christmas tree" distribution over the trunk
  - Pityriasis rosea often begins with a "herald patch," which is slightly larger than the other lesions
  - This self-limited eruption spontaneously regresses in 6 to 12 weeks
- Secondary syphilis: small erythematous and hyperkeratotic scaly macules, papules, and plaques are located on the trunk, extremities, palms, and soles
  - The patient may report history of a "chancre" (ulcer of primary syphilis) in the previous 2 to 10 weeks

- The treatment of nummular eczema is nonemergent
- Localized lesions can be treated with topical corticosteroids: a mid-potency to super-high-potency topical corticosteroid may be applied to the lesions bid for 2 weeks; should not be applied to the face, axillae, or groin
  - Mid-potency: prednicarbate (Dermatop®) 0.1% ointment or cream; triamcinolone acetonide (Aristocort®) 0.1% ointment or cream
  - High-potency: fluocinonide (Lidex®) 0.05% ointment or cream; clobetasol propionate (Temovate®) 0.05% ointment or cream; halobetasol propionate (Ultravate®) 0.05% ointment or cream, betamethasone dipropionate 0.05% in optimized ointment (Diprolene®)
  - Although topical corticosteroids are indicated for use for a few weeks, emphasize the side effects of prolonged use of corticosteroids such as skin atrophy
  - Consider the use of tacrolimus 0.1% (Protopic®) ointment bid, which may be used for prolonged periods with no risk of atrophy
- Generalized lesions can be treated with a combination of topical corticosteroids or crude coal tar and either ultraviolet B light (UVB) therapy or psoralens plus ultraviolet A (PUVA) light therapy

- Treat any secondary infections (*Staphylococcus aureus* most common)
  - Dicloxacillin: 500 mg bid for 10 days (adults); 12.5 to 25 mg/kg/day (children <40 kg)
  - Cephalexin (Keflex®): 500 mg bid for 10 days (adults); 25 to 50 mg/kg/day (children)
  - *Penicillin-allergic*: erythromycin 500 mg bid for 10 days (adults); 40 mg/kg/day for 10 days (children)

MANAGEMENT/FOLLOW-UP

- Patients who are treated with topical corticosteroids should be followed up by a primary care physician or a dermatologist in 2 weeks to assess progress and evaluate for skin atrophy
- Patients who require more advanced forms of treatment, such as ultraviolet therapy or combination therapy, should be seen by a primary care physician or a dermatologist within 2 to 4 weeks for therapy

ICD-9-CM Code

692.9

ORF

- There is usually a history of contact with animals, such as sheep, goat, or musk oxen, which can carry the orf virus and transmit it to humans
- Patients report the development of one or few isolated lesions, most commonly on the dorsum of a finger over a period of days to weeks
- Patients may have associated fevers and/or lymphadenopathy
- Patients may have a history of similar lesions in the past that spontaneously improved over a period of weeks

- The patient present with one or a few lesions

- The most common location is the dorsal aspect of the right index finger, but any cutaneous surface may be affected (Fig. 65-1)
- The lesions progress through six stages:
  ○ Papular: red, elevated lesion
  ○ Targetoid: nodule with a central red portion, a white middle ring, and a red outer portion
  ○ Acute: elevated, rapidly growing, weeping lesion (Fig. 65-2)
  ○ Regenerative: a thin dry crust on the surface of the lesion that may have black dots on the surface as well
  ○ Papillomatous: small papillomas develop over the surface of the lesion
  ○ Regressive stage: thick crust over the surface of the lesion with a decrease in size of the papillomas
- The patient may have associated fever, lymphadenopathy, and/or lymphangitis
- There have been no underlying diseases found as a predisposition to developing orf

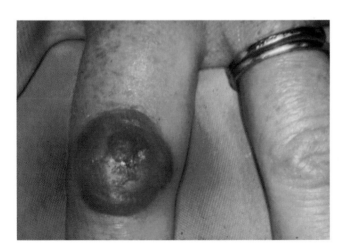

FIGURE 65-1 *The target phase shows a white circle with central and peripheral erythema.*

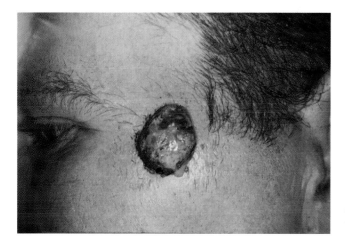

FIGURE 65-2 *In the acute phase there is a weeping of the surface overlying an elevated tumor.*

DIAGNOSIS

- Clinical suspicion should be confirmed by microscopic examination of a biopsy specimen

DIFFERENTIAL DIAGNOSIS

- Herpetic whitlow: this infection is caused by the herpes simplex virus
  - These lesions often occur most frequently on the fingers of health care workers exposed to patients with oral and/or genital herpetic infections
  - Whitlows appear as papules, vesicles, or erosions
- *Mycobacteria marinum* infection: this infection is caused by a mycobacterium that occurs in swimming pools and fish tanks
  - It presents as a violaceous papule at the site of inoculation, which progresses to a verrucous plaque over a few weeks
  - The most common sites include the hands
  - Lesions are usually solitary, but sporotrichoid (lymphangitic) spreading may be seen
- Fungal infections: infections with blastomycosis, coccidioidomycosis, and sporotrichosis can produce similar clinical presentations and may be distinguished histopathologically and by culture

- Milker's nodule: this infection presents as a single erythematous nodule on a finger that gets transmitted to humans by direct contact with infected cattle
  - The infectious nodule undergoes the same progression of stages as do the lesions in orf virus infection

TREATMENT

- The treatment of orf is nonemergent
- The lesions will spontaneously heal in about 5 weeks; thus no treatment is required
- Patients may choose to have the lesion excised for more rapid resolution
- Any suspected superficial infection should be treated appropriately

MANAGEMENT/FOLLOW-UP

- The patient should be seen by either the primary care physician or a dermatologist within 1 week of the emergency department visit to evaluate progression of the lesion

ICD-9-CM Code

051.2

PARAPSORIASIS

- In actuality, parapsoriasis is a group of related and unrelated diseases
- Gradual development of scaly and oval-shaped patches that are mainly found on the trunk and flexural areas
- Patient may report pruritus within the lesions
- Often patients have been treated for their condition with marginal response
- These conditions are present for weeks, months, or years prior to diagnosis

- Oval or irregularly shaped thin scaling plaques that are well-marginated are visible
- Lesions of large plaque parapsoriasis (LPP) generally measure >5 cm in diameter, whereas lesions of small plaque parapsoriasis (SPP) are <5 cm in diameter (Figs. 66-1 to 66-3)
- Red or salmon-colored lesions usually located on trunk and/or flexural areas of the skin

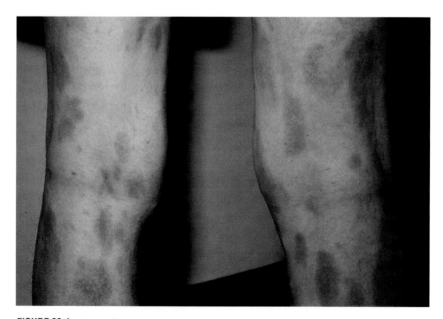

FIGURE 66-1   *Large plaque parapsoriasis (LPP).*

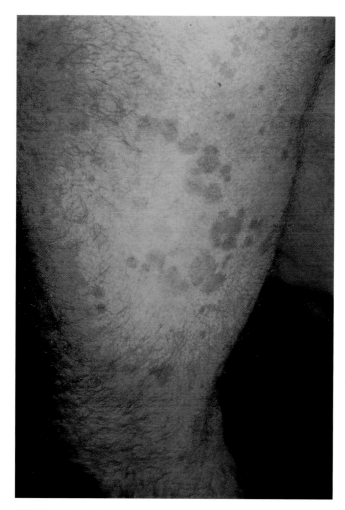

FIGURE 66-2 *Small plaque parapsoriasis (SPP).*

- Surface of the lesions appears finely wrinkled and may become atrophic
- Digitate dermatosis is a distinctive variant of SPP that appears as yellow- to red-colored thin plaques distributed over lines of cleavage on the skin; gives the appearance of a hug that left "fingerprints" on the trunk

DIAGNOSIS

- Clinical findings require confirmation by examination of a skin biopsy

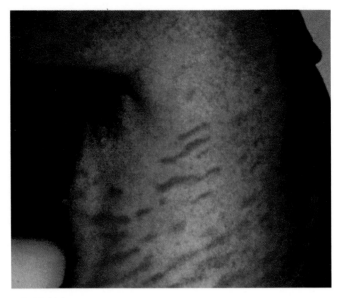

FIGURE 66-3 *Small plaque parapsoriasis (SPP).*

- Mycosis fungoides: LPP may be indistinguishable and may be the same condition as mycosis fungoides, both clinically and histologically
  - This chronic cutaneous T-cell lymphoma presents with scaly patches and plaques that may be located on any cutaneous surface
  - Thick plaques are more likely mycosis fungoides than parapsoriasis
- Atopic dermatitis: poorly defined erythematous patches and plaques in which acute lesions appear edematous and chronic lesions appear lichenified
  - Atopic dermatitis is often associated with allergic rhinitis and asthma
- Psoriasis: this inflammatory skin disease is characterized by thick, erythematous papules and plaques with silvery scales that has a predilection to include the elbows, knees, scalp, ears, umbilicus, and gluteal cleft

- Pityriasis rosea: erythematous to pink scaly papules and plaques classically in a "Christmas tree" distribution over the trunk
  - It may begin with a "herald patch," which is slightly larger than the other lesions
  - This is a self-limited eruption that spontaneously regresses in 6 to 12 weeks
- Secondary syphilis: presents with erythematous and hyperkeratotic scaly plaques located on the trunk, extremities, palms, and soles
  - Patients may report a history of a chancre of primary syphilis in the previous 2 to 10 weeks

- The treatment of all forms of parapsoriasis is nonemergent
- Large plaque parapsoriasis may actually be mycosis fungoides, and treatment requires aggressive therapy, with the goal of suppressing progression to mycosis fungoides
  - Localized lesions can be treated with topical corticosteroids: a mid-potency to super-high-potency topical corticosteroid may be applied to the lesions bid for 2 weeks; should not be applied to the face, axillae, or groin
    - Mid-potency: prednicarbate (Dermatop®) 0.1% ointment or cream; triamcinolone acetonide (Aristocort®) 0.1% ointment or cream
    - High-potency: fluocinonide (Lidex®) 0.05% ointment or cream; clobetasol propionate (Temovate®) 0.05% ointment or cream; halobetasol propionate (Ultravate®) 0.05% ointment or cream, betamethasone dipropionate 0.05% in optimized ointment (Diprolene®)
  - Emphasize that the side effect of prolonged use of corticosteroids is skin atrophy

  - Generalized lesions should be treated with a combination of topical corticosteroids and either ultraviolet B light (UVB) therapy or psoralen phtotochemotherapy (PUVA)
- SPP may be left untreated; however, most patients opt for treatment for symptom improvement and/or cosmetic concerns
  - Topical corticosteroids and/or UVB therapy is the treatment of choice (see above)

- Patients who are treated with topical corticosteroids should be followed up by a primary care physician or dermatologist within 2 weeks to assess progress
- Patients who require more advanced forms of treatment, such as UV therapy or combination therapy, should be seen by a primary care physician or a dermatologist within 1 to 2 weeks for therapy

ICD-9-CM Code

696.2

PEDICULOSIS (LICE)

HISTORY

- Patients present with a history of pruritus of the scalp, body, or pubic area
- The condition is most common in children of school age, and affected children may report sharing hats, combs, or brushes
- Patients may report a history of contact with someone who had pediculosis

PHYSICAL EXAMINATION

- Lice: head, body, or pubic lice are identified with either the naked eye or a hand lens (Figs. 67-1 to 67-3)
  - Lice are often difficult to find in the scalp or on the body, but pubic lice are usually easier to locate

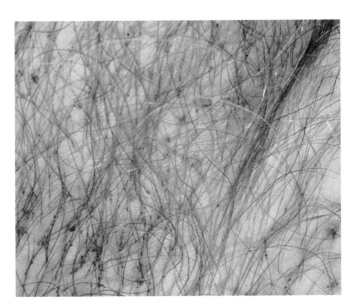

FIGURE 67-1 *Pediculosis pubis in the pubic area.*

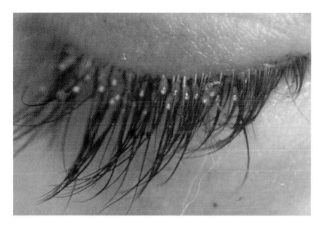

FIGURE 67-2   *Pediculosis pubis on the eyelashes.*

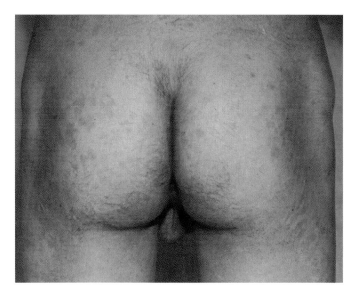

FIGURE 67-3   *Pediculosis pubis on the buttocks.*

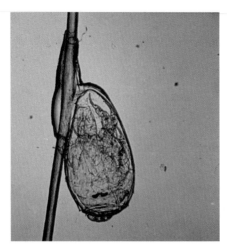

FIGURE 67-4 *Pediculosis pubis showing an egg attached to a hair shaft.*

- Nits: oval gray-white egg capsules are often firmly cemented to hair shafts (Fig. 67-4)
  - If the patient has been infested recently, the nits will be close to the scalp
  - With long-standing infestation, the nits may be several centimeters away from the scalp
- Due to chronic scratching, the patient may have excoriations, lichenification, and/or superficial infections of the skin

DIAGNOSIS

- In pediculosis capitis, infestation of the scalp is caused by the head louse *Pediculus humanus capitis*

  - The diagnosis is confirmed when lice and/or nits are found on the scalp; the beard and/or eyelashes may be affected
- In pediculosis pubis, infestation of the pubic area and/or hair-bearing regions of the body is caused by the crab or pubic louse, *Phthirus pubis*
  - The diagnosis is confirmed/made when lice and/or nits are found in these areas

- In pediculosis corporis, infestation of the body, primarily hair-bearing sites, is caused by the body louse, *Pediculus humanus corporis*
  - The diagnosis is confirmed made when lice and/or nits are found in these areas
- The diagnosis is based on site of infestation, as one cannot otherwise clinically differentiate between body and hair louse subspecies
  - The pubic louse or crab louse is readily distinguished from the others
- A louse can be examined by light microscopy to evaluate this six-legged wingless insect that is 1 to 4 mm in length
- Nits are 0.5-mm oval-shaped, gray-white eggs that can be seen by plucking the hair, placing it on a slide, and viewing the eggs under a microscope

- Seborrheic dermatitis (dandruff): in this common condition, scaling and redness are seen over the scalp and/or face
  - Crusts and scale are not "cemented" to the hair shaft as are nits, but freely moveable hair casts may be visible
- Debris from hair gels and other hair care products: these can simulate the appearance of nits; however, the former is easily removed from the hair shaft

TREATMENT

- Treatment is designed to kill the nits and the adult lice on the patient as well as to clean all contaminated bedding, clothing, and personal hygiene products
  - All household contacts of a person infested should be examined and treated if necessary
  - All people treated for pediculosis should machine wash with detergent and dry or dry clean all clothing, bedding, towels, and hats
  - Any combs or brushes should be soaked in rubbing alcohol or Lysol® 2% solution for 1 hour
  - The floor and furniture should be vacuumed thoroughly as well

- Pediculosis capitis
  - Permethrin (Nix®) 1% cream rinse is available over the counter and has low mammalian toxicity
    - The hair should be washed with regular shampoo, rinsed with water, and towel-dried
    - Permethrin cream rinse should then be applied to coat the hair and scalp, left on for 10 minutes, and then washed off with water
    - This agent may not be used on the eyebrow and eyelash area
    - Apply petrolatum to the eyebrows or eyelash areas twice daily for 8 days, followed by gentle removal of nits
    - A fine-toothed nit comb, which can be obtained over the counter, should be used to comb the nits out of the hair after treatment
    - A second treatment may be required if adult nits are observed after a week of application
  - Pyrethrin (RID®) 0.3% shampoo is available over the counter; has low mammalian toxicity
    - The agent should be applied to damp hair, left on for 10 minutes, and then washed off with warm water
    - This agent may not be used on the eyebrow and eyelash area
    - Apply petrolatum to the eyebrows or eyelash areas twice daily for 8 days, followed by gentle removal of nits

- A fine-toothed nit comb accompanies the product and should be used to comb the nits out of the hair after treatment
- Since the product is not totally ovicidal, a second application is recommended 7 to 10 days later to kill newly hatched nymphs from eggs that survived the first treatment
- Other pyrethrin shampoos, gels, and lotions are available over the counter
  - ○ Malathion (Ovide®) 0.5% is available only by prescription
    - This agent is applied to the involved skin or hair for 8 to 12 hours and is then washed off
    - This agent may be used on the eyebrow and eyelash area
    - Note that this is the single most effective agent now available
    - The hair should then be rinsed with water and dried
    - A fine-toothed nit comb should be used to comb the nits out of the hair after treatment
    - If live lice are seen 7 days after treatment, a second treatment should be performed
    - This agent is not recommended for use on infants, young children, pregnant or lactating women, or patients with seizure disorders or other neurologic diseases
  - ○ Lindane (Kwell®) 1% shampoo is available only by prescription
    - The patient should lather the hair and scalp thoroughly with the shampoo and leave on for 4 minutes
    - This agent may be used on the eyebrow and eyelash area
    - The hair should then be rinsed with water and dried
    - A fine-toothed nit comb should be used to comb the nits out of the hair after treatment
    - If live lice are seen 7 days after treatment, a second treatment should be performed
    - This agent has a potential for central nervous system toxicity if overused, so 60 ml should be prescribed for 2 uses per person, without any refills
    - This agent is not recommended for use on infants, young children, pregnant or lactating women, or patients with seizure disorders or other neurologic diseases
- Pediculosis pubis
  - ○ Any of the above-listed medications may be used
  - ○ Recommend application to all affected areas including the mons pubis and perianal regions, as well as the chest, axillae, thighs, and trunk in hairy individuals
  - ○ Sexual contacts should be treated
  - ○ Other general measures mentioned above, including washing of clothing, should be followed as well

- Pediculosis corporis
  - Lindane (Kwell®) 1% lotion can be applied from head to toe, left on for 8 hours, and then washed off with water; reapply in 1 week
  - Malathion (Ovide®) 0.5% can be applied from head to toe, left on for 8 hours, and then washed off with water; reapply in 1 week
  - Sexual contacts should also be treated
  - Other general measures mentioned above, including washing of clothing, should be followed as well

- Patients should be followed up by their primary care physician or dermatologist in 1 week to assess progress and to determine whether another treatment will be needed

ICD-9 Code

132.9

CHAPTER 68

PEMPHIGUS VULGARIS AND PEMPHIGUS FOLIACEUS

HISTORY

- Both are autoimmune disorders with autoimmunity to the surface glycoproteins of suprabasal keratinocytes that result in painful blisters and erosions
- Pemphigus vulgaris
  - Presents with painful, flaccid blisters and erosions that are abrupt in onset anywhere on the skin surface, including mucous membranes
    - Mucous membrane disease may be present for months before skin lesions develop
  - The usual age of onset of disease is 50 to 60 years old, but it may occur at any age
- Pemphigus foliaceus
  - Presents as painful, scaly, crusted lesions that are often confined to the head, neck, and upper trunk areas
  - The disease may be localized for years or may progress rapidly
  - An endemic form of the disease is seen in Brazil, often occurring in children and young adults, and is called fogo selvagem
  - Less commonly seen on mucous membranes
  - The usually age of onset is 50 to 60 years old, but it can occur at any age

PHYSICAL EXAMINATION

- Pemphigus vulgaris
  - Painful, flaccid vesicles and erosions anywhere on the body, but often starts in intertriginous zones of skin on normal-appearing skin or on an erythematous base (Figs. 68-1 to 68-4)
  - The Nikolsky and Asboe-Hansen signs may be present
    - Nikolsky sign: in patients with active blisters, light lateral sliding pressure with a gloved finger will separate normal-looking epidermis, producing an erosion
    - Asboe-Hansen sign: light lateral pressure on the blister edge spreads the blister into clinically normal skin
  - Often occurs on mucous membranes and most commonly occurs on oral mucosa, although the conjunctiva, anus, penis, vagina, and labia may be involved
- Pemphigus foliaceus
  - One sees scaly, crusted erosions, often on an erythematous base, in the head, neck, and upper trunk areas
  - Primary lesions of flaccid vesicles may be difficult to find on examination
  - This condition rarely involves mucous membranes

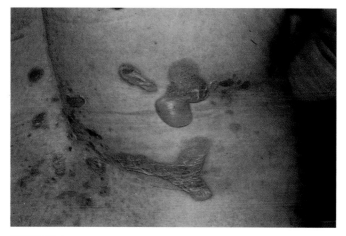

FIGURE 68-1 *Pemphigus vulgaris: flaccid blisters.*

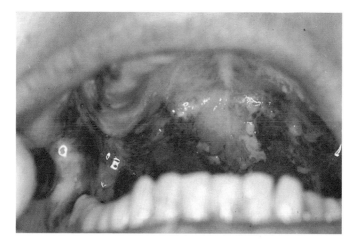

FIGURE 68-2 *Pemphigus vulgaris: oral erosions.*

DIAGNOSIS

- The definitive diagnosis requires examination of skin biopsy specimens for routine staining and also for direct immunofluorescence
- Indirect immunofluorescence studies may also be positive in these diseases and may correlate with disease activity

DIFFERENTIAL DIAGNOSIS FOR BOTH CONDITIONS

- Skin involvement
  - Bullous pemphigoid: generally presents with large, tense vesicles and bullae; a smaller proportion has mucous membrane involvement
  - Hailey-Hailey disease (benign familial pemphigus): this chronic genodermatosis presents with vesicles and more

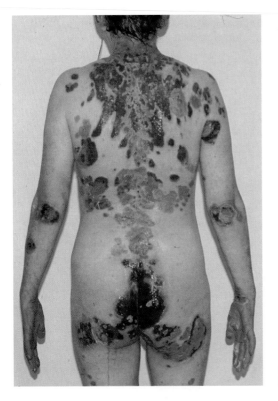

FIGURE 68-3 *Extensive erosions due to blistering in pemphigus vulgaris.*

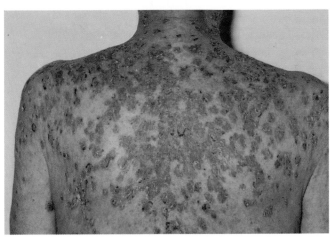

FIGURE 68-4 *Pemphigus foliaceus on upper back.*

commonly crusted erythematous plaques in intertriginous areas
- Erythema multiforme: this reaction pattern may produce large vesicles, but typical targetoid lesions are usually demonstrated

- Dermatitis herpetiformis: this autoimmune blistering disorder generally is so pruritic that vesicles have been removed by fingernails prior to examination, and widespread erosions are absent

- Bullous impetigo: this infectious disease is more common in children and presents with vesicles or bullae containing clear to yellow fluid, usually located on the trunk, extremities, face, or intertriginous areas
- Mucous membrane involvement
- Acute herpetic stomatitis: may present as acute, painful vesiculation and erosions of the mucous membranes of the mouth
  - The skin or mucosa is erythematous and edematous and has small to large grouped vesicles with central umbilications
  - As lesions mature, vesicles may coalesce, become vesiculopustules and then erosions
  - Tzanck smear preparation examination is positive for viropathic findings
- Erythema multiforme: as noted above, this reaction pattern may produce large vesicles including in the mucosae, but typical targetoid lesions are usually demonstrated elsewhere
- Cicatricial pemphigoid: this slowly progressive scarring autoimmune disease presents with erosions of any mucous membrane including the mouth, nose, eyes, and anogenital areas
- Aphthous ulcers: presents with shallow, small painful erosions
- Lichen planus: this chronic condition can present only with mucous membrane erosions that may be symptomatic or nonsymptomatic

- Mainstay of treatment for both pemphigus vulgaris and foliaceus is systemic corticosteroid agents, such as prednisone; occasionally, pemphigus foliaceus can be treated with topical corticosteroids
  - High doses such as 2.0 mg/kg/day of prednisone are often used initially to control the eruption, but dose is decreased to a lower level relatively quickly over weeks to months depending on the response

- Other immunosuppressants, such as cyclophosphamide (Cytoxan®), azathioprine (Imuran®), cyclosporine (Neoral®), or methotrexate (Rheumatrex®), are sometimes required for control and may also be added as corticosteroid-sparing medications
- Other reported therapies include intramuscular gold, antimalarial agents, dapsone, and extracorporeal photochemotherapy

- Pemphigus vulgaris
  - Requires close monitoring by the primary care physician, preferably with the assistance of a dermatologist until the disease is under control
  - Significant morbidity and mortality may be associated with this disease
  - Untreated pemphigus vulgaris may have a 90% 2-year mortality rate
  - Patients severely affected may require admission for intensive care unit management and should be managed analogously to burn patient
  - If ocular involvement or oropharyngeal or ophthalmologic involvement is suspected, the patient may require comanagement with otolaryngology and ophthalmology
- Pemphigus foliaceus
  - This condition is usually less severe and easier to control and is associated with less morbidity and mortality then pemphigus vulgaris
  - Requires close monitoring by a dermatologist until disease is controlled and then regular follow-up thereafter

ICD-9-CM Code

694.4 Pemphigus vulgaris and foliaceus

CPT Code

11100 Biopsy

PERIORAL DERMATITIS

HISTORY

- This skin disease usually occurs in females of childbearing age and is located around the mouth, but may be on other areas of face as well
- The condition has relatively rapid onset within a few days
- Some patients may be using topical corticosteroid agents to treat this condition
- The patient may notice a cyclical exacerbation around the menstrual cycle

PHYSICAL EXAMINATION

- Grouped, acneiform, firm, pinhead-sized erythematous papules with some fine scaling laterally in the nasolabial folds, chin, or upper lip, sparing the rim of the lip at the vermilion border (Figs. 69-1 and 69-2)
- Atypical presentations can also involve the glabella, eyelids, and forehead

DIAGNOSIS

- The diagnosis is mainly clinical, with an acneiform-appearing eruption concentrated around the mouth or eyes as a relatively classic presentation

DIFFERENTIAL DIAGNOSIS

- Rosacea: usually in a different distribution on the face (over the cheeks and nose) and associated with telangiectasias, pustules, and prominent background erythema (some consider perioral dermatitis a form of rosacea)
- Seborrheic dermatitis: may have similar distribution in nasolabial folds, but usually seen as poorly defined, scaly patches and plaques rather than discrete papules on the scalp and other areas of the face, such as around the eyebrows and nose
- Contact dermatitis: usually comprising poorly defined, scaly patches with possible vesiculation noted, often in the same distribution as perioral dermatitis
- Acne vulgaris: usually scattered more diffusely on the face and diagnosed by the presence of comedones, inflammatory papules, pustules, and nodules

TREATMENT

- The treatment of perioral dermatitis is nonemergent
- Topical
  - If topical corticosteroids are being used, taper medication and then discontinue
    - Stopping them abruptly may lead to exacerbation

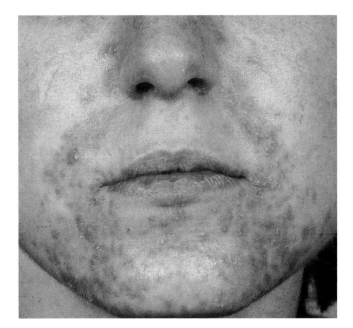

FIGURE 69-1 *Perioral dermatitis.*

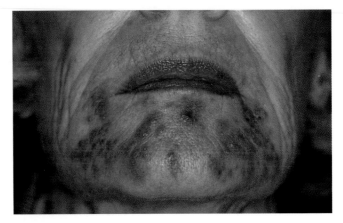

FIGURE 69-2 *Perioral dermatitis.*

- ○ Topical metronidazole (Metrogel®), clindamycin (Cleocin®), or erythromycin (Erygel®) can be used bid for several months until eruption is controlled or resolved
- Oral
  - ○ Oral antibiotics, such as tetracycline (Sumycin®) 250 to 500 mg by mouth bid or doxycycline (Vibramycin®) 50 to 100 mg by mouth bid for an adult; requires several months of use to see improvement
  - ○ Oral erythromycin 250 to 500 mg by mouth bid may be useful in pregnant females but may be less effective
- May often combine both topical and oral treatments for a short period, with tapering later of the oral antibiotic

- Therapy will be needed for at least 3 to 4 months to be sure of adequate control; based on response, could begin to taper medications at that time
- Follow-up recommended with either primary care physician or dermatologist within 4 to 8 weeks after starting therapy

- Eruption may resolve spontaneously or persist for several years with intermittent flaring, but has a good prognosis

ICD-9-CM Code

695.3

CPT Code

None

PHYTOPHOTODERMATITIS

HISTORY

- The patient presents with rapid onset of bullae on an exposed surface, such as on the neck or extremities, in bizarre configurations suggesting an exogenous source without associated pruritus
- Patients may report a history of recent contact with furocoumarin-containing plants, such as limes, lemons, oranges, celery, parsnip, grass, or dill
- Ultraviolet A (UV-A) exposure is subsequently required to induce the phototoxic, non–immune-mediated reaction that causes this dermatitis
- Often seen in farm workers, nursery personnel, florists, gardeners, bartenders, celery harvesters, and grocery clerks

PHYSICAL EXAMINATION

- Small and large bullae associated with minimal erythema on exposed surfaces in odd configurations that may be unilateral or bilateral (Figs. 70-1 and 70-2)
- Once healing has begun, one may see linear, hyperpigmented streaks on the skin

DIAGNOSIS

- History and physical examination alone will guide to this diagnosis

DIFFERENTIAL DIAGNOSIS

- Allergic contact dermatitis: usually very pruritic, and one sees small vesicles associated with erythema in linear, bizarre configurations
- Porphyria cutanea tarda: produces noninflammatory vesicles, bullae, or erosions distributed symmetrically on sun-exposed areas, associated with hypertrichosis, scarring, milia formation, and liver dysfunction
- Bullous pemphigoid: this autoimmune disease produces tense, pruritic bullae on an erythematous base in an older person on both exposed and covered areas

TREATMENT

- The main treatment measure should be to avoid infection, as bullae heal by keeping areas clean and dry
- Mid- to high-potency topical corticosteroid agents for 1 to 2 weeks may speed resolution
  - Mid-potency: prednicarbate (Dermatop®) 0.1% ointment or cream; triamcinolone acetonide (Aristocort®) 0.1% ointment or cream

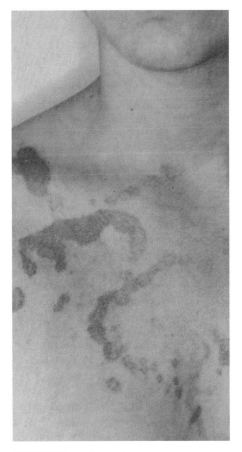

FIGURE 70-1 *Berloque phytophotodermatitis.*

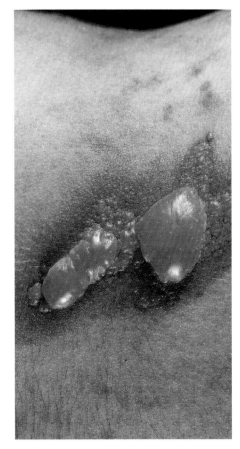

FIGURE 70-2 *Berloque phytophotodermatitis.*

    ◦ High-potency: fluocinonide (Lidex®) 0.05% ointment or cream; clobetasol propionate (Temovate®) 0.05% ointment or cream; halobetasol propionate (Ultravate®) 0.05% ointment or cream, betamethasone dipropionate 0.05% in optimized ointment (Diprolene®)
- The condition usually resolves in approximately 1 week

- Avoidance of the offending agent in combination with ultraviolet exposure will help to prevent future episodes
- No specific follow-up is needed

ICD-9-CM Code

692.72

CHAPTER 71

PIGMENTED PURPURIC ERUPTIONS

HISTORY

- Schamberg's disease: presents with brown-red, occasionally itchy spots on lower legs, usually in male patients, but females may be affected as well; occurs in children or adults
- Lichenoid purpura of Gougerot and Blum: presents with asymptomatic brown-red spots and bumps on legs in males aged 40 to 60 years, but may affect females as well
- Purpura annularis telangiectoides (Majocchi's disease): presents with round, asymptomatic, brown-red lesions anywhere on the body in adolescent and young adult patients; has equal sex predilection

PHYSICAL EXAMINATION

- Schamberg's disease: irregular patches of orange-brown, "cayenne pepper" spots on the anterior aspects of the lower legs (Fig. 71-1)
- Lichenoid purpura of Gougerot and Blum: erythematous, orange to purpuric macules and papules around the ankles, spreading to the lower body, that may become confluent
- Purpura annularis telangiectoides: 1- to 3-cm annular or targetoid plaques, telangiectasias, and "cayenne pepper" spots

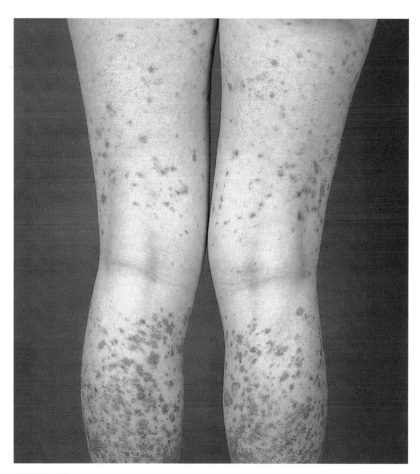

FIGURE 71-1 *Pigmented purpuric dermatosis: Majocchi's purpura.*

- These are clinical diagnoses
- If there is any question, examination of a skin biopsy may be necessary to distinguish from small vessel vasculitis

DIFFERENTIAL DIAGNOSIS

- Small vessel vasculitis: may be difficult to distinguish if lesions are extensive and of abrupt onset, but in Schamberg's disease, the nonpalpable nature of the lesions may be helpful
  - Small vessel vasculitis is usually more purpuric and may ulcerate
- Traumatic purpura: a common condition on the lower extremities in which patients usually provide a history of trauma and linear lesions of nonpalpable or palpable purpura may be seen
- Statis dermatitis: patients have significant brown discoloration of skin on the lower aspects of the anterior legs that may feel firm and bound-down
- Thrombocytopenia: should be considered in any patient with purpura, and laboratory investigation may be necessary

- Patients may be treated with topical corticosteroids, such as prednicarbate (Dermatop®) 0.1% ointment or cream; triamcinolone acetonide (Aristocort®) 0.1% ointment or cream bid to affected skin; hydrocortisone valerate (Westcort®) 0.2% cream or ointment, twice per day to the affected areas
- Compression support hose (30 to 40 mm Hg) should also be prescribed and recommended to help decrease serum leakage from blood vessels

- Patients should be referred to their primary care physician or dermatologist within the next 2 to 4 weeks for follow-up
- All three of these diagnoses may have a chronic course

ICD-9-CM Code

287.2

CPT Code

11100   Biopsy

PITTED KERATOLYSIS

HISTORY

- Patient usually complains of itching and foul-smelling feet
- They may also complain of sliminess of the foot skin, with the foot sticking to the socks
- This condition affects men, women, adults, and children equally and tends to be much worse in warm climates

PHYSICAL EXAMINATION

- Superficial erosions or pits of the plantar surface and occasional palmar surfaces are visible (Fig. 72-1)
  - Many small pits may coalesce into larger distinct erosions
  - This condition is predominantly found on pressure-bearing areas and in the web spaces between toes

DIAGNOSIS

- This is a diagnosis based on history and clinical findings
- The causative organism is a *Corynebacterium* species or *Micrococcus sedentariusm*; and these organisms invade the stratum corneum that has been softened by sweat and moisture
  - A Gram's stain of scraping from the involved areas will show coccoid and filamentous organisms with branching and septae

DIFFERENTIAL DIAGNOSIS

- Tinea pedia: usually one will see diffuse, scaly, poorly defined patches with a white, fine, powdery scale, often in a moccasin distribution, with associated white, macerated plaques in the interdigital web spaces and no prominent pitting
  - Examination of a KOH preparation reveals hyphae
- Erythrasma: usually one will see hyperkeratotic patches in the web spaces that exhibit a coral-red fluorescence under Wood's lamp examination with no pitting of the soles

TREATMENT

- Appropriate hygiene of the feet should be encouraged, keeping them as dry as possible
- Absorbent foot powders (Zeasorb® AF powder or Micatin® powder) once per day to the feet may be beneficial
- Topical antibiotic agents, such as erythromycin (Cleocin® solution, Clindets®) or erythromycin (Emgel®) applied bid will help the condition
- Topical benzoyl peroxide 4% to 10% (e.g., Benzac AC® or Brevoxyl®) in gel or wash form bid is also bactericidal and is safe topically

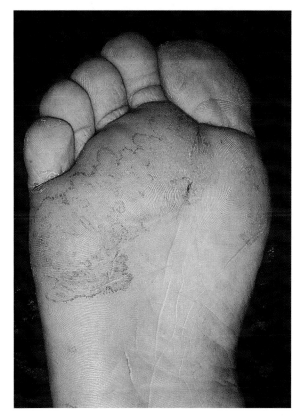

FIGURE 72-1 *Pitted keratolysis.*

- The patient should follow up with the primary care physician or a dermatologist in 1 to 2 months

- The condition is recurrent but is easily treated

ICD-9 Code

686.9

PITYRIASIS ROSEA

- Patient notes a scaly rash that has been present for for 1 to 8 weeks
- Pruritus may be severe in some cases but is usually mild
- Patients may be able to identify the first lesion, the "herald patch," which is larger and more pronounced than the others
- The eruption generally reaches maximum intensity in about 2 weeks and usually resolves spontaneously in approximately 6 to 8 weeks
- Pityriasis rosea affects men and women equally and can occur at any age, but the most commonly affected patients are between the ages of age 10 and 40 years
- Usually there is no prodrome, but patients occasionally report malaise, headache, nausea, loss of appetite, fever, joint pain, and lymphadenopathy before the onset of the eruption
- Pityriasis rosea is more common during the spring and autumn months, suggesting that the disease is related to an infectious agent, such as a virus or bacteria

- The eruption initially consists of an oval to round plaque with a central, scaly, salmon-colored area and a darker red peripheral zone with a collarette of fine scale distributed on the trunk (Figs. 73-1 to 73-4)
- This "herald patch" may be mistaken for a tinea infection, and microscopic examination of a KOH preparation is negative
- Two days to 2 months later, the patient develops a generalized, symmetric eruption of smaller plaques and papules with similar morphology to the herald patch
  - Lesions are generally confined to the trunk, neck, and extremities, sparing the distal extremities and the face
- Due to the distribution and orientation of lesions along relaxed skin tension lines, the eruption may appear to have a "Christmas tree pattern"
- Atypical pityriasis rosea involving only the face, neck, or distal extremities or involving only intertriginous areas may occur

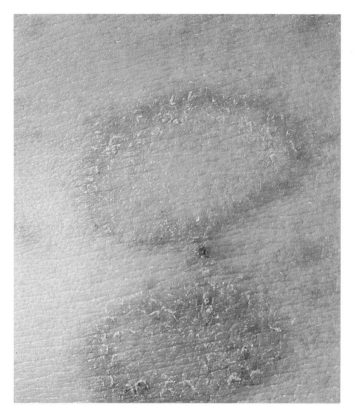

FIGURE 73-1 *Pityriasis rosea: double herald patch.*

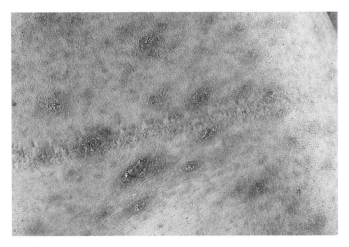

FIGURE 73-2 *Pityriasis rosea: generalized eruption.*

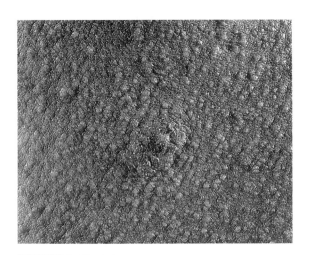

FIGURE 73-3 *Pityriasis rosea.*

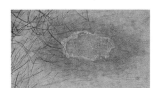

FIGURE 73-4 *Pityriasis rosea.*

- The diagnosis is based primarily on the history and physical examination
- No blood test is helpful, but if there is any doubt, serologic testing for syphilis should be performed

- Nummular eczema: can be confused with pityriasis rosea, but usually has fewer lesions that are more papulovesicular and not necessarily confined to the trunk and proximal extremities
- Guttate psoriasis: this condition, without a "herald patch," often has more intensely erythematous macules and papules with thicker, white scale that covers the entire lesion
- Tinea corporis: usually 1 to 10 lesions are seen, each of which demonstrates central clearing, compared with numerous small pityriasis rosea lesions that are confluent
  ○ Examination of a KOH preparation will readily distinguish the two conditions
- Drug eruption: There have been rare reported pityriasis rosea-like drug eruptions, and clinical history of recent drug exposure may help distinguish the two
- Secondary syphilis: often involves the palms, soles, and mucous membranes and lacks a herald patch; lesions are usually less erythematous than pityriasis rosea lesions
  ○ Any doubt about differentiation should prompt serology for syphilis, which may help to distinguish the two diseases

- The treatment of pityriasis rosea is nonemergent
- The eruption is usually self-limited, and, if patients are not symptomatic, no specific treatment is needed
- Symptomatic treatment may be prescribed, including topical mid-potency steroids, such as triamcinolone cream (Aristocort®) applied bid for 2 to 4 weeks
- Ultraviolet B (UVB) phototherapy may also help to decrease itching

- Usually the eruption is self-limited and resolves in approximately 6 weeks, although it may last 12 weeks
- No specific follow-up is needed unless the condition does not resolve or the patient becomes highly symptomatic

ICD-9 Code

696.3

CHAPTER 74

PITYRIASIS RUBRA PILARIS

HISTORY

- The patient presents with gradual or rapid onset of a red, scaly erythrodermic rash that usually starts on the face and scalp, progresses from head to toe, and may involve all areas of body, including palms and soles
- Both acquired and autosomal dominant inherited forms exist
  - The inherited form usually appears in childhood
  - The acquired form may occur at any age but is usually seen in middle-aged adults
- The condition may be quite pruritic in some patients

PHYSICAL EXAMINATION

- Examination of the face and scalp reveal red, scaly patches and plaques, sometimes with very thick hyperkeratosis
- The trunk and extremities show scaling orange-red to yellowish plaques with sharp borders separated by islands of normal skin ("islands of sparing") that may expand, coalesce, and eventually cover the entire body, including the face (Fig. 74-1)
  - At this point, the patient appears to have an exfoliative erythroderma

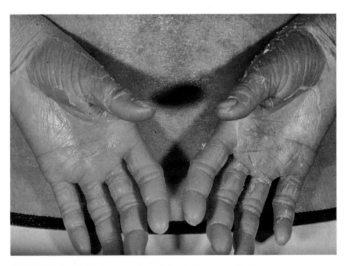

FIGURE 74-1 *Follicular papules of pityriasis rubra pilaris.*

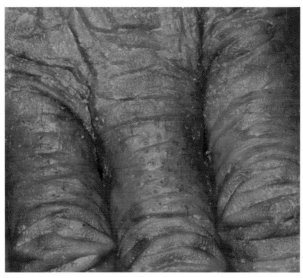

A.

FIGURE 74-2 *Hyperkeratotic palmar lesions.*

- Prominent involvement of hands with hyperkeratotic, waxy appearing palms and soles
  - The dorsum of the hands have follicular-based, hyperkeratotic papules that appear as follicular plugs with surrounding erythema (Fig. 74-2)
- Nails show yellow-brown discoloration, subungual hyperkeratosis, nail plate thickening, and some nail pitting

DIAGNOSIS

- The history and clinical exam may be suggestive, but examination of a skin biopsy specimen is usually needed to distinguish between other disorders, especially in erythrodermic patients

DIFFERENTIAL DIAGNOSIS

- Psoriasis: pityriasis rubra pilaris may mimic psoriasis closely both clinically and histologically, especially early in disease
  - Psoriasis may be more plaque-like and without cephalocaudal progression or "islands of sparing," and psoriasis never produces waxy appearing palms and soles
- Atopic dermatitis: usually composed of less well-defined, scaling patches and plaques that are more erythematous in color than pityriasis rubra pilaris
  - The patient may also have a history of atopy including asthma and allergic rhinitis
  - Atopic dermatitis never produces waxy appearing palms and soles

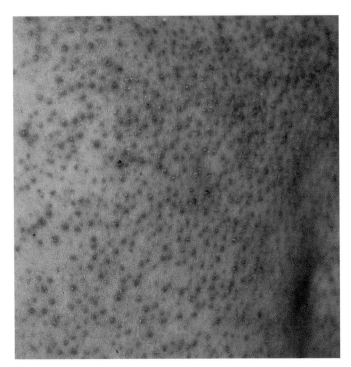

B.

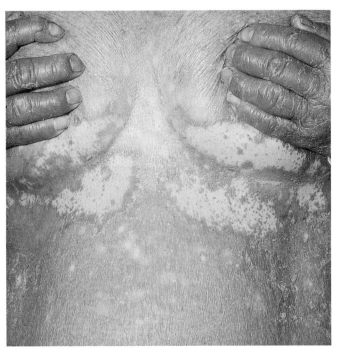

C.

- Drug eruption: usually a drug eruption is more truncal in distribution, without clear "islands of sparing," and is composed of pruritic, erythematous, poorly defined scaling patches, or it may be morbilliform in nature
  - One is generally able to elicit a history of new medication addition
  - It would be rare for drug eruptions to produce waxy appearing palms and soles

TREATMENT

- Treatment of pityriasis rubra pilaris is nonemergent
- Systemic treatments, such as oral acitretin (Soriatane®) or weekly oral methotrexate (Rheumatrex®), may be required in the more severe, difficult-to-treat cases
  - These agents are not appropriate for prescribing in the emergency department; acetretin is not safe to use in women of childbearing age who drink alcohol or are anticipating pregnancy within the next 3 years of their life
- Keratolytic solutions and creams (lactic acid, or urea-containing creams) bid may be helpful for hyperkeratotic plaques, especially on hands and feet

- Topical mid-potency corticosteroid ointments, such as triamcinolone (Aristocort®) 0.1% cream or ointment applied bid may also be helpful for nonfacial areas

MANAGEMENT/FOLLOW-UP

- This disease is exceptionally difficult to treat, and the familial type (juvenile onset) often persists throughout life, while the acquired type may have remissions
- The patient should be seen within one week by a dermatologist for evaluation and formulation of a treatment strategy

ICD-9-CM Code

696.4

CPT Code

11100   Biopsy

CHAPTER 75

POLYMORPHOUS ERUPTION OF PREGNANCY

HISTORY

- A primigravid patient presents late in the second or third trimester of pregnancy with intensely pruritic lesions on the abdomen, often in "stretch marks," in the periumbilical area, as well as buttocks and upper thighs
- The disease may also occur on the arms, forearms, and legs and occurs rarely in multiparous women
- Patients may complain of not being able to sleep at night due to itching

PHYSICAL EXAMINATION

- Erythematous papules, excoriations, and urticaria-like papules and plaques are present in the periumbilical area, often in the striae distensae
- Similar lesions may be seen on the buttocks and upper thigh and rarely on the arms, forearms, and legs (Fig. 75-1)
- Vesicles and bullae are absent
- The face is almost always spared

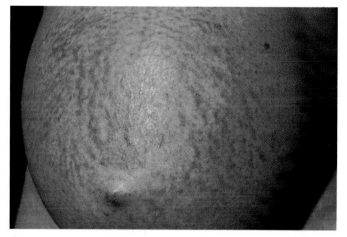

A.

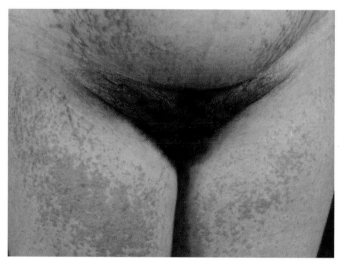

B.

FIGURE 75-1 *Pruritic urticarial papules and plaques of pregnancy.*

- This is a clinical diagnosis supported by history and physical examination
- Examination of a skin biopsy specimen is not generally needed, but this should be performed if vesicles or bullae are seen, to exclude herpes (pemphigoid) gestationis

DIFFERENTIAL DIAGNOSIS

- Herpes (pemphigoid) gestationis: this autoimmune disease of pregnancy may have a similar distribution but usually has vesicles or bullae and may involve the palms, soles, chest, back, and face
  - Examination of a skin biopsy specimen, possibly including a direct immunofluorescence study, will distinguish the two
- Erythema multiforme: discrete lesions scattered diffusely, often involving the palms and soles
  - It is usually more of an erythematous, dusky color with a targetoid appearance
- Drug eruption: the history may help if new pharmacologic agents were initiated within the preceding several weeks; few drug eruptions present with the amount of pruritus seen in polymorphous eruption of pregnancy
  - Drug eruptions are not usually localized to the abdomen and striae distensae
- Urticaria: may closely mimic polymorphous eruption of pregnancy but tends to have more widely distributed, transient, larger lesions not localized to the striae distensae
- Cholestasis of pregnancy: patients present with severe pruritus but without skin findings except excoriations
  - The diagnosis is confirmed by demonstrating elevated liver transaminases and elevated bilirubin

- Reassurance that the disease will resolve around the time of delivery may help patients cope with this condition
- Mid-potency topical corticosteroid agents such as prednicarbate (Dermatop®) 0.1% ointment or cream or triamcinolone acetonide (Aristocort®) 0.1% ointment or cream may decrease the pruritus sensations
- Ultraviolet B phototherapy can be beneficial for severely affected patients, as can systemic corticosteroid therapy

- The eruption tends to resolve spontaneously after delivery and usually does not recur with subsequent pregnancies
- No specific follow-up is needed unless the disease is severe
- Fetal morbidity or mortality does not appear to be increased in this disease, unlike some other eruptions of pregnancy

ICD-9-CM Code

692.9

POLYMORPHOUS LIGHT ERUPTION

HISTORY

- Patient presents in spring or early summer with a new, pruritic eruption on exposed areas of skin that is relatively rapid in onset, occurring 30 minutes to a few hours after sun exposure
- The condition usually begins within the first 3 decades of life and affects women 2 to 3 times more often than men
- A family history of a similar eruption may be noted, and patients often refer to their condition as "sun poisoning"
- Patients should not have a history of rheumatologic diseases including lupus and rheumatoid arthritis

PHYSICAL EXAMINATION

- One observes pruritic papules, papulovesicles, and/or plaques symmetrically on any sun-exposed area, including the face (Fig. 76-1)
- One may also see eczematous, insect bite-like, and erythema multiforme-like lesions

DIAGNOSIS

- The diagnosis is largely based on history and physical exam
  - Any concern about differentiating this condition from systemic lupus erythematosus should prompt laboratory evidence excluding lymphopenia, glomerulonephritis, and other sequelae of systemic lupus erythematosus
  - Examination of a skin biopsy specimen may be needed to distinguish polymorphous light eruption from other diseases, such as subacute cutaneous lupus and other photosensitive conditions

DIFFERENTIAL DIAGNOSIS

- Subacute cutaneous lupus: patients present with erythematous papules, plaques, and annulae on both sun- and non–sun-exposed skin in association with positive tests for antinuclear antibody, SS-A, and SS-B studies
  - Examination of a skin biopsy specimen helps to establish the diagnosis definitively
- Jessner's lymphocytic infiltrate: this uncommon condition tends to be more persistent than polymorphous light eruption, and the differentiation is based on difference in histopathologic findings
- Solar urticaria: the eruption may appear similar to polymorphous light eruption, but the history is significantly different, with eruption beginning after only a few minutes of sun exposure and resolving after 1 to 2 hours

TREATMENT

- If untreated, with no additional ultraviolet exposure, most lesions resolve within 1 week of onset

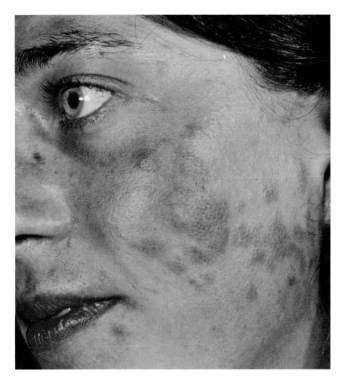

FIGURE 76-1 *Polymorphous light eruption.*

- Treatment can shorten the duration of the disease
  - Mildly affected patients can be treated with mid- to high-potency corticosteroids bid for 1 week
    - Mid-potency: triamcinolone acetonide (Aristocort®) 0.1% ointment or cream
    - High-potency: fluocinonide (Lidex®) 0.05% ointment or cream; clobetasol propionate (Temovate®) 0.05% ointment or cream; halobetasol propionate (Ultravate®) 0.05% ointment or cream, betamethasone dipropionate 0.05% in optimized ointment (Diprolene®)
- Systemic corticosteroid therapy, such as prednisone intitiated at a dose of 1 mg/kg/day tapered over 1 week, may be necessary in severely affected patients but should only be prescribed in healthy, young patients without significant comorbidities
- Patients may benefit from reducing exposure to ultraviolet light and from ongoing solar protection including hats, protective clothing, and a broad-spectrum sunscreen with a maximum sun protection factor (SPF) of 30

- Other alternatives for chronic management of severe disease include hydroxychloroquine (Plaquenil®)

- The patient should follow up with their primary care physician or dermatologist within 2 weeks after diagnosis
- If there is any concern that the patient may have an autoimmune disease, consider more urgent follow-up for evaluation
- Patient may need to start the "hardening" process (careful slow exposure to UV light) in the early spring every year if patient usually becomes severely affected with eruption

ICD-9 Code

692.72

CPT Code

11100   Biopsy

PORPHYRIA CUTANEA TARDA

HISTORY

- Patients present with nonpainful blisters and sores forming on extensor surfaces of hands, arms, and face associated with scarring in the areas and very fragile skin
- Patients generally present in the spring and summer
- Patients may also notice increased hair growth on face
- Two types are known:
  - Type I is acquired and may be related to liver damage from a wide variety of conditions, including alcoholism, hepatitis B or hepatitis C infection, or excessive iron or estrogen ingestion
  - Type II is familial and has a mixed or variable autosomal dominant pattern
- The condition is due to a deficiency of uroporphyrinogen decarboxylase in both types
- This condition occurs throughout the world and is the most common of all porphyrias
- Porphyria cutanea tarda is found most often in men in the third and fourth decades of life
- The condition is exacerbated by sunlight in the visible spectrum (peak sensitivity is 410 nm or the Soret band)

PHYSICAL EXAMINATION

- One sees vesicles, bullae, and superficial erosions on sun-exposed areas of the face, arms, and occasionally the dorsum of the feet, with the most common site being the dorsum of the hands and forearms (Figs. 77-1 to 77-3)
- Scarring and milial cysts are noted in areas of involvement if the patient has had previous flares
- On the face, one may see hypertrichosis, most commonly in the temple, preauricular, and mandibular areas
- Hypopigmentation and hyperpigmentation may also be visible
- Patients can eventually develop a scarring alopecia of the scalp

DIAGNOSIS

- The diagnosis is a clinical one based on the history of skin fragility combined with characteristic lesions, but the diagnosis should be confirmed with laboratory evaluation
- Definitive diagnosis requires a quantitative 24-hour urine porphyrin evaluation

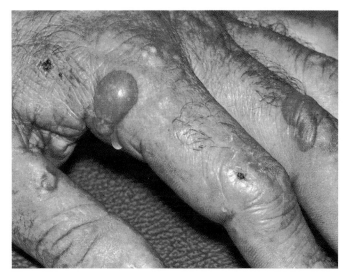

FIGURE 77-1 *Porphyria cutanea tarda.*

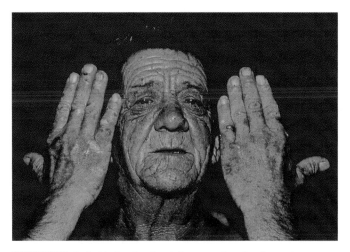

FIGURE 77-2 *Periorbital and malar violaceous coloration, hyperpigmentation, and hypertrichosis.*

- Further investigation of hepatic damage may be required, with liver transaminases and hepatitis studies, as well as a complete blood count, serum iron level, total iron binding capacity, and ferritin levels
- Microscopic examination of a skin biopsy of skin is usually required to eliminate other mimics

DIFFERENTIAL DIAGNOSIS

- Variegate porphyria: lesions that are clinically similar to those of porphyria cutanea tarda but associated with neurovisceral symptoms, like acute intermittent porphyria

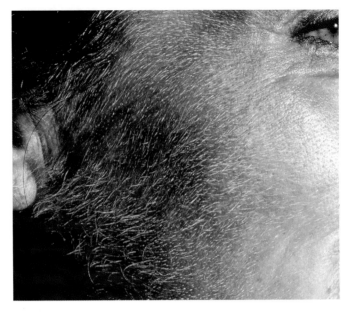

FIGURE 77-3   *Hypertrichosis in a female with porphyria cutanea tarda.*

- ○ A history of acute abdominal attacks of pain associated with seizures or paralysis will help
  - Porphyrin studies of the serum, urine, and feces will aid in distinguishing these conditions
- ○ Pseudoporphyria: this drug-induced condition (often due to furosemide, nalidixic acid, nonsteroidal antiinflammatory drugs, and pyridoxine, or occasionally seen in a setting of chronic renal failure in patients receiving hemodialysis) is quite difficult to distinguish from porphyria cutanea tarda
  - Patients with pseudoporphyria do not have elevated porphyrin levels
- Epidermolysis bullosa acquisita: this autoimmune disease can produce an identical clinical presentation, but other porphyria cutanea tarda hallmarks, such as hypertrichosis, photodistribution, and elevated urinary porphyrins are not present
- Scleroderma: patients with long-standing porphyria cutanea tarda may have changes of the hands and arms that are reminiscent of scleroderma
  - ○ However, the hypertrichosis, milial cysts, and bulla, as well as increased porphyrin levels, are diagnostic of porphyria cutanea tarda and are not present in scleroderma
- Dermatitis herpetiformis: vesicles and superficial erosions may appear in a similar distribution on the arms, but this is not a photodistributed dermatosis
  - ○ This condition is usually nonscarring and is highly pruritic, with different histopathologic findings and normal porphyrin levels

- Treatment of porphyria cutanea tarda is nonemergent
- Avoid all medications associated with drug-induced porphyria cutanea tarda
- The mainstay of therapy is phlebotomy, which is effective because it depletes the excessive hepatic iron stores
  - Approximately 500 ml of blood is removed weekly or every other week until the hemoglobin decreases to 10 g/dl
  - The first evidence of improvement is decreased skin fragility, followed later by cessation of new vesicle development
- Antimalarial agents, such as hydroxy-chloroquine 200 mg twice per week, may be used as alternative therapy
  - Antimalarial agents can induce a chemical hepatitis
  - This may help liberation of excessive iron stores from the liver and may enhance rapid removal of drug-porphyrin complex from the liver

MANAGEMENT/FOLLOW-UP

- Patient will need to be evaluated and treated over the long term for their disease
- Referral to a dermatologist is suggested within a 2-week period

ICD-9-CM Code

277.1

PRESSURE ULCER

- The patient initially has a red, tender area with subsequent asymptomatic or painful ulceration over a bony prominence, such as the sacrum, malleoli, ischial tuberosities, heels, elbows, trochanters, and occiput of the scalp
- This condition can occur at any age and there is an equal distribution between sexes
- The condition is most likely to be found in patients who have difficulties with mobility including patients with orthopedic and neurologic diseases (e.g., obtunded patients or spinal cord injury patients) as well as those who are bed-ridden or wheelchair-bound
- Risk factors include inadequate nursing care, diminished sensation, immobility, hypotension, fecal or urinary incontinence, fractured bones, and poor nutritional status
- The most likely cause is chronic pressure-induced ischemia of the tissue at the site

PHYSICAL EXAMINATION

- The recognized stages of decubitus ulcers include:
  - Stage I: nonblanchable erythema of intact skin with poorly defined margins (Fig. 78-1)
  - Stage II: partial-thickness skin loss involving epidermis, dermis, or both; ulcer is superficial and may appear as an abrasion, blister, or shallow crater that is irregular in shape
  - Stage III: full-thickness skin loss involving damage to or necrosis of subcutaneous tissue that may extend down to fascia (Figs. 78-2 and 78-3)
  - Stage IV: full-thickness loss with extensive destruction, tissue necrosis, or damage to muscle, bone, or supporting structures; may see undermining and sinus tracts
- Purulence and erythema at edges of ulcer suggest infection

DIAGNOSIS

- The history and clinical exam are suggestive of something
- If margins of ulcer are verrucous or suggest infection or malignancy, a skin biopsy should be performed
- If patient is febrile, one may need studies such as a blood culture and complete blood count with platelets, as well as wound or tissue culture

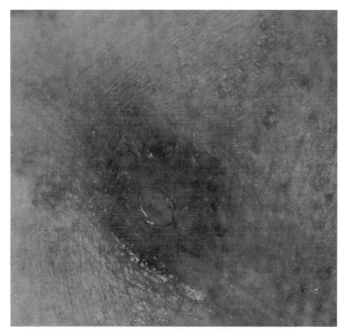

FIGURE 78-1   *Early sacral pressure sore.*

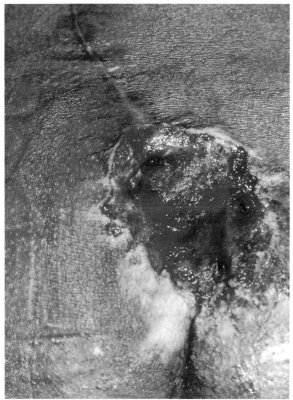

FIGURE 78-2   *Large, full-thickness sacral pressure sore.*

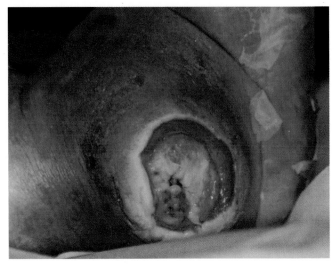

FIGURE 78-3 *Deep pressure sore.*

- Infectious ulcer, such as deep fungal, chronic viral, or atypical mycobacterial infection: usually the history and physical exam will help distinguish these
  - If one is suspicious of infection, wound and tissue cultures should be performed
- Vasculitic ulcer: this is usually seen in areas lacking pressure, and livedo reticularis and palpable purpura may be present to help guide the clinical impression
- Thermal burn: the history will almost always be definitive; burns have a very asymmetric, exogenous appearance and are not necessarily over bony prominences
- Carcinoma, such as basal cell or squamous cell carcinoma: not typically located over bony prominences and has indurated borders
  - Examination of a skin biopsy specimen will help distinguish these
- Pyoderma gangrenosum: usually rapid in onset and painful, with a shaggy, loose, undermined, erythematous to violaceous border
  - Ulcers are not typically seen over bony prominences

- Meticulous cleansing is necessary in the area to avoid accumulation of feces and urine around the site, especially if a sacral ulcer is noted, which may predispose to infection and worsening of ulceration
- Patients who are unable to ambulate or rotate the body should be manually turned every 2 to 3 hours to avoid continuous pressure in one localized area
- Attempt to maintain good nutritional status since this will aid in healing
- Topical antibiotics, such as silver sulfadiazine, under moist sterile gauze or under semiocclusive or hydrocolloid dressings, may be helpful for early erosions; other topical antibiotics that can be used for cleansing include Dakin's solution, acetic acid, povidone-iodine solution, and hydrogen peroxide
- Hydrogel bandages such as DuoDerm® may be necessary for ulcerations that are slow to heal
- For deeper ulcers, surgical management with debridement may be necessary, in addition to local wound care and hydrocolloid or foam dressings

PRESSURE ULCER

- Complications such as bacteremia and osteomyelitis will need management with systemic antibiotics

- Decubitus ulcers may take months to heal
  - For superficial, shallow ulcers, the patient should be seen at least monthly by the primary care physician, dermatologist, or general or plastic surgeon while continuing local wound care at home
  - Home health nursing may be required
  - For deeper, more extensive ulcers, the patient may need monitoring every few weeks by a plastic or general surgeon
    - Intermittent debridement may be necessary in the office while continued local wound care is performed at home

ICD-9-CM Code

707.0

HISTORY

- Patient notices small, red, itchy "bumps" filled with fluid, usually after sweating in a hot, humid environment and occlusion of the skin
- The condition is more often seen in infants but may also be seen in children and adults
- The condition occurs when occlusion of sweat ducts causes sweat extravasation into the epidermis, leading to inflammation and itching

PHYSICAL EXAMINATION

- One may see small, erythematous papulovesicles on the occluded areas and superficial excoriation
- The most common locations are the forehead, upper trunk, and volar aspects of the upper arms
- In miliaria crystallina, one may only see very superficial clear flaccid vesicles that are easily ruptured with minimal pressure or rubbing (Fig. 79-1)

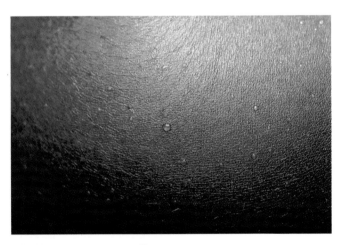

FIGURE 79-1 *Miliaria crystallina.*

- The diagnosis is easily made by the history and clinical appearance of lesions

DIFFERENTIAL DIAGNOSIS

- There are no clinical mimics of this condition

TREATMENT

- No specific treatment is warranted beyond encouraging patients to maintain a cool, dry environment and allow adequate air circulation to the affected skin

- Eruption usually resolves within a day after moving to a cooler environment and removing occlusion
- Symptomatic improvement of pruritus may occur with the use of 1% hydrocortisone cream

MANAGEMENT/FOLLOW-UP

- The patient may follow up with the primary care physician or dermatologist as needed

ICD-9-CM Code

705.1

PRURIGO NODULARIS

HISTORY

- Patient presents with very itchy "bumps" exclusively where they can reach, sparing the central portion of the back
- The condition has been present for months to decades prior to presentation
- This condition can affect any age, but it is more common in middle-aged and older adults
- Patients may have a history of atopic dermatitis or other disease that causes pruritus
- Emotional stress may also contribute to the severity of the disease

PHYSICAL EXAMINATION

- Lesions are firm, lichenified, sometimes excoriated, erythematous papules or nodules ranging from 0.5 to 2 cm in size (Fig. 80-1)
- Lesion number may range from a one to hundreds of lesions

- Many times patients can be observed scratching during the encounter
- The skin is normal between lesions, and there is no evidence of other pruritic disorders such as scabies

DIAGNOSIS

- Diagnosis is easily suggested by history of intense pruritus and numerous lesions with similar morphology and age
- Occasionally, a skin biopsy may be needed to exclude other conditions including pemphigoid nodularis (a variant of bullous pemphigoid)
- If there is any concern about a systemic etiology to the disease, an evaluation for systemic diseases including liver and renal function tests, thyroid-stimulating hormone, and other tests is appropriate

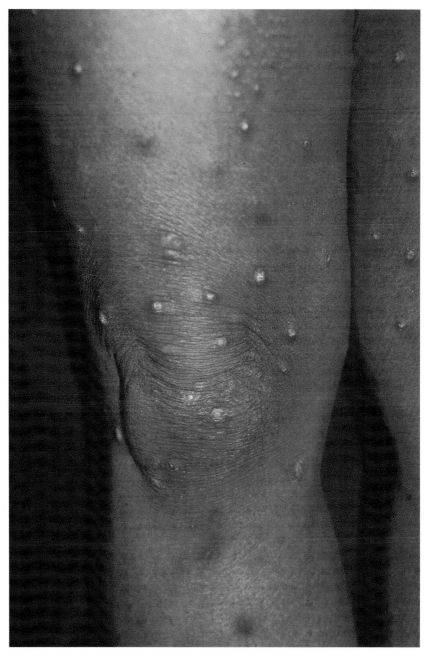

FIGURE 80-1 *Prurigo nodularis.*

- Perforating disorders (e.g., perforating folliculitis): may have similar morphology, but these lesions often have a central keratotic plug that may be manually removed, resulting in bleeding
  - Pruritus may also be intense with these conditions
- Hypertrophic lichen planus: usually less nodular but may be very pruritic; oral involvement with Wickham's striae of the buccal mucosa may be helpful in diagnosing lichen planus
- Keratoacanthoma: this is almost always singular and painful, whereas prurigo nodules are multiple and pruritic
- Squamous cell carcinoma: usually patients do not have widespread numerous lesions, and they are not necessarily pruritic
- Nodular scabies: may mimic prurigo nodularis closely but can usually be distinguished because patients have typical scabies lesions elsewhere

- The treatment of this condition is non-emergent
- If there is a readily identifiable underlying metabolic cause of pruritus, this should be identified and treated
- Potent topical corticosteroids are the mainstay of therapy, including fluocinonide (Lidex®) 0.05% ointment or cream; clobetasol propionate (Temovate®) 0.05% ointment or cream; halobetasol propionate (Ultravate®) 0.05% ointment or cream, betamethasone dipropionate 0.05% in optimized ointment (Diprolene®)
  - These agents may also be applied under occlusion with plastic wrap or bandages to enhance penetration and decrease scratching behavior
- Individual troublesome lesions may be frozen with liquid nitrogen cryotherapy or injected with 0.2 to 0.5 ml of 10 mg/ml of triamcinolone acetonide (Kenalog®)

- Ultraviolet phototherapy can help decrease cutaneous inflammation and is a helpful approach
- Topical capsaicin may also be helpful with pruritus by depleting substance P from the neurons involved, but patients often do not tolerate it due to a burning sensation
- The most effective treatment is thalidomide 50 to 200 mg qhs, but this is not appropriate to prescribe in the emergency department setting

- Patients should be followed by their primary care physician or dermatologist every few months
- If systemic therapy is started, frequent monitoring is required

ICD-9-CM Code

698.3

PRURITUS ANI

- Patient presents with unpleasant, itching sensation localized to the perianal area
- Many patients are in the fifth to sixth decades of life, but the condition can occur in younger and older patients
- Patients may have a history of atopic disease and/or diathesis or urinary or fecal incontinence
- Many patients excessively scrub their perianal skin, use copious amounts of harsh soaps, and use large numbers of over the counter medicaments on the area
- Many patients have multifactorial disease

PHYSICAL EXAMINATION

- Most commonly, one finds only mild to marked erythema (Fig. 81-1)
- Additionally, one may see perianal erosions, excoriations, and lichenification

DIAGNOSIS

- The diagnosis is based on history and physical exam, without evidence of other primary dermatosis, such as psoriasis, seborrheic dermatitis, or infection
- Very rarely will a skin biopsy be required

DIFFERENTIAL DIAGNOSIS

- Tinea cruris: well-demarcated, erythematous, scaly patches with scaling collarette and central clearing
  - Examination of a KOH preparation of the scale should be positive for hyphae
- Candidiasis: brightly erythematous patches and plaques with satellite pustules are visible in the perianal area
  - Examination of a KOH preparation of the scale should be positive for pseudo-hyphae or yeast
- Condyloma: verrucous papules may cause perianal itching and can be readily identified by clinical examination
- Psoriasis: macerated, erythematous, occasionally scaly, well-demarcated patches and plaques with no satellite pustules
  - Patients often have a history of psoriasis and have psoriasis elsewhere on body
- Seborrheic dermatitis: poorly defined, erythematous, scaly patches possibly with evidence of seborrheic dermatitis elsewhere on the body
- Atopic dermatitis: poorly defined, erythematous, scaly patches in the perineal area, but also at other locations on the body, such as antecubital and posterior tibial fossae

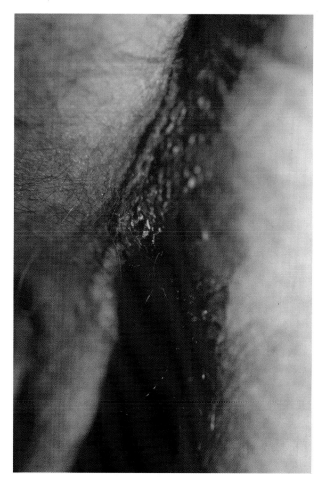

FIGURE 81-1 *Pruritus ani.*

- Contact dermatitis: chronic irritation of the area with harsh and repetitive cleansing techniques or application of potential allergens including many over the counter antibiotic medications may produce contact dermatitis with erythema, scale, small vesicles, and, in chronic disease, lichenification
- *Enterobius vermicularis* (pinworm) infection: usually found in children; nocturnal itching is a prominent feature, with perianal erythema visible
  - An adhesive tape test should be positive for eggs of the organism
- Other infections: erythematous, poorly defined patches that may be painful to the touch; etiologic agents include *Staphylococcus, Streptococcus,* and *Corynebacterium*

TREATMENT

- Treatment includes discussing with the patient the necessity of avoiding chronically rubbing the area and strict maintenance of hygiene
  - Gentle cleansing with a soft washcloth and water only may be used to remove rectal seepage in the area
  - No soap or cleansers of any kind should be employed
- Patients should discontinue the use of all topical over the counter agents to the area

- Zinc oxide ointment or other barrier creams (Desitin® or A&D ointment®) may be helpful
- Hydrocortisone 1% to 2.5% ointment or hydrocortisone with pramoxine (Pramasone® 2.5% ointment) ointment may be used bid to the area intermittently to help with itching and inflammation
- Antihistamines may be helpful at night, such as hydroxyzine 12.5 to 25 mg orally at bedtime as needed for an adult, to help reduce scratching during sleep

MANAGEMENT/FOLLOW-UP

- The patient will need to be seen within 4 weeks by the primary care physician or dermatologist

ICD-9 Code

698.0

CPT Code

None

PSORIASIS

HISTORY

- Psoriasis vulgaris presents with slowly progressive, scaling, erythematous papules and plaques, often on the elbows and knees, scalp, and umbilical and gluteal cleft skin
  - Patients complain of pruritus and may also complain of a "nail fungus"
- Guttate psoriasis is a less common variant of psoriasis, and patients may have a recent history of a *Streptococcal* pharyngitis with subsequent rapid and alarming onset of small, scaling, widespread, erythematous macules and papules
- Pustular psoriasis is a less common variant of psoriasis and is an acute, widespread sterile pustular eruption occurring in patients who may or may not have a history of psoriasis that may be associated with systemic symptoms such as fever, malaise, arthralgias, and laboratory abnormalities

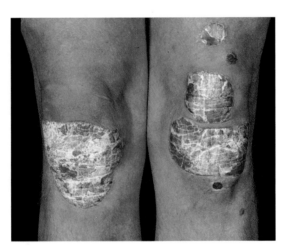

FIGURE 82-1 *Psoriasis.*

such as elevated liver transaminases, elevated erythrocyte sedimentation rate, and elevated white blood cell count

- Psoriasis occurs in 2% to 4% of the population and has equal sex prevalence
- One-third of patients have family members with psoriasis or psoriatic arthritis

- Psoriasis vulgaris: round to oval, erythematous, hyperkeratotic plaques with silvery scale occurring most commonly over elbows, knees, scalp, and lumbar and gluteal areas, as well as in the periumbilical area (Figs. 82-1 and 82-2)

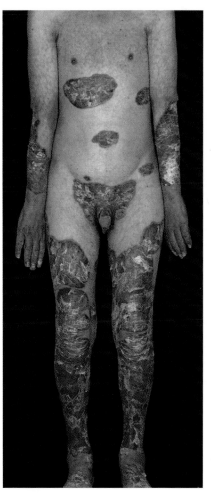 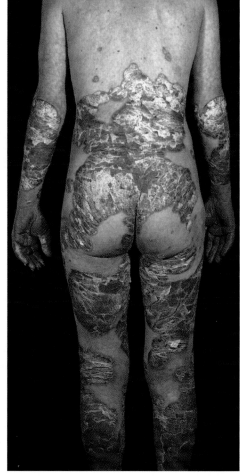

FIGURE 82-2 *Chronic stationary psoriasis.*

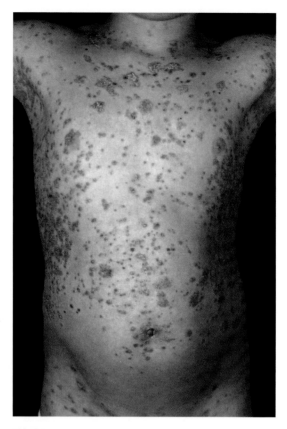

FIGURE 82-3 *Eruptive guttate psoriasis.*

- ○ Disease may also occur in a widespread distribution
- ○ Nail involvement with tiny pits, the oil drop sign (a look reminiscent of a small drop of oil underneath the nail plate), and nail thickening
- ○ Koebner phenomenon is occasionally found, in which psoriatic lesions of the skin disease are induced by skin trauma
- Guttate psoriasis: small, round to teardrop-shaped, erythematous, hyperkeratotic macules and papules that appear psoriasiform, usually on the upper trunk and proximal extremities (Fig. 82-3)
- Pustular psoriasis: widespread brightly erythematous skin with a generalized eruption of sterile pustules 2 to 3 mm in diameter disseminated over the trunk and extremities

- ○ Pustules that may form confluent "lakes" of pus
- ○ Pustules under the nail bed may lead to loss of the entire nail
- ○ Because of the appearance of exfoliative erythroderma, patients may be febrile, hemodynamically unstable, and develop high-output heart failure

DIAGNOSIS

- In psoriasis vulgaris, the history, family history, distribution of the eruption, and morphology of the lesions help guide the diagnosis of psoriasis

- Guttate psoriasis: a history of recent *Streptococcal* pharyngitis and the clinical morphology of the lesions will aid the diagnosis
- Pustular psoriasis: fever, generalized erythroderma, and disseminated pustules in a patient with a history of psoriasis is highly characteristic of a pustular flare of psoriasis
  - Examination of a skin biopsy specimen may help differentiate pustular psoriasis from its mimics

DIFFERENTIAL DIAGNOSIS

Psoriasis Vulgaris

- Atopic dermatitis: poorly defined erythematous patches and plaques that usually begin in early infancy; adult onset is uncommon
  - Acute lesions appear edematous; chronic lesions appear thickened, with accentuation of skin markings (lichenified)
  - This condition is often seen in association with allergic rhinitis and/or asthma
- Tinea corporis: scaly erythematous plaques with central clearing affecting the skin of the body that can be confirmed by KOH preparation examination
- Seborrheic dermatitis: a chronic dermatosis associated with redness and scaling on areas where sebaceous glands are prominent, such as the scalp ("dandruff"), face, and chest
  - Lesions are yellowish red, greasy scaling macules and papules of various sizes
- Lichen planus: can mimic psoriasis, but lichen planus lesions tend to be more violaceous (purple) and polygonal, have much less scale, and are frequently found with oral lesions
- Mycosis fungoides: a chronic cutaneous T-cell lymphoma presenting with scaly patches, plaques, and tumors that may be located on any cutaneous surface
- Pityriasis rosea: erythematous to pink scaly papules and plaques classically in a "Christmas tree" distribution over the trunk

  - Pityriasis rosea begins with a "herald patch," which is slightly larger than the other lesions
  - This self-limited eruption regresses spontaneously in 6 to 12 weeks
- Secondary syphilis
  - Erythematous and hyperkeratotic scaly plaques located on trunk, extremities, palms, and soles
  - Patient may report a history of a "chancre" (ulcer of primary syphilis) in the previous 2 to 10 weeks
  - Condyloma lata: soft, flat-topped pink to tan papules on the perineum and perianal areas

Guttate Psoriasis

- Lichen planus (see above description)
- Pityriasis rosea (see above description)
- Pityriasis lichenoides et varioliformis acuta: generally presents in children and young adults as small scaling macules and papules with occasional visible crusts
  - Spontaneous resolution of lesions is commonly observed, with subsequent replacement by newer lesions
  - The diagnosis is a clinical one supplemented by examination of a skin biopsy specimen
- Secondary syphilis (see above description)
- Tinea corporis (see above description)

Pustular Psoriasis

- Pustular drug eruption: these eruptions can present as an exfoliative erythroderma with minute pustules in temporal association with initiation of treatment with a new medication
  - Examination of a skin biopsy specimen may help differentiate psoriasis from drug eruptions
- Subcorneal pustular dermatosis: this inflammatory skin disease may present with much less erythema than psoriasis, but hundreds to thousands of minute pustules are characteristic
- Examination of a skin biopsy specimen may help differentiate psoriasis from subcorneal pustular dermatosis

- Psoriasis treatment is only emergent for pustular psoriasis, and treatment varies considerably depending on the type and location of the disease
- Psoriasis vulgaris: the mainstay of therapy is various topical medications
  - Topical corticosteroid agents are most commonly combined with a topical noncorticosteroidal medication
  - Topical corticosteroid agents cause less burning than many of the noncorticosteroid agents when applied to the skin, but they do cause atrophy when repeatedly applied over months or years
    - High-potency agents may be appropriate for bid use on the nonintertriginous trunk and extremities for 4 weeks; examples include fluocinonide (Lidex®) 0.05% ointment or cream; clobetasol propionate (Temovate®) 0.05% ointment or cream; halobetasol propionate (Ultravate®) 0.05% ointment or cream, betamethasone dipropionate 0.05% in optimized ointment (Diprolene®)
    - Mid-potency agents may be sufficient for nonfacial and nonintertriginous skin in mild to moderate severity disease; examples include triamcinolone acetonide (Aristocort®) 0.1% ointment or cream; prednicarbate (Dermatop®) 0.1% ointment or cream; hydrocortisone valerate (Westcort®) 0.2% cream or ointment bid to affected skin
    - Low-potency agents are best used on the face and intertriginous areas; examples include hydrocortisone 0.5% to 2.5% ointment or cream bid or Desonide (DesOwen®) 0.05% cream or ointment bid
  - Hydrocortisone 2.5% ointment should be used twice per day as needed for intertriginous sites
  - Topical corticosteroids are often combined with other topical medications, including calcipotriene (Dovonex®), tar preparations (Estar® gel), anthralin (Drithocreme®), or tazarotene (Tazorac®)
    - Because of the high relative efficacy, greatest cosmetic acceptance, and relatively low level of irritation, calcipotriene (Dovonex®) cream, ointment, and solution is the corticosteroid-sparing treatment of choice
    - Patients should initiate treatment with a topical corticosteroid appropriate for their site and severity of disease and use calcipotriene bid at the same time as the corticosteroid
    - Whenever feasible, patients should discontinue the topical corticosteroid agent and continue the calcipotriene
    - In addition to calcipotriene, tacrolimus 0.1% (Protopic®) ointment can be used in place of corticosteroids on the face and intertriginous are as over the long term and may decrease corticosteroid requirements
- Disseminated psoriasis vulgaris occupying more than 10% total body surface area will not generally clear with topical agents alone, and clearance will require phototherapy (ultraviolet B light), photochemotherapy (oral or topical psoralen plus ultraviolet A light), systemic acitretin (Soriatane®), systemic cyclosporine (Neoral®), or systemic methotrexate (Rheumatrex®)
  - These phototherapeutic and medication options have much greater potential for efficacy than topical agents and have much greater risk of toxicity
    - They are not appropriate for initiation in the emergency department setting

- Psoriasis is a treatable but not a curable condition, so all patients should be followed by the primary care physician or dermatologist
- Patients with severe erythrodermic psoriasis may require hospital admission for stabilization prior to initiating intensive outpatient treatment

- If patients have mild disease, they are appropriate candidates for referral to their primary care physician or dermatologist
- If patients have moderate to severe disease, they are appropriate candidates for referral to a dermatologist

ICD-9-CM Code

696.1

CHAPTER 83

PYODERMA GANGRENOSUM

HISTORY

- The patient presents with a progressively enlarging painful pustule or papulonodule that may rapidly break down to form an ulcer
- Patients may have a history of previous similar lesions
- Many patients have a history of predisposing systemic diseases, including ulcerative colitis, Crohn's disease, arthritis (rheumatoid and other), monoclonal gammopathy, hematologic malignancy (myelogenous), or Behçet's disease, or they may currently be treated with granulocyte/macrophage colony-stimulating factor (GM-CSF)
- Most cases are idiopathic
- The disease may occur at any age, with equal sex distribution
- If lesions are very acute, the patient may also have systemic symptoms of fever and toxicity

PHYSICAL EXAMINATION

- One sees an ulcer with a raised, violaceous, inflammatory, undermined border and a boggy, necrotic base; lesions may be solitary or arise in clusters (Figs. 83-1 and 83-2)
- Any part of the body, including the face, may be involved simultaneously, but mucous membranes are usually spared
- Lesions may be noted in areas of trauma, such as surgical sites; this is called pathergy
- Ulcers heal with thin, atrophic, cribiform scars

DIAGNOSIS

- This is primarily a diagnosis based on the history and clinical findings, but examination of a skin biopsy specimen is necessary to exclude other diagnoses
- Other evaluations for systemic diseases may be indicated, such as gastrointestinal evaluation, complete blood count, rheumatoid factor levels, serum protein electrophoresis, etc., especially if history is suggestive

DIFFERENTIAL DIAGNOSIS

- Atypical mycobacterial infection: lesions are usually more chronic, but a similar ulcer may be present and is more likely to be confused with an older lesion of pyoderma gangrenosum
  - Examination of a skin biopsy specimen with special stains for acid-fast bacilli and tissue culture is necessary to establish this diagnosis
- Deep fungal infection: blastomycosis, cryptococcosis, histoplasmosis, sporotrichosis, and coccidiomycosis may have chronic ulcerations that are similar to pyoderma gangrenosum
  - Examination of a skin biopsy specimen with special stains for fungus and fungus culture are necessary to establish this diagnosis

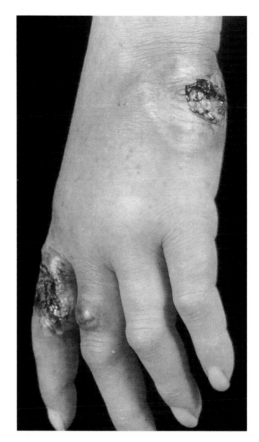

FIGURE 83-1 *Lesions of pyoderma gangrenosum.*

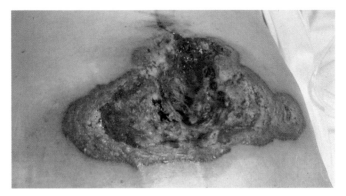

FIGURE 83-2 *Rapidly enlarging pyoderma gangrenosum triggered by laparotomy.*

- Ulcerative squamous cell or basal cell carcinoma: these lesions are chronic and usually differ in history and physical examination from pyoderma gangrenosum
  ○ Definitive diagnosis is obtained through examination of skin biopsy specimens
- Sweet's syndrome: may closely mimic early lesions of pyoderma gangrenosum and the histopathology of these two diseases are almost identical
  ○ The main differences are the associated symptoms and lesional distribution of Sweet's syndrome (see that chapter)
- Traumatic or stasis ulcer: these may also be considered in the differential diagnosis, but they are chronic and lack the erythematous to violaceous undermined borders

TREATMENT

- If lesions are large, treatment may be emergent
- With isolated lesions that are small (<1 cm) and few in number (<4), topical or intralesional corticosteroids such as triamcinolone acetonide (Kenalog®) 10 mg/ml may be injected into the borders of the lesions
- Systemic corticosteroids are the most effective treatment and dramatically halt the progression of lesions; doses as high as 2.0 to 4 mg/kg/day may initially be necessary
  ○ Much lower doses, such as 1 mg/kg/day, are often effective

- Patients will most likely require oral corticosteroids for several months to years; these are tapered very slowly
- Corticosteroid-sparing agents are often required to taper the corticosteroid agents as quickly as possible
  - Dapsone or sulfasalazine may be helpful and are used in combination with oral corticosteroids
    - Patients must be monitored carefully for side effects and complications
  - Cyclosporine (Neoral®) at doses from 6 to 10 mg/kg/day is highly effective either alone or in combination with systemic corticosteroid agents
    - Patients must be monitored carefully for side effects and complications
- Other systemic medications may be used, including methotrexate (Rheumatrex®), azathioprine (Imuran®), mycophenolate mofetil (CellCept®), and cyclophosphamide (Cytoxan®)
  - Patients must be monitored carefully for side effects and complications
- Aggressive debridement should be avoided if possible due to the likelihood of pathergy
- Topical tacrolumus (Protopic®) 0.1% ointment may be used on the bordeks to decrease systemic agent requirements

- All patients will need to be followed regularly by a clinician familiar with treating pyoderma gangrenosum, usually a dermatologist since this is a condition that waxes and wanes, with recurrence at other sites likely in the future
- If the patient has signs and symptoms of inflammatory bowel disease, skin lesions may worsen in parallel with bowel disease exacerbation
- Significant scarring and disfigurement may occur

ICD-9-CM Code

686.01

CPT Code

11100   Biopsy
11900   Intralesional injection

PYOGENIC GRANULOMA

HISTORY

- The patient complains of a red bump that may be painful and bleeds spontaneously after minor trauma
- The papule may have been present for days to several months and is growing rapidly
- This condition is most common in children, but it may be seen at any age

PHYSICAL EXAMINATION

- One sees a bright to dusky red, dome shaped or pedunculated papule or nodule, often with superficial erosion and crusted blood (Fig. 84-1)
- Common locations include the fingers, lips, mouth, trunk, and toes

DIAGNOSIS

- The history and physical exam are suggestive of the diagnosis
- Submission of a skin biopsy specimen for microscopic examination should be performed as part of the ablative or excisional treatment procedure

DIFFERENTIAL DIAGNOSIS

- Malignant melanoma: melanomas are usually brown or black, and pyogenic granulomas lack these colors
- Bacillary angiomatosis: this infectious disease occurs most commonly in immuno-compromised hosts such as AIDS patients and presents with multiple enlarging friable erythematous papules
- Basal cell carcinoma: these tumors are flesh-colored and are rarely brightly erythematous
- Metastatic carcinoma: these are usually rapidly growing dome-shaped papules and nodules

TREATMENT

- Treatment beyond obtaining hemostasis is nonemergent
- Removal of the lesion is generally curative
  - This can be accomplished by using a scalpel or razor blade to remove the papule and submitting the lesion for histopathologic examination, followed by light curettage and electrodesiccation

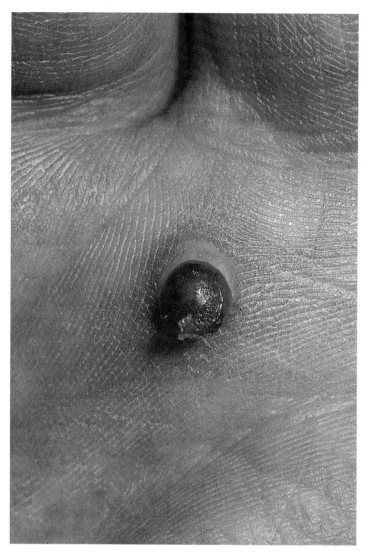

FIGURE 84-1 *Pyogenic granuloma.*

○ Surgical excision (and submitting the lesion for histopathologic examination) may also be performed

MANAGEMENT/FOLLOW-UP

• Follow-up is required within 1 week for removal of the lesion
• Lesions may occasionally recur

RAYNAUD'S DISEASE AND PHENOMENON

HISTORY

- Patients complain of episodic attacks of numbness and whiteness of digits when exposed to cold temperatures
  - After rewarming, the digits become bright red, and throbbing pain may occur
- The cause is unknown, but it is felt to be related to local vasospasm in the digits
- Raynaud's disease is an idiopathic, primary form of the disease that occurs in patients 15 to 40 years of age with a strong 4:1 female to male predominance
- Raynaud's phenomenon is a secondary form of the disease and is most commonly associated with connective tissue diseases, such as scleroderma, lupus erythematosus, dermatomyositis, and rheumatoid arthritis, but it may occur in people who use vibratory tools at work
- Several drugs may also induce Raynaud's phenomenon, such as propranolol, a beta-adrenoreceptor blocker, and ergotamine
- The disease is also associated in some cases with hypothyroidism, cryoglobulins, macroglobulins, and polycythemia

PHYSICAL EXAMINATION

- Examination may be normal in patients with primary disease, and attacks may be hard to induce

- During an attack, one sees well-demarcated blanching or cyanosis of the digits (Fig. 85-1)
  - Digits distal to the line of ischemia are cold, while the proximal digit is warmer and red
  - With warming, the previously blanched digits become cyanotic to red as secondary reactive hyperemia develops and pain occurs
- Patients with recurrent severe problems may have trophic changes with tense and atrophic skin, nail deformities, sclerodactyly, and ischemic ulcerations

DIAGNOSIS

- Diagnosis is usually made by history
- Further evaluation is usually not necessary, but if patients have a history suggestive of rheumatologic disease, then consider obtaining antinuclear antibody levels, complete blood count with platelets, erythrocyte sedimentation rate, and rheumatoid factor and cryoglobulin levels

DIFFERENTIAL DIAGNOSIS

- Acrocyanosis: the hands and feet are involved, in addition to the digit, with nonepisodic persistent color change

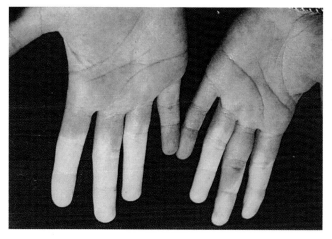

FIGURE 85-1   *A vasospastic attack in a patient with Raynaud's phenomenon.*

TREATMENT

- Treatment of Raynaud's disease or phenomenon is nonemergent
- Consider informing the patient of the necessity of wearing multiple layers of clothing; avoiding direct cold contact with the digits is very important
- Cessation of tobacco smoking should be encouraged
- Efficacy has been reported for several pharmacologic agents
  ○ Calcium channel blockers, such as long-acting nifedipine (Procardia XL®) or diltiazem (Cardizem® CD), may be helpful in decreasing the frequency, duration, and severity of the attacks
  ○ Topical nitrates such as nitroglycerin (Nitro-Bid®) ointment 2% may be applied in thin laters bid for patients with severe disease
  ○ Prazosin (Minipress®) has also been reported to be helpful

MANAGEMENT/FOLLOW-UP

- Patients with more severe disease should be seen within the next 1 to 2 weeks by their primary care physician, dermatologist, or rheumatologist
- If a primary disease process is leading to secondary Raynaud's phenomenon, treatment of the primary disease may help with some of the signs and symptoms of Raynaud's phenomenon
- This can be a chronic problem, and a small proportion of patients may have digital auto-amputations or chronic trophic changes

ICD-9-CM Code

443.0

ROCKY MOUNTAIN SPOTTED FEVER

HISTORY

- Abrupt onset of high fever reaching as high as 40°C with a characteristic petechial eruption in an acutely ill patient
- Two-thirds of patients have a history of a tick bite, with travel to endemic areas, such as the Southeast US
- Common symptoms include chills, headache, myalgias, arthralgias, malaise, hearing loss and vertigo, photophobia, nausea, diarrhea, vomiting, and anorexia
- Sinus tachycardia, hypotension, or shock may be present
- Mental status changes such as irritability, restlessness, tremor, or confusion are not uncommon
- Fever may persist for up to 2 weeks
- Cutaneous eruption may not begin until 1 to 5 days after the onset of systemic symptoms

PHYSICAL EXAMINATION

- Systemically ill patient
- Initial eruptions are pink and macular, blanching on pressure; these are found first on the wrists and ankles; in 6 to 18 hours these lesions begin to involve the palms and soles and then extend proximally (Figs. 86-1 and 86-2)
- These begin to become more red and papular on the second day and evolve into petechiae and purpura
- When severe, ecchymoses, necrotic ulcerations, and distal gangrene can be seen in the toes, fingers, earlobes, nose, scrotum, or vulva
- Signs of sepsis
- The eruption may not be present in 10% to 20% cases
- Splenomegaly is present in 50% cases

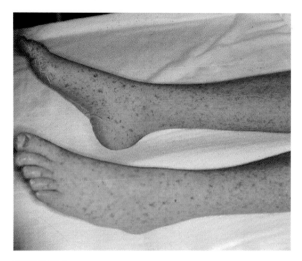

FIGURE 86-1 *Rocky Mountain spotted fever in the legs and ankles.*

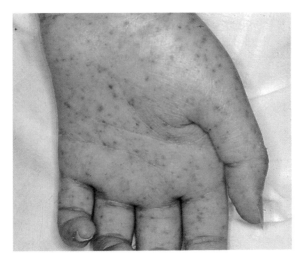

FIGURE 86-2 *Rocky Mountain spotted fever in the hands and wrists.*

DIAGNOSIS

- Clinical presentation
- Indirect fluorescent antibody test (1:64): most specific
- Indirect hemagglutination test: most sensitive
- Direct fluorescent antibody test of skin biopsy tissue: most rapid but insensitive
- Polymerase chain reaction test may be available

DIFFERENTIAL DIAGNOSIS

- Acute bronchitis
- Drug eruption
- Enteroviral infection
- Gastroenteritis
- Gonococcemia
- Hepatitis
- Idiopathic thrombocytopenic purpura
- Infectious mononucleosis
- Influenza
- Kawasaki's disease
- Leptospirosis
- Measles
- Meningococcemia
- Pneumonia
- Rubella
- Sepsis
- Secondary syphilis
- Thrombotic thrombocytopenic purpura
- Typhoid fever
- Vasculitis

- Oral doxycycline 100 mg bid for 7 days in adults and 2–4 mg/kg bid for 7 days in children
- For severely ill patients requiring admission:
    - Doxycycline 100 mg IV q12hr in adults and 2–4 mg/kg q12hr in children
    - Chloramphenicol 50 mg/kg/day (given intravenously q6hr)
    - Cefotaxime may also be given if menigococcemia is also suspected
    - Antibiotic therapy should be continued for 3 days after fever has resolved
- Supportive therapy in the form of IV hydration and treatment of shock, renal failure, etc.

- Fatal in 20% to 80% of untreated cases
- Management of severe multisystem involvement of the vasculitis is most important
- Complications such as bronchopneumonia, otitis media, eighth nerve deafness, parotitis, congestive heart failure, acute renal failure, glomerulonephritis, and internal hemorrhages can be seen
- The cutaneous eruption, once resolved, can leave postinflammatory pigment changes that may persist for months

ICD-9 Code

082.0

ROSACEA

HISTORY

- Patients present with flushing and red "bumps" on the face; usually seen in fair-skinned people, with women affected three times as often as men
- Rosacea can also be associated with connective tissue hypertrophy and sebaceous gland hyperplasia of the nose, called rhinophyma
- The disease most commonly presents in the third and fifth decades of life
- The etiology is not clear, but individuals may identify factors that exacerbate rosacea including consumption of alcoholic beverages, hot beverages, exercise, spicy foods, and ultraviolet radiation exposure
- Patients may have ocular complaints, such as redness or scratchiness of the eyes, that are independent of the severity of facial rosacea and may precede the skin findings by several years
- Recent topical corticosteroid use may exacerbate the condition

PHYSICAL EXAMINATION

- Disease may initially begin as episodic flushing and blushing that eventually becomes persistent and blanchable erythema
- On the central facial area, principally the nose, cheeks, chin, forehead, and glabella, one sees erythematous papules and pustules, erythema, and telangiectasias (Fig. 87-1)
  - The amount of erythema is more marked than one would expect in acne vulgaris
- In later stages, patients may develop large nodules and tissue hyperplasia with rhinophyma (Fig. 87-2)
- With ocular involvement, the most common finding is inflamed margins of the eyelids with scales and crusts
  - Pain and photophobia may be present

DIAGNOSIS

- Usually history and physical exam will lead to the diagnosis

DIFFERENTIAL DIAGNOSIS

- Acne vulgaris: patients may have a similar distribution of rosacea, but there are often comedones in acne, and the amount of erythema in acne vulgaris is much less than that seen in rosacea
- Seborrheic dermatitis: patients present with erythematous, poorly defined scaly patches, as opposed to the erythematous papules and pustules in rosacea
- Lupus erythematosus: presents with photodistributed malar erythema, but there are no papules and pustules as in rosacea

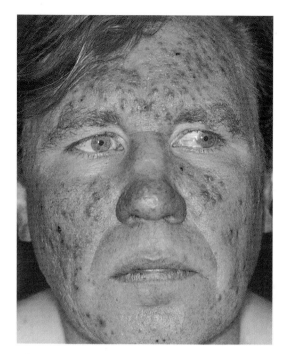

FIGURE 87-1 *Rosacea, stage II.*

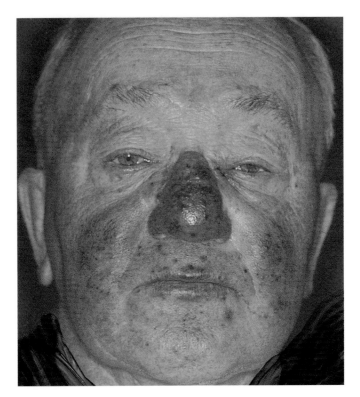

FIGURE 87-2 *Rosacea, stage III.*

- Treatment of rosacea is nonemergent
- Treatment has a greater effect on the papules and pustules, less effect on the associated erythema, and virtually no effect on telangiectasias or flushing
- All harsh cleansers and abrasive agents to the skin should be discontinued
  - Only very mild soaps or cleansers should be used, including Cetaphil®, Aquanil®, or Dove®
- For mild rosacea, topical antibiotic agents such as topical metronidazole (Metrogel® or Noritate®) or topical clindamycin (Climdagel®) may be applied bid to the affected skin areas
  - Maximum improvement is not seen until 3 to 4 months
- Additionally helpful topical agents include tretinoin (Retin A®) 0.025% cream or 0.1% microgel

- For moderate to severe cases of rosacea, oral antibiotics including tetracycline (Sumycin®) 250 to 500 mg bid, doxycycline (Dynacin®) 50 to 100 mg bid, or erythromycin (E-Mycin®) 250 to 500 mg bid may be necessary

- Milder forms of rosacea may be managed by the patient's primary care physician or dermatologist within 4 weeks of evaluation
- Patients with ocular symptoms associated with rosacea should have an eye examination by an ophthalmologist

ICD-9-CM Code

695.3

CHAPTER 88

ROSEOLA INFANTUM

HISTORY

- Sudden onset of fever (up to 40.6°C) in children 6 to 24 months of age due to infection with human herpesvirus (HHV) 6 or 7
- Fever persists for 3 to 5 days, usually with no other symptoms, and child appears well
- Mild pharyngitis, tympanic injection, and nodal enlargement are sometimes present
- Characteristic eruption develops on the day of defervescence or 1 to 2 days later
- Characteristic eruption fades without desquamation within hours to a few days

- Most cases are asymptomatic and self-limited; complications include febrile seizures and rarely encephalitis, hemophagocytic syndrome, hepatitis, and immune thrombocytopenic purpura

PHYSICAL EXAMINATION

- Discreet, irregular, 2- to 4-mm rose-pink macules and papules, sometimes with a white halo (Fig. 88-1)
- These macules and papules blanch on pressure

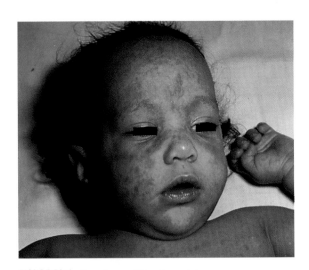

FIGURE 88-1   *Exanthem subitum (roseola).*

- The eruption usually begins on the trunk and spreads to the neck and extremities
- Palpebral edema (heavy eyelids) are commonly seen

- Clinical exam is usually sufficient for diagnosis
  - Supportive laboratory findings include transient leukopenia with relative lymphocytosis and atypical lymphocytes on complete blood count
- If an exact diagnosis is critical, one may determine acute and convalescent titers of HHV6 by immunofluorescent antibody test, ELISA, or neutralizing antibody test
  - An alternative is to order a polymerase chain reaction test to detect HHV6 from peripheral blood

- Other viral exanthems are too numerous to mention and may differ only in subtle ways from roseola; a few include:
  - Enterovirus
  - Rubella
  - Adenovirus
  - Coxsackievirus
  - Rotavirus
  - Measles

- Scarlet fever: associated with streptococcal disease and the constellation of oropharyngeal findings with a positive streptococcal test
- Drug reactions: patients should have a history of a new drug having been administered within 1 to 3 weeks prior to the onset of the eruption; constitutional symptoms are uncommon with drug eruptions

- Supportive therapy with antipyretics such as ibuprofen or acetaminophen

- Most cases are asymptomatic and self-limited
- Complications include febrile seizures and rarely encephalitis, hemophagocytic syndrome, hepatitis, and immune thrombocytopenic purpura
- If any complications occur, patients should be seen by their primary care physician

ICD-9 Code

057.8

RUBELLA (GERMAN MEASLES)

HISTORY

- Most commonly seen in an unvaccinated child presenting in the spring months with irritability, malaise, sore throat, mild conjunctivitis, headache, lymphadenopathy, and fever, followed in 1 to 7 days by a characteristic eruption
- In younger children, the prodromal symptoms can be absent
- The eruption fades after 2 to 3 days
- In older children and adults, arthritis may begin as the rash fades, lasting ro 1 to 2 weeks

PHYSICAL EXAMINATION

- Exanthem begins on the face as pink macules that become confluent and spreads centrifugally, downward to the trunk and extremities (Fig. 89-1)
- Striking lymphadenopathy may be palpated in the suboccipital, postauricular, anterior, and posterior cervical nodes
- Pinpoint petechiae may be present on the soft palate
- Eruption absent in 25% patients
- Arthralgias and mild arthritis is more common in females

DIAGNOSIS

- Clinical exam
- Rubella hemagglutination inhibiting antibody soon after the start of the rash and repeated 2 weeks later

DIFFERENTIAL DIAGNOSIS

- Other viral exanthems are too numerous to mention and may differ only in subtle ways from roseola; a few include:
  ○ Enterovirus
  ○ Rubella
  ○ Adenovirus
  ○ Coxsackievirus
  ○ Rotavirus
  ○ Measles
- Scarlet fever: associated with streptococcal disease and the constellation of oropharyngeal findings and positive streptococcal testing
- Drug eruption: patients should have a history of a new drug having been administered within 1 to 3 weeks prior to the onset of the eruption; constitutional symptoms are uncommon with drug eruptions
- Kawasaki's disease: five of the six major criteria are generally present, including 1) presentation with 5 days or more of a spiking fever up to 40°C in infants and children; 2) acute nonsuppurative cervical lymphadenopathy; 3) changes in peripheral extremities, including edema and erythema, progressing to desquamation; 4) bilateral conjunctival injection; 5) oral mucosal disease, including oropharyngeal erythema, erythematous to fissured lips, and "strawberry" tongue; 6) scalatiniform eruption
- Rubeola: erythematous macules and papules that begin at the forehead and behind the ears and then spread cephalocaudally to the neck, upper extremities, trunk, and then lower extremities with buccal and labial mucosa erythema, as well as Koplik spots in the oral mucosa, usually opposite the second molars

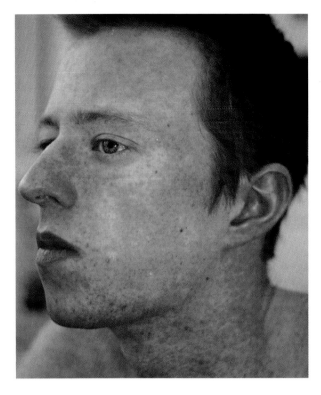

FIGURE 89-1 *Rubella.*

- Toxic shock syndrome: the association of an infection (in a febrile patient) with flexurally accentuated early macular or maculopapular exanthem that becomes diffuse and that may resemble scarlet fever
  - The distribution always involves extremities; erythematous palms and soles and erythema of the mucous membranes with conjunctival injection are commonly observed
  - There may be clinical evidence of hypotension, peripheral edema, and muscle tenderness

TREATMENT

- Treatment is symptomatic only
- Prophylaxis is the standard therapy in developed countries
  - The rubella vaccine is given at age 12 to 15 months and again at 4 to 6 years
  - Women of childbearing age should avoid pregnancy for 3 months after immunization due to a theoretic risk of fetal infection

MANAGEMENT/FOLLOW-UP

- A self-limited disease, usually with no sequelae
- Rare cases of encephalitis, thrombocytopenic purpura, and peripheral neuritis
- The congenital rubella syndrome is a devastating condition in which multiple congenital defects occur in infants who acquire rubella during intrauterine life
  - Testing of pregnant females for hemagglutination-inhibition antibodies can determine whether they are immune or susceptible to German measles

ICD-9-CM Code

056.9

RUBEOLA [MEASLES]

HISTORY

- Children 3 to 6 years of age are affected most commonly
- Patients experience a 3- to 5-day-long pro-drome of coryza, dry cough, conjunctivitis, photophobia, and fever followed by the characteristic cutaneous eruption
- Patients may have fever as high as 40°C
- There is a seasonal incidence in the United States, with the highest incidence from October through March
- Other symptoms noted may include nausea, vomiting, diarrhea, headache, and malaise

- Nonvaccinated children, especially Black and Hispanic children in inner cities, have a higher risk

PHYSICAL EXAMINATION

- Erythematous macules and papules that be-gin at the forehead and behind the ears and then spread cephalocaudally to the neck, upper extremities, trunk, and then lower extremities (Figs. 90-1 and 90-2)
- Patients may display buccal and labial mu-cosa erythema

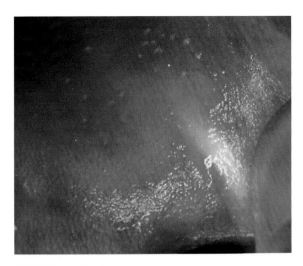

FIGURE 90-1   *Measles.*

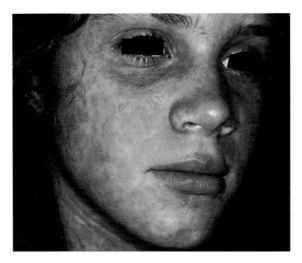

FIGURE 90-2 *Measles.*

- Koplik spots in the oral mucosa are usually opposite the second molars and appear as small red papules with a central bluish-white speck
- Purpura may occur if thrombocytopenia is present and may be associated with bleeding of the respiratory passages or gastrointestinal tract
- Other findings may include lymphadenopathy, splenomegaly, and conjunctival injection
- Findings of encephalitis may rarely occur and may be a sign of potentially lethal disease

DIAGNOSIS

- Clinical presentation is generally sufficient for diagnosis
- Complement fixing, neutralizing, and hemagglutination-inhibiting detection of antibody in serum can be performed for unusual cases

- Other viral exanthems are too numerous to mention and may differ only in subtle ways from roseola; a few include:
  ○ Enterovirus
  ○ Rubella
  ○ Adenovirus
  ○ Coxsackievirus
  ○ Rotavirus
- Scarlet fever: associated with streptococcal disease and the constellation of oropharyngeal findings and positive streptococcal testing
- Drug eruption: patients should have a history of a new drug having been administered within 1 to 3 weeks prior to the onset of the eruption; constitutional symptoms are uncommon with drug eruptions
- Roseola infantum: the eruption of roseola does not have a sandpaper-like characteristic, there are no oropharyngeal findings suggestive of streptococcal infection, and patients with roseola are usually feeling better at the time of the skin eruption
- Kawasaki's disease: five of the six major criteria are generally present, including 1) presentation with 5 days or more of a spiking fever up to 40°C in infants or children; 2) acute nonsuppurative cervical lymphadenopathy; 3) changes in peripheral extremities, including edema and erythema, progressing to desquamation; 4) bilateral conjunctival injection; 5) oral mucosal disease, including oropharyngeal erythema, erythematous to fissured lips, and "strawberry" tongue; 6) scalatiniform eruption
- Rubella: the exanthem begins on the face as pink macules that become confluent and spreads centrifugally, downward to the trunk and extremities, associated with lymphadenopathy in the suboccipital, postauricular, anterior, and posterior cervical nodes; pinpoint petechiae may be present on the soft palate
- Toxic shock syndrome: the association of an infection (in a febrile patient) with flexurally accentuated early macular or maculopapular exanthem that becomes diffuse and that may resemble scarlet fever
  ○ The distribution always involves extremities; erythematous palms and soles and erythema of the mucous membranes with conjunctival injection are commonly observed
  ○ There may be clinical evidence of hypotension, peripheral edema, and muscle tenderness

- Prevention through immunization is the "treatment" of choice
- Supportive therapy in the form of bed rest, hydration, antipyretics, and antitussive agents
- Immune serum globulin (intramuscular dose of 0.25 ml/kg) may attenuate or prevent measles if given within 6 days of exposure

- The condition is usually self-limited, lasting about 10 days
- Measles is contagious from 3 to 5 days prior to onset of symptoms to 5 to 6 days after the onset of the rash

- Serious complications may occur that are potentially fatal
  - Encephalitis occurs in 1 in 890 people
  - Bacterial superinfections include pneumonia and otitis media
  - Bleeding of the respiratory passages or gastrointestinal tract
- Patients with any evidence of complications need emergent treatment

ICD-9-CM Code

055.9

CHAPTER 91

SARCOIDOSIS

HISTORY

- Young adult, usually under 40 years of age, with variable presentation depending on organ involvement
- One-third of patients complain of nonspecific symptoms such as fever, weight loss, and fatigue
- In the United States, Blacks and females are more likely to develop sarcoidosis
- Pulmonary involvement may be evidenced by subacute symptoms of cough, chest pain, or dyspnea, or patients may be asymptomatic
- Cutaneous involvement, present in 20% to 35% of cases, has a variable morphology (see below)
- Ocular involvement may be shown by redness of the eyes, watering, cloudy vision, or photophobia
- Organ-specific symptoms may indicate the involvement of other organ systems, including the central nervous system (CNS) as well as the endocrine, gastrointestinal (GI), musculoskeletal, cardiovascular, and renal systems
  - CNS: cranial nerve, meninges, hypothalamus, pituitary gland involvement
  - Endocrine: pituitary gland and hypothalamus involvement
  - GI: granulomas in the mucosal wall, pancreas, and liver
  - Cardiovascular: conduction disturbances, arrhythmias, congestive heart failure, sudden death, valvular involvement, pericardial disease, and myocardial infarction
  - Musculoskeletal: arthritis affecting knees, ankles, elbows, wrists, and/or small joints of the hands; cystic bony lesions in the hands/feet
  - Renal: granulomatous infiltration of the renal parenchyma or renal arteries

PHYSICAL EXAMINATION

- Cutaneous sarcoidosis has both specific and nonspecific cutaneous manifestations
  - Specific lesions
    - Lupus pernio: chronic, violaceous, indurated papules on the face, particularly the nose, lips, and ears
    - Skin plaques: indurated, violaceous plaques on the limbs, back, or buttocks; plaque centers can be pale and atrophic; usually symmetrical; plaques can be scaly, as in psoriasis
    - Skin papules: waxy, translucent papules 2 to 6 mm, with a flat top; commonly occur on the face, particularly around the eyes. (Fig. 91-1)

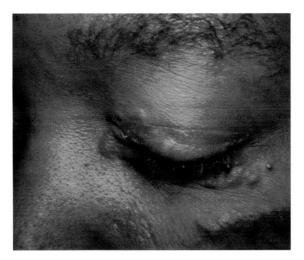

FIGURE 91-1 *Sarcoidosis.*

- Subcutaneous nodules: oval, firm nodules on the trunk/extremities; they are painless
- Scar involvement: sarcoidosis may infiltrate scar tissue on any cutaneous surface; scars become violaceous and swollen.
  - Nonspecific lesions
    - Erythema nodosum: tender, red nodules on the anterior lower extremities; usually a hallmark of acute sarcoidosis, in women of child-bearing age

- Alopecia
- Erythroderma
- Ichthyosis
- Dystrophic calcifications
- Lymphadenopathy
- Splenomegaly

DIAGNOSIS

- Clinical presentation
- Skin biopsy demonstrating noncaseating granulomas
- Negative stains/cultures for other organisms such as deep fungal or mycobacterial
- Radiologic evidence of pulmonary involvement (hilar adenopathy, pulmonary infiltrates, fibrosis, bullae)
- Hypercalcemia
- Elevated serum angiotensin-converting enzyme

DIFFERENTIAL DIAGNOSIS

- Cutaneous sarcoidosis
  - Granuloma annulare
  - Syphilis
  - Rheumatoid nodules
  - Erythema nodosum
  - Cutaneous tuberculosis
  - Ichthyosis
  - Atypical mycobacteria
  - Leprosy
  - Blastomycosis
  - Brucellosis
  - Coccidiomycosis
  - Borreliosis
- Pulmonary sarcoidosis
  - Pneumoconiosis
  - Drug reactions
  - Hypersensitivity pneumonitis
  - Idiopathic pulmonary fibrosis
  - Histiocytosis
  - Systemic lupus erythematosus
  - Scleroderma

- Treatment is generally nonemergent unless there is acute, major organ system compromise
- Glucocorticoid treatment
  - Prednisone 10 to 20 mg bid, tapered to 10 mg/day or every other day
  - Intralesional injections of triamcinolone acetonide 2 to 5 mg/ml weekly
  - Topical glucocorticoid creams or lotions 3 to 4 times per day
- Antimalarials (can be used in combination with glucocorticoids)
  - Chloroquine 250 mg bid for 6 months
  - Hydroxychloroquine 200 mg bid for periods longer than 6 months
  - Ophthalmologic exam needed to prevent retinopathy

- Immunosuppressive agents
  - Methotrexate
  - Azathioprine
  - Chlorambucil
  - Allopurinol
  - Levamisole
  - Colchicine

MANAGEMENT/FOLLOW-UP

- All patients need follow-up with the primary care physician and a specialist expert in managing the specific organ system involvement

ICD-9 Code

135

SCABIES

HISTORY

- Patients complain of severe itching, especially at night, and may have a history of other family members with an itchy rash
- Scabies is acquired by close skin-to-skin contact, and transmission by sexual contact is possible
- The etiologic agent is a mite, *Sarcopotes scabiei* var. *hominis,* which lives just below the stratum corneum of the epidermis
- Crusted (Norwegian) scabies is a type of scabies that is a highly contagious condition due to the large number of mites present and the prominent crusted scale and tends to occur in patients who are in the neonatal period, the physically debilitated, and the immunocompromised (e.g., AIDS and cancer patients)

PHYSICAL EXAMINATION

- Most frequently scabies presents with small erythematous papules and excoriated lesions bilaterally on the extremities, especially on the hands, in the finger web spaces, and on the sides of the fingers, as well as flexor surfaces such as wrists, elbows, penis, breasts, and anterior axillary folds (Fig. 92-1)
  - In infants, the palms, soles, ankles, wrists, face, scalp, and trunk are commonly involved
    - Palm and sole vesicles, vesiculopustules, and bullae may be seen
  - In children and young adults, lesions may be found on the wrists, the sides of the fingers, the finger web spaces, the feet, and and the ankles
    - The gluteal cleft may be involved, but patients rarely forward the history of itching in this location
    - In men, the penis and scrotum may have highly inflammatory papules and nodules (Fig. 92-2)
- The pathognomonic lesion is a burrow, usually 0.5 to 1.5 mm in width and 5 to 15 mm in length, slightly raised, with scaling, meandering lines
  - The distal end of the burrow harboring the mite may have a tiny vesicle
  - Burrows may be numerous but are detected in only 40% of patients
- Secondary features due to chronic scratching behavior may confuse the clinical picture, including eczematous changes, secondary infections such as impetigo, and numerous excoriations
- Crusted (Norwegian) scabies appears as hyperkeratotic patches and plaques in a generalized distribution, with hyperkeratotic debris under the fingernails
  - The most amazing examination scabies preparations may be obtained from patients with crusted scabies, inasmuch as there are often thousands of mites

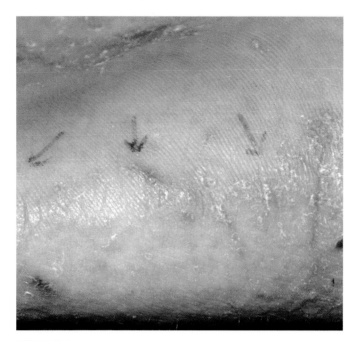

FIGURE 92-1 *Scabies on the palm.*

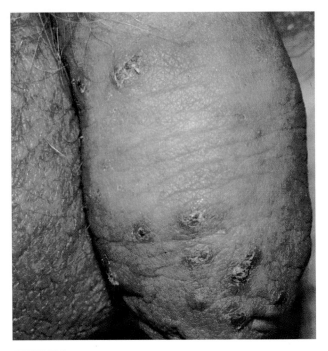

FIGURE 92-2 *Sabies on the penis and scrotum.*

- The diagnosis is primarily based on the history and physical examination
- To confirm the diagnosis, one can prepare a scabies preparation by gently scraping the skin of a burrow with a small scalpel blade, apply the materials and mineral oil to a microscope slide, and then demonstrate the mites, feces (scybala), or eggs microscopically

DIFFERENTIAL DIAGNOSIS

- Atopic dermatitis: may also be very pruritic, but usually has poorly defined, erythematous patches on the flexor surfaces; lacks burrows, and a scabies preparation is negative
- Papular urticaria: most commonly associated with arthropod bites, and there are no burrows
- Dermatitis herpetiformis: a blistering disease that usually involves the extensor surfaces and is quite pruritic, but burrows are lacking

TREATMENT

- Topical treatments with scabicides are the most common forms of treatment, and some treatments can be associated with toxicities that are worthy of mention
- The entire family should be treated once, and, given the known failure rates, re-treatment in 1 week is reasonable
  - Permethrin (Elimite®) 5% is a synthetic pyrethroid that has low toxicity and is the treatment of choice

- The patient should apply a thin layer on the body, covering all surfaces of the skin, including the groin and web spaces, from the neck down; this layer should be washed off after 10 hours
- If scalp involvement is present, 100% body surface area coverage may be required
- Although permethrin is not approved for use in infants younger than 2 years of age or pregnant women, it is the safest treatment available for these groups
  ○ Lindane (Kwell®) 1% is applied like permethrin, but is left on for 8 hours and then rinsed off thoroughly
    - 10% of the lindane applied to the skin is absorbed, and prolonged or excessive use can cause neurotoxicity
    - This agent should generally not be used in infants or young children, pregnant or nursing women, or patients with seizure disorders
  ○ Malathion (Ovide®) is a highly effective scabicide, but it is not indicated for this use in the United States

- Malathion has the potential to be absorbed and is neurotoxic, so it should generally not be used in infants or young children, pregnant or nursing women, or patients with seizure disorders
  ○ Oral ivermectin, indicated as an antiparasitic medication, may be given as a single oral dose of 200 µg/kg
    - This agent is not indicated as a scabicide, and caution should be exercised in its use

MANAGEMENT/FOLLOW-UP

- Materials of daily contact, such as clothing, bedding, etc., should be washed in water with laundry detergent and machine-dried
- Items of daily contact, such as seat cushions, that cannot effectively be laundered should be placed in a sealed plastic bag for 1 to 2 weeks

ICD-9 Code

133.0

SCARLET FEVER (SCARLATINA)

HISTORY

- Children, generally 2 to 10 years old, presenting with fever, nausea, vomiting, chills, abdominal pain, and malaise 2 to 5 days after the onset of streptococcal pharyngitis or other streptococcal infections including postsurgical or postpartum infections and cellulitis
- Sore throat is a usual symptom when associated with streptococcal pharyngitis
- The characteristic cutaneous eruption develops 24 to 48 hours after onset of the pharyngeal symptoms

PHYSICAL EXAMINATION

- Patients appear ill and febrile
- Beefy red tonsillar enlargement, tonsillar exudates, and tender submandibular adenopathy when streptococcal pharyngitis is present
- Initial "white strawberry" tongue followed by bright "red strawberry" tongue (Fig. 93-1)
- Punctate erythema is found on the palate
- A sandpaper-like exanthem of diffuse, blanchable erythema covered with 1- to 2-mm confluent red papules, begins on the head and neck and then moves to the trunk and then extremities.
  - Exanthem lasts for 4 to 5 days, followed by desquamation, starting from the head and neck and spreading to the trunk and extremities
  - The characteristic desquamation is an aid to clinical diagnosis (Fig. 93-2)
- The cheeks are flushed, without discreet papules, and there is circumoral pallor
- The palms and soles are spared, but areas of pressure such as the buttocks and sacrum and antecubital skin may be markedly involved
- Linear petechiae (Pastia's lines) are present in the antecubital fossae and/or axillary folds in severe cases
- Generalized lymphadenopathy is usually present
- Splenomegaly is sometimes present

DIAGNOSIS

- Clinical examination with laboratory confirmation
- Positive streptococcal culture of the throat or positive rapid streptococcal test
- Other supportive laboratory findings include eosinophilia, leukocytosis, and microscopic hematuria

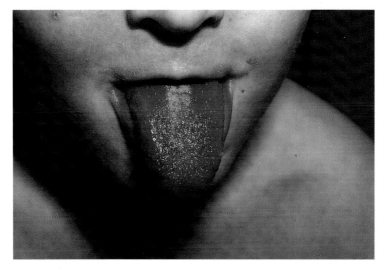

FIGURE 93-1   *Scarlet fever.*

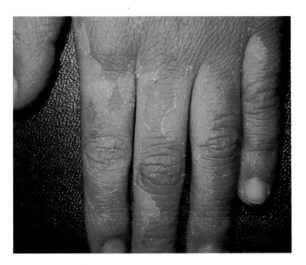

FIGURE 93-2   *Scarlet fever.*

- Drug eruption: patients should have a history of a new drug having been administered within 1 to 3 weeks prior to the onset of the eruption; constitutional symptoms are uncommon with drug eruptions
- Roseola infantum: the eruption of roseola does not have a sandpaper-like characteristic, there are no oropharyngeal findings suggestive of streptococcal infection, and patients with roseola are usually feeling better at the time of the skin eruption
- Kawasaki's disease: five of the six major criteria are generally present, including 1) 5 days or more of a spiking fever up to 40°C at presentation in infants and children; 2) acute nonsuppurative cervical lymphadenopathy; 3) changes in peripheral extremities, including edema and erythema, progressing to desquamation; 4) bilateral conjunctival injection; 5) oral mucosal disease, including oropharyngeal erythema, erythematous to fissured lips, and "strawberry" tongue; 6) scalatiniform eruption

- Rubella: the exanthem begins on the face as pink macules that become confluent and spreads centrifugally, downward to the trunk and extremities, associated with lymphadenopathy in the suboccipital, postauricular, anterior, and posterior cervical nodes; pinpoint petechiae may be present on the soft palate
- Toxic shock syndrome: the association of an infection (in a febrile patient) with flexurally accentuated early macular or maculopapular exanthem that becomes diffuse and may resemble scarlet fever
  - The distribution always involves extremities; erythematous palms and soles and erythema of the mucous membranes with conjunctival injection are commonly observed
  - There may be clinical evidence of hypotension, peripheral edema, and muscle tenderness

- Penicillin V 400,000 units po 4 times/day for 10 days for adults and children weighing more than 60 lbs; 200,000 to 400,000 units po tid to qid for 10 days for children weighing less than 60 lbs
- Erythromycin 500 mg po bid for 10 days for adults; 30 to 50 mg/kg/day divided qid for 10 days in children (should not exceed 1 g/day in children)
- Supportive antipyretics such as ibuprofen or acetaminophen

- Patients should follow up with the primary care physician within several days
- The febrile illness lasts for 4 to 5 days
- Skin desquamation may continue for several weeks
- The course is rapidly attenuated with systemic penicillins

ICD-9-CM Code

034.1

SCLERODERMA

- Patients may complain of slow onset of thickening or tightening of the skin, which may be localized or diffuse, as well as pain and blanching of digits when exposed to cold (Raynaud's phenomenon) and difficulty swallowing; some forms of scleroderma have other, more severe systemic manifestations
- Classification
  - Morphea is a variant of scleroderma that is limited to the skin only, with no internal involvement; it is usually seen in localized plaques
    - Variants include localized morphea, generalized morphea, linear morphea, and subcutaneous morphea (morphea profunda)
    - Patients lack any history of internal manifestations including Raynaud's phenomenon, sclerosis of the fingers with sclerodactyly, and internal organ involvement
    - Women are affected three times as often as men, and the disease is more common in white populations
  - Systemic sclerosis can be classified into two different subsets: limited systemic sclerosis and diffuse systemic sclerosis
    - Limited systemic sclerosis includes patients with CREST syndrome (calcinosis cutis, Raynaud's phenomenon, esophageal dysmotility, sclerodactyly, and telangiectasias); they are usually women who are older than patients with diffuse systemic sclerosis
    - Often patients have a positive anti-centromere antibody
    - Late in the disease course, patients may develop pulmonary hypertension and other systemic involvement, but patients usually outlive their disease
  - Diffuse systemic sclerosis often starts as Raynaud's phenomenon and swelling of the hands and feet that are acute in onset, but it progresses to tightening of the skin, with a hide-bound feel diffusely except for the back and buttocks
    - Patients may note periarticular pain
    - Nail fold telangiectasias, destruction of the nail fold, and early internal organ involvement, including systemic hypertension related to renal disease, pulmonary fibrosis, and myocardial fibrosis
    - Patients often have a positive anti-topoisomerase 1 antibody (Scl-70)
    - Women are affected four times as often as men, and Black women are more often affected
- Classification into one of these groups is important prognostically, since patients with localized disease and CREST have a more limited course, whereas patients with diffuse systemic sclerosis can have a rapidly progressive, fatal course if untreated

- Localized morphea: well-circumscribed, indurated, sclerotic plaques with erythematous borders and an ivory color noted centrally; commonly few in number and often found on the trunk and extremities (Fig. 94-1) see chapter 61
- Generalized morphea: plaques that are similar to those of localized morphea but much more numerous; found on trunk, abdomen, buttocks, and legs
- Subcutaneous morphea: deep, bound-down, sclerotic plaques without significant overlying color change
- Linear morphea: a singular, unilateral band similar in appearance to localized morphea, often on the lower extremities; one specific form occurs on the frontal or frontoparietal area of head and is called *coup de sabre*
- Systemic sclerosis findings depend on the sites involved
  - Patients often have sclerodactyly, and ulcerations are noted on the fingertips associated with Raynaud's phenomenon
  - In diffuse systemic sclerosis, thickening and edema of the skin will spread to the upper extremities, trunk, face, and finally the lower extremities; thickening and sclerosis of facial skin may lead to an expressionless face, as well as decreased ability to open the mouth widely (Figs. 94-2 and 94-3)
  - Mat-like, box telangiectasias may also be seen on the face and upper trunk as well as peri-nail-fold telangiectasias

DIAGNOSIS

- Requires a punch or incisional skin biopsy to confirm the disease
- Lab work including complete blood count with platelets, renal function tests, antinuclear antibody, chest x-ray, barium swallow, and possibly anticentromere antibody and anti-Scl-70 antibody levels, needs to be performed in systemic sclerosis
- In localized morphea, checking a Lyme titer may be necessary, since *Borrelia burgdorferi* can cause a condition in the skin that is similar to morphea; history of a tick bite might prompt this testing

DIFFERENTIAL DIAGNOSIS

- Scleroderma-like syndromes: have been noted in patients exposed to toxic rapeseed oil and L-tryptophan; an exposure history may be helpful in distinguishing these
- Chronic graft-versus-host disease: can cause a clinical picture similar to scleroderma, and history of bone marrow transplantation is very important here

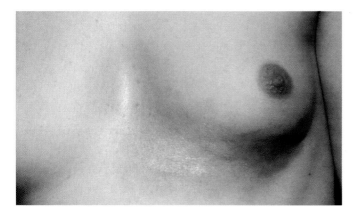

FIGURE 94-1 *Morphea.*

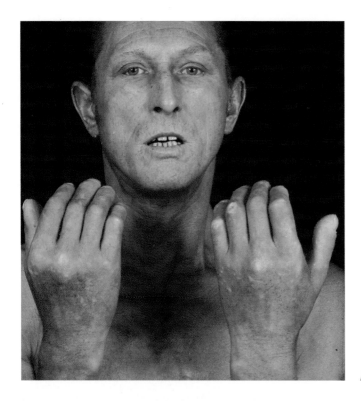

FIGURE 94-2 *Scleroderma.*

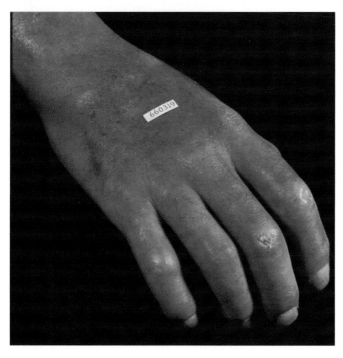

FIGURE 94-3 *Scleroderma.*

- Acrodermatitis chronica atrophicans: a lesion similar to localized morphea, usually on an extremity and caused by a tick bite infected with *Borrelia burgdorferi*
- Radiation dermatitis: can cause a picture that is similar to morphea; history is helpful
- Panniculitis: some forms may mimic localized morphea

TREATMENT

- Unless patients are hemodynamically unstable because of congestive heart failure, treatment of all forms of morphea and scleroderma is nonemergent
- Beyond management of hemodynamic compromise, other aspects of care may be managed on an outpatient basis
- Once the diagnosis of morphea has been established:
  ○ Consider a trial of 4 weeks of bid topical therapy with potent corticosteroids such as fluocinonide (Lidex®) 0.05% ointment or cream; clobetasol propionate (Temovate®) 0.05% ointment or cream; halobetasol propionate (Ultravate®) 0.05% ointment or cream, betamethasone dipropionate 0.05% in optimized ointment (Diprolene®)
  ○ Intralesional corticosteroid injection such as triamcinolone acetonide (Kenalog®) 2.5 to 5.0 mg/ml to the borders of the lesion; inject along the border using about 0.1 ml with each injection
  ○ Other agents with anecdotal reports of success include antimalarial agents, diphenylhydantoin, colchicine, methotrexate, and systemic corticosteroids
  ○ Long-term management of the patient's limited skin mobility with physical and occupational therapy may be necessary to prevent permanent contractures of the large and small joints of the extremities
- Once the diagnosis of CREST syndrome or systemic sclerosis has been established:
  ○ Immunosuppressive systemic treatments are generally required, such as azathioprine, chlorambucil, methotrexate, cyclophosphamide, systemic glucocorticoids, D-penicillamine, or extracorporeal photopheresis
  ○ Patients need management of their Raynaud's phenomenon with behavioral changes and possibly with calcium-channel blockers or nitroglycerin paste
  ○ Gastroesophageal reflux management associated with their esophageal dysmotility may be required
  ○ Long-term management of the patient's limited skin mobility with physical and occupational therapy may be necessary to prevent permanent contractures of the large and small joints of the extremities

MANAGEMENT/FOLLOW-UP

- Morphea will require follow-up within 2 to 4 weeks with the primary care physician or dermatologist
  ○ Morphea tends to be localized and usually self-limited, although in some cases significant morbidity may be associated with scarring
- All CREST and systemic sclerosis patients should be followed closely by their primary care physician in concert with a multidisciplinary management team including rheumatology, dermatology, gastroenterology, nephrology, and cardiology specialists
  ○ Limited systemic sclerosis (CREST) rarely progresses to diffuse systemic sclerosis and is a chronic, slowly progressive disease
  ○ Diffuse systemic sclerosis may be rapidly progressive and life-threatening

ICD-9 Code

701.0 Morphea
710.1 Scleroderma

CPT Code

11100 Biopsy

CHAPTER 95

SEBORRHEIC DERMATITIS

- Patient complains of flaking, redness, and itchiness of the scalp and ears, around the eyebrows, around the nose, and in the center of the chest
- Patients with neurologic diseases such as Parkinson's disease and the immunocompromised such as those with AIDS may have more severe disease
- Can occur at any age, but has two age peaks, infancy and the fourth to the seventh decades of life
- Disease tends to be worse in the winter
- Men are more often affected than women

PHYSICAL EXAMINATION

- Mild to marked greasy scaling and erythema in poorly defined patches on the scalp, eyebrows, nasolabial folds, external ear canals, retroauricular folds, and central chest over the sternum (Figs. 95-1 to 95-3)
- The petaloid variant begins as follicular and perifollicular redness and scaling that spreads to form clearly outlined, round to circinate patches, resembling petals of a flower
- Some patients may also have an associated blepharitis of the upper and lower eyelids

DIAGNOSIS

- This is a clinical diagnosis

DIFFERENTIAL DIAGNOSIS

- Psoriasis: presents as a chronic condition with brightly erythematous scaly plaques typically found on the scalp, elbows, knees, and periumbilical and gluteal cleft areas
- Acrodermatitis enteropathica (zinc deficiency)
- Allergic or irritant contact dermatitis: may present anywhere there is a topical exposure to irritants or allergens; the amount of erythema is much greater than is seen with seborrheic dermatitis
- Atopic dermatitis: frequently presents with scalp itching and subtle scaling and erythema, indistinguishable in appearance from seborrheic dermatitis
  - Other clues to atopic dermatitis such as itching involvement of the neck and antecubital and popliteal fossae may be helpful
- Tinea capitis and tinea facei: these conditions are due to fungal infection and present with reasonably well-circumscribed patches of erythema, broken hairs, and scaling with occasional central clearing

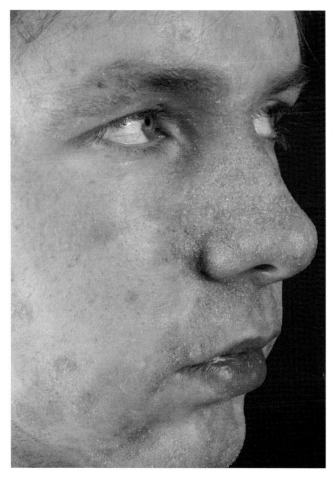

FIGURE 95-1 *Seborrheic infantile dermatitis with involvement of the nasolabial folds, cheeks, eyebrows, and nose.*

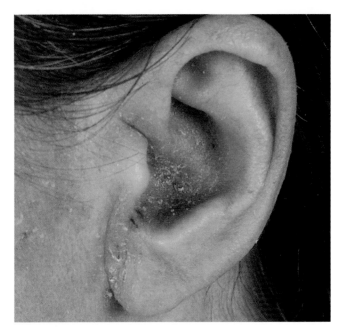

FIGURE 95-2 *Seborrheic dermatitis of the earlobe.*

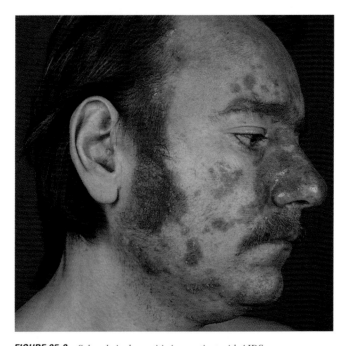

FIGURE 95-3 *Seborrheic dermatitis in a patient with AIDS.*

- Perioral dermatitis: this acneiform disease presents most commonly in young women with a perioral distribution of brightly erythematous papules

- Treatment of seborrheic dermatitis is nonemergent
- This is a long-term disease over which patients need to exert control, but this condition is not curable
- Shampoos containing selenium sulfide (Selsun Blue®), zinc pyrithione (Head & Shoulders®), and ketoconazole (Nizoral®), salicylic acid (T-Sal®), or tar (T-Gel®) are the safest long-term treatment and should be used two to seven times per week as tolerated
  - These agents may also be used on the face, ears, and chest
- Low-potency topical corticosteroids such as hydrocortisone 1% solution (Scalpicin®) or cream (Cortizone 10®, Lanacort®) may be used on the scalp, face, or chest once to twice per day as needed
  - Stronger topical corticosteroids such as desonide (DesOwen®) 0.05% cream, lotion or ointment bid or fluocinolone oil (Derma-Smoothe/FS® oil) bid may be helpful for periods of not longer than 4 weeks
  - Corticosteroid-sparing agents such as tacrolimus (Protopic®) 0.1% ointment has no known ability to cause skin atrophy even when applied chronically and may be applied bid to affected skin areas
- Ketoconazole (Nizoral®) cream or clotrimazole (Lotrimin®) cream may also be helpful on the face and chest as corticosteroid-sparing agents
- Patients with seborrheic blepharitis: patients benefit from warm compresses and gentle debridement with cotton swabs one or more times per day
  - Baby shampoo diluted with water may also be helpful as a cleansing agent
  - Other topical agents including hydrocortisone 1% ointment or desonide (DesOwen®) 0.05% lotion or ointment may be applied bid for 2 to 4 weeks

- Patients may have follow-up with the primary care physician or dermatologist for this condition within 4 weeks

ICD-9-CM Code
690.10

CHAPTER 96

SEBORRHEIC INFANTILE DERMATITIS (CRADLE CAP)

- Parents of infants who are a few months old will often notice greasy-looking scale and redness of the scalp or intertriginous folds, with occasional involvement of the central face, chest, and neck
- The eruption on the scalp is often called "cradle cap"

- One observes greasy scaling in erythematous patches on the scalp, face, retroauricular folds, pinnae of the ears, and neck, with occasional similar eruptions of the axillae, anogenital area, and groin (Fig. 96-1)

- The diagnosis is usually made clinically based on history and physical exam

- Atopic dermatitis: usually presents more diffusely on the body with less-well-defined patches and accentuation of the neck and the antecubial and popliteal fossae; patient may have a history of asthma or allergic rhinitis

- Psoriasis: this may be difficult to distinguish from seborrheic dermatitis, but psoriasis is rare in newborns aand presents with much more erythema than in seborrheic dermatitis
- Scabies: does not usually present with confluent scaling and symmetric erythema, and characteristic burrows and pustules are commonly found
- Langerhans cell histiocytosis: extremely severe seborrheic infantile dermatitis seen in conjunction with failure to thrive and hepatosplenomegaly should suggest consideration of Langerhans cell histiocytosis
  - A skin biopsy is necessary to distinguish between these two
- Tinea capitis and corporis: tinea infections are uncommon in infants, but they can occur
  - Although tinea infections should be more brightly erythematous with scaling and central clearing, examination of a KOH preparation may help distinguish between these two diseases
- Leiner's disease: a rare variant of seborrheic dermatitis in infants; a sudden confluence of lesions progresses to a diffuse scaling and redness of the skin (erythroderma) associated with severe illness including anemia, diarrhea, and vomiting
  - Secondary bacterial infection may occur
  - The familial form of the disease is associated with C5 complement deficiency, leading to ineffective opsonization of bacteria

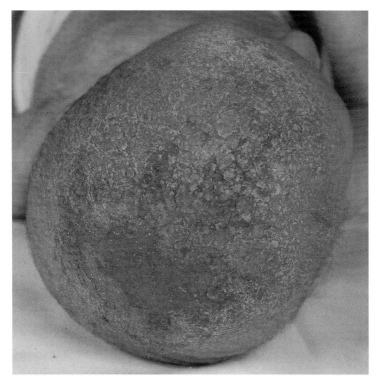

FIGURE 96-1 *Seborrheic infantile dermatitis of the scalp.*

- Treatment of seborrheic infantile dermatitis is nonemergent
- Shampoos containing selenium sulfide (Selsun Blue®), zinc pyrithione (Head & Shoulders®), ketoconazole (Nizoral®), or salicylic acid (T-Sal®) can help and may be used two to seven times per week as tolerated
- Low-potency topical corticosteroids such as hydrocortisone 1% cream or ointment (Cortizone 10®, Lanacort®) may be applied to the scalp, face, axillae, or elsewhere once to twice per day as needed
- Ketoconazole (Nizoral®) cream or clotrimazole (Lotrimin®) cream may also be helpful as a corticosteroid-sparing agent
- Scalp: mild baby shampoos and very mild topical glucocorticoids (1% hydrocortisone cream or lotion) may be helpful, as well as very mild salicylic acid preparation (3% to 5%) to debride scales; however, one must be careful to avoid overdosage and salicylism in an infant
- Intertriginous area: very mild topical glucocorticoids (1% hydrocortisone) may be helpful; if fungal superinfection occurs, use topical antifungal agents (nystatin or imidazole preparations)

- The disease usually continues for several weeks to months
- Patient may have follow-up with primary care physician or dermatologist within 4 weeks

ICD-9-CM Code

690.12

SEBORRHEIC KERATOSIS

HISTORY

- Patient complains of "warts" or "moles" that may be flesh-colored or brown and itchy; often concerned that lesion is increasing in size and changing color
- Patient may note that his/her parents had numerous similar lesions
- Seborrheic keratoses are very common benign skin tumors often seen in people over 30 years old; an individual patient may develop multiple lesions, numbering into the hundreds
- Several clinic variants exist, including common seborrheic keratosis, melano-acanthoma, dermatosis papulosa nigra, and stucco keratosis

PHYSICAL EXAMINATION

- Start out as flat, well-demarcated, brown-colored macules that progress to uneven, dull, verrucous-surfaced, "stuck-on," and greasy-appearing plaques; multiple follicular plugs with follicular prominence may be noted (Figs. 97-1 and 97-2)
- Can be found anywhere on the body, except mucous membranes; usually not found on the palms and soles

DIAGNOSIS

- Diagnosis is usually made clinically, with typical appearance and history
- Occasionally, biopsy may be required to rule out malignant melanoma in changing lesions

DIFFERENTIAL DIAGNOSIS

- Verruca vulgaris: these lesions usually have spires of scales extending upward, occur in younger patients, and are not usually multiple
- Malignant melanoma: does not usually have scaly surfaces and usually displays border irregularity, color variation, and asymmetry
- Atypical nevus: these have many of the features of melanoma, but all features (border irregularity, color variation, and asymmetry) are more subtle than those found with melanoma
- Solar lentigo: these benign lesions lack scale and have no clinical atypia
- Actinic keratosis: are often more rough in

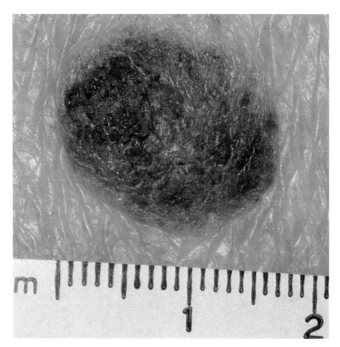

FIGURE 97-1 *Seborrheic keratosis.*

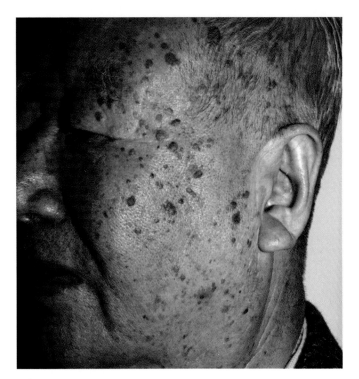

FIGURE 97-2 *Multiple small seborrheic keratoses.*

feel and usually lack the brown color of seborrheic keratoses

- Squamous cell carcinoma: is usually nonpigmented, has an indurated base, and is present on sun-exposed skin

- No treatment is required
- Lesions that are easily irritated or cosmetically bothersome may be treated with liquid nitrogen cryotherapy, superficial electrodesiccation, or laser therapy
- Any lesion that is not typical of a seborrheic keratosis should be considered a candidate for a skin biopsy to exclude malignant melanoma

- No specific management or follow-up is required
- Intermittent treatment for cosmetically sensitive lesions or easily irritated lesions may be necessary

ICD-9-CM Code

702.19 Benign
702.11 Irritated/inflamed

CPT Code

17000 Destruction of lesion (1 lesion)
17003 Destruction of each additional lesion (2 to 14 lesions)
17004 Destruction of 15 or more lesions (do not also code 17000)

SQUAMOUS CELL CARCINOMA

HISTORY

- Patients report a slowly enlarging skin lesion that has been present for months to years
- Although it can occur on any cutaneous surface, sun-exposed areas of the arms, hands, neck, face, and scalp are affected most commonly
- Patients may report pain or bleeding within the lesion
- Patients who have undergone organ transplants and are on immunosuppressive therapy have a tendency to develop numerous squamous cell carcinomas

PHYSICAL EXAMINATION

- Invasive squamous cell carcinoma presents as skin-colored to erythematous, tender, indurated papules, plaques, or nodules, with scaling on the surface and possible ulceration (Figs. 98-1 to 98-3)
- Superficial squamous cell carcinoma: tender, erythematous, scaly plaque with a sharply defined border
- Squamous cell carcinomas may occur on mucosal sites as well, including the lips and oral and genital mucosae (Fig. 98-4)

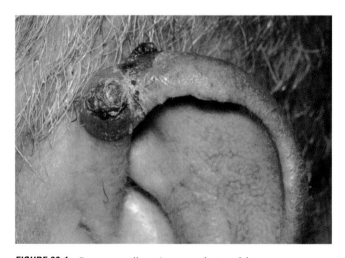

FIGURE 98-1 *Squamous cell carcinoma on the top of the ear.*

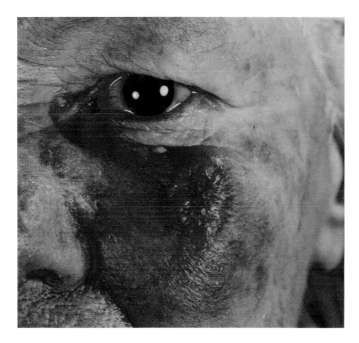

FIGURE 98-2 *Squamous cell carcinoma on the cheek.*

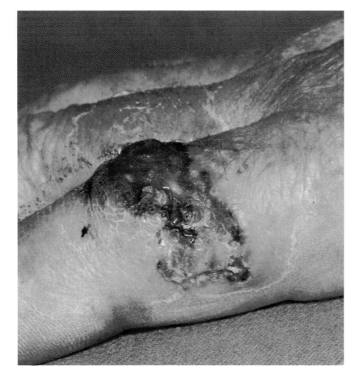

FIGURE 98-3 *Squamous cell carcinoma on the finger.*

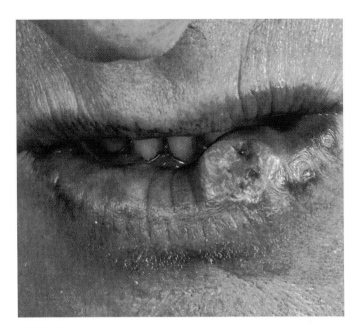

FIGURE 98-4   *Squamous cell carcinoma on the lower lip.*

- Squamous cell carcinoma may also develop at sites of old burn scars, preexisting skin disorders such as lichen sclerosis et atrophicus, or areas of prior therapeutic radiation

- The diagnosis is a clinical one that should be confirmed by skin biopsy examination

- Keratoacanthoma: a rapidly enlarging skin tumor that most commonly occurs on sun-exposed areas of the skin
  - Often presents as a dome-shaped papule with a central keratotic plug
- Verrucae vulgaris (warts): skin-colored lesions that vary in size and shape and can appear on any cutaneous surface
  - One may see "black dots" on the surface
- Basal cell carcinoma: a slowly evolving, pearly, erythematous papule that may occur on any cutaneous surface of the skin, but most commonly is on sun-damaged skin
- Prurigo nodularis: a keratotic flesh-colored to erythematous papule or nodule that occurs due to chronic picking or scratching of the skin

- The treatment of squamous cell carcinoma is nonemergent
- Squamous cell carcinoma does have a small metastatic potential, so prompt treatment is recommended
- Surgical excision is recommended for the treatment of invasive squamous cell carcinoma
- Superficial squamous cell carcinoma may be treated with either cryosurgery, curettage and electrodessication, topical fluorouracil, topical imiquimod, or surgical excision

- Patients who are suspected to have a squamous cell carcinoma should be referred to their primary care physician or a dermatologist for a skin biopsy and further management

ICD-9-CM Codes

173.0 Skin of lip
173.1 Eyelid, including canthus
173.2 Skin of ear and external auditory canal
173.3 Skin of other and unspecified parts of face
173.4 Scalp and skin of neck
173.5 Skin of trunk, except scrotum
173.6 Skin of upper limb, including shoulder
173.7 Skin of lower limb, including hip
173.8 Other specified sites of skin
173.9 Skin, site unspecified

STAPHYLOCOCCAL SCALDED SKIN SYNDROME (RITTER'S DISEASE)

HISTORY

- This condition is most common during the first 2 years of life and is rare in adults
- Patients may have signs and symptoms of staphylococcal infections common in this aged population, including impetigo, infected umbilical stumps in neonates, otitis media, purulent conjunctivitis, or nasopharyngeal infection
- Patients have sudden onset of fever, irritability, cutaneous tenderness, and characteristic cutaneous eruption and blister formation
- Fluid and electrolyte abnormalities and sepsis have been described

PHYSICAL EXAMINATION

- Patients appear ill, irritable, and febrile (Figs. 99-1 to 99-3)
- The appearance of the eruption depends on its duration
  - Initially, a scarlatiniform exanthem (staphylococcal scarlet fever syndrome) or broad sheets of tender erythema may appear with accentuation of the periorificial and intertriginous areas
  - Within 24 to 48 hours flaccid blisters and superficial sloughing may occur

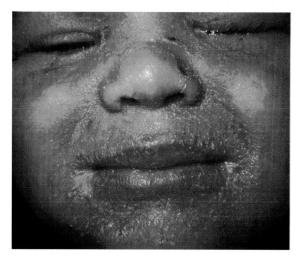

FIGURE 99-1 *Staphylococcal scalded skin syndrome.*

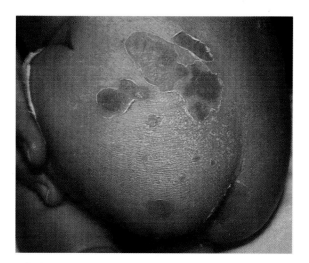

FIGURE 99-2 *Staphylococcal scalded skin syndrome.*

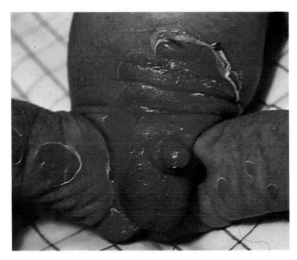

FIGURE 99-3 *Staphylococcal scalded skin syndrome.*

- ○ The eruption quickly becomes generalized, and flaccid bullae may develop
  - - Note that the pathology is nid-epidermal, so full-thickness slough-ing does not occur
- ○ The Nikolsky sign may now be present
  - - In patients with active blisters, light lateral sliding pressure with a gloved finger will separate normal-looking epidermis producing an erosion
- ○ Skin desquamation follows
- • Mucous membranes are normal

- • This is a clinical diagnosis based on the history and physical examination and is confirmed by a positive staphylococcal culture
- • An emergent skin biopsy specimen interpretation may aid the diagnosis

- Kawasaki's disease: five of the six major criteria are generally present, including 1) presentation with 5 days or more of a spiking fever up to 40°C in infants and children; 2) acute nonsuppurative cervical lymphadenopathy; 3) changes in peripheral extremities, including edema and erythema, progressing to desquamation; 4) bilateral conjunctival injection; 5) oral mucosal disease, including oropharyngeal erythema, erythematous to fissured lips, and "strawberry" tongue; 6) scarlatiniform eruption
- Toxic shock syndrome: the association of an infection (in a febrile patient) with flexurally accentuated early macular or maculopapular exanthem that becomes diffuse and may resemble scarlet fever
  - The distribution always involves extremities; erythematous palms and soles and erythema of the mucous membranes with conjunctival injection are commonly observed
  - There may be clinical evidence of hypotension, peripheral edema, and muscle tenderness
- Toxic epidermal necrolysis: the patient population is older, the mucous membranes are generally involved, and the sloughing that occurs is much more severe (full epidermal thickness)
- Drug eruption: may present as an erythroderma, but a source of staphylococcal infection will not be found, and a history of recent drug exposure is obtained

- The treatment of staphylococcal scalded skin syndrome is emergent
- Intravenous penicillinase-resistant anti-staphylococcal antibiotics such as nafcillin 75 to 100 mg/kg/day in divided doses, or, for patients who are mildly affected, dicloxacillin 50 mg/kg/day divided into qid dosing
- Supportive care may be required with bland ointments such as Vaseline® or Aquaphor®
- If necessary, fluid and electrolyte monitoring and replacement may be required

- Widespread desquamation is followed by complete healing in 5 to 7 days
- The mortality rate is low, but death can be caused by pneumonia or sepsis

ICD-9-CM Code

038.10

- The patient complains of a nonhealing sore, usually on the distal lower extremity, and may have a history of stasis dermatitis or "poor circulation in the legs"
- Patients may also complain of aching and swelling of the legs that is made worse when "feet hang down"
- The condition is more common in females, usually in a middle-aged or elderly patient
- A history of thrombophlebitis is occasionally found
- Patients often have incompetent valves in the veins, leading to dysfunction of the calf muscle pump
- Patients may note previous minor trauma at the site prior to ulcer development

PHYSICAL EXAMINATION

- Irregularly shaped ulcer with punched-out appearance on a background of pitting edema (Fig. 100-1)
  - Ulcers have granulation tissue at the base and often have white or yellow purulent exudate

- Surrounding cellulitis may occasionally be noted and may lead to further lymphedema
- Ulcers are usually located on the medial lower calf, especially over the malleolus
- Similar ulcers have been noted in other dependent areas of the body
- Patients should have palpable pedal pulses to exclude arterial insufficiency as a cause of their disease
- Other changes of stasis dermatitis, such as small brown macules indicative of hemosiderin deposition, may be noted

DIAGNOSIS

- The diagnosis is made clinically by history and physical exam
- Rarely, examination of a skin biopsy specimen is needed to exclude vasculitis, infection, or squamous cell carcinoma
- If cellulitis is noted, wound cultures may also be necessary to evaluate the organism causing secondary infection
- Doppler vascular studies may also be helpful to evaluate valvular competence

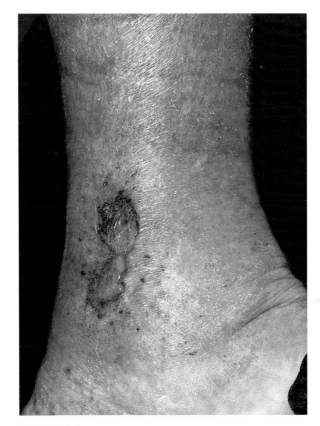

FIGURE 100-1 *Venous insufficiency.*

- Arterial insufficiency ulcers: patients lack evidence of stasis changes of the legs and have poorly palpable pedal pulses or no pedal pulses
  - Patients may also have poor capillary refill, decreased hair growth on the distal legs, decreased sensation, and dependent erythema
- Vascultis diseases: polyarteritis nodosa and nodular vasculitis may produce nonhealing ulcers, but there usually is a marked component of palpable purpura and purpura surrounding the ulcer or ulcers
- Squamous or basal cell carcinoma: these cancers may arise on the legs and give rise to chronic ulcers, but the borders are usually quite indurated
  - Any suspicious ulcer should be considered a candidate for a diagnostic skin biopsy
- Infections with atypical mycobacteria and fungal organisms: infections with these organisms usually have papules, nodules, and crusted erosions that are most commonly multiple
  - Differentiation may require a diagnostic skin biopsy
- Pyoderma gangrenosum: this inflammatory condition demonstrates brightly erythematous to violaceous borders, and the border of an advancing ulcer shows undermining

- If there is no evidence of cellulitis, treatment of venous ulcers is nonemergent
- Local wound care is imperative to assist wound healing, with dressing changes dependent on the type of dressing, and treatment of secondary infection as needed
- The mainstay of therapy is the control of peripheral edema and improvement of venous circulation
  - Application of graduated compression hose, Unna's boots, and corrective surgery for venous insufficiency are all ways of reducing venous hypertension
  - Maintaining a moist healing environment for the wound using colloidal dressings such as DuoDerm® may help speed resolution
- Allergic contact dermatitis frequently complicates venous ulcers and is usually related to applied topical preparations
- Skin graft procedures may also be helpful if the wound base can support a graft
- Any secondary infection should be treated with appropriate systemic antibiotic agents

- Patients should be followed by their primary care physician or a dermatologist as often as weekly until the ulcer is healed
- Patients who have a past medical history of venous ulcer formation are at increased risk of developing another in the future
- Squamous cell carcinomas developing in chronic venous ulcers are well described

ICD-9 Code

454.0

CPT Code

11100   Biopsy

CHAPTER 101

STRIAE ATROPHICAE (STRIAE DISTENSAE, STRETCH MARKS)

HISTORY

- Often seen in patients who are or have been pregnant, morbidly obese patients, patients treated with systemic corticosteroid therapy, or patients with chronic liver disease or Cushing's disease
- Lesions often noted on abdomen, flanks, and upper aspect of upper and lower extremities

PHYSICAL EXAMINATION

- See pink to purple, atrophic, jagged, linear plaques on the abdomen, flanks, and upper and lower extremities (Fig. 101-1)

DIAGNOSIS

- The diagnosis is clinical diagnosis

DIFFERENTIAL DIAGNOSIS

- The clinical picture usually is classic and leaves little room for differential diagnosis

TREATMENT

- The treatment of striae is nonemergent
- No specific treatment is necessary or effective
- The appearance usually improves with time, weight loss, removal of systemic corticosteroid therapy, or normalization of cortisol levels

MANAGEMENT/FOLLOW-UP

- No specific follow-up is needed for striae distensae
- Closer monitoring by the patient's primary care physician may be required if underlying systemic disease is present (i.e., Cushing's disease)

ICD-9 Code

701.3

CPT Code

None

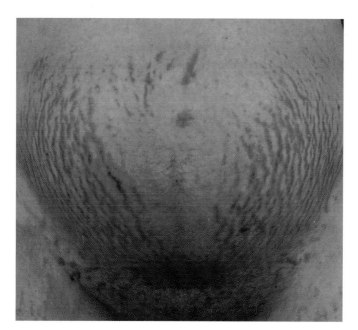

FIGURE 101-1 *Striae distensae.*

CHAPTER 102

SUNBURN

HISTORY

- Sunburn is seen in light-skinned Caucasians with acute onset pruritic or tender, photodistributed eruption following ultraviolet light exposure
  - Onset within the 24 hours after the ultraviolet exposure
- A history of phototoxic medications is important to elicit
  - Medications such as sulfonamides, tetracyclines, chlorothiazides, phenothiazines, furosemide, nalidixic acid, amiodarone, and naproxen are known to be phototoxic
- A history of artificial sunlamp use is important
- Headache, fever, chills, and weakness are not uncommon symptoms

PHYSICAL EXAMINATION

- Photodistributed confluent erythema with edema; skin may be tender or pruritic (Fig. 102-1)
- When severe, vesicles and bullae are seen on painful skin
- Patient may appear toxic, with rapid heart rate

DIAGNOSIS

- Clinical exam

DIFFERENTIAL DIAGNOSIS

- Photodrug eruption (includes phototoxic reactions and photoallergic reactions)
- Systemic lupus erythematosus
- Erythropoietic protoporphyria

TREATMENT

- Topical
  - Cool wet dressings
  - Topical anesthetic agents (e.g., benzocaine, lidocaine)
- Systemic
  - Aspirin
  - Indomethacin
- Burn unit admissions are rarely required for severe/widespread burns calling for fluid replacement and prophylaxis of infection

MANAGEMENT/FOLLOW-UP

- Burns that are severe but do not require hospitalization may require follow-up with the patient's primary care physician or dermatologist
- Hats, protective clothing, and sunscreens for future prevention

ICD-9 Code

692.71

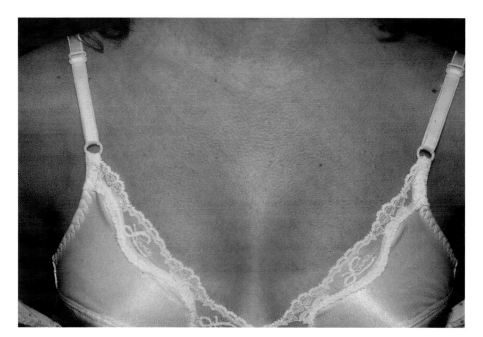

FIGURE 102-1 *Sunburn.*

CHAPTER 103

SWEET'S SYNDROME

- Sudden onset of fever preceding or accompanying the development of characteristic painful skin lesions, along with leukocytosis
- Variable associated symptoms including prodrome of malaise, arthralgia, myalgia, fever, headache, and gastrointestinal symptoms
- More common in women aged 20 to 60
- Associations with malignancies (especially hematologic), inflammatory bowel disease, and medications (all-trans retinoic acid, estradiol, minocycline, trimethoprim sulfamethoxazole, and granulocyte colony-stimulating factor)

PHYSICAL EXAMINATION

- Sharply demarcated, tender red patches, plaques, or nodules (usually larger than 1 cm) that appear vesiculated but do not express fluid (Fig. 103-1)
  - One lesion or multiple asymmetrically distributed lesions may occur
  - Involvement of the upper extremities, face, and neck is most common
  - Conjunctivitis or episcleritis may occur

- Lesions evolve to become dusky plum color
  - Lesions may coalesce to form confluent plaques that have sharp borders
  - These may become bullous or may ulcerate in severe cases
- Pathergy (development of lesions in areas of skin trauma) may occur
- Palms, soles, and mucous membranes are spared

DIAGNOSIS

- Clinical exam plus skin biopsy demonstrating dense neutrophilic infiltrate in the lower dermis
- Peripheral leukocytosis and elevated sedimentation rate may be observed, urinalysis may find proteinuria, and liver transaminases may be elevated
- Consider a chest x-ray if there are any pulmonary symptoms

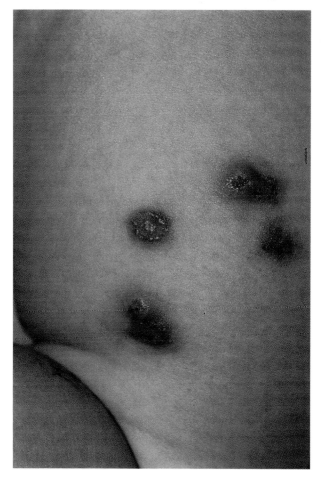

FIGURE 103-1 *Sweet's syndrome (acute febrile neurotrophic dermatosis).*

- Atypical mycobacterial infection: usually more chronic in nature but may have similar ulcer and is more likely to be confused with older lesion of Sweet's syndrome
  - A skin biopsy with special stains for acid-fast bacilli and tissue culture are necessary
- Deep fungal infection: blastomycosis, cryptococcosis, histoplasmosis, sporotrichosis, and coccidiomycosis may have acute lesions that are similar to Sweet's syndrome
  - A skin biopsy with special stains for fungi and tissue culture is necessary
- Pyoderma gangrenosum: may mimic Sweet's syndrome, but often patients with pyoderma gangrenosum have a history of inflammatory bowel disease and have fewer lesions
- Erythema multiforme: oral ulcerations associated with constitutional symptoms, a typical rash or targetoid lesions, and involvement of other mucosal sites such as the genitalia and conjunctivae
- Behçet's disease: recurrent oral and genital ulceration associated with eye disease, arthritis, vasculitis, and other skin lesions

- Patients need to be diagnosed accurately prior to treatment; if they have no systemic symptoms, then treatment is nonemergent
- Treatment may be emergent if lesions are exceptionally painful or if patients have signs of severe internal disease
- Prednisone 1 mg/kg/day tapered over 6 weeks
- Intralesional corticosteroid injection with triamcinolone acetonide (Kenalog®) 3.0 to 10 mg/ml) for isolated tender lesions
- Other miscellaneous treatments for long-term management include:
  - Oral SSKI 300 to 900 mg/day for 2 weeks
  - Colchicine 1.5 mg/day for 1 week, followed by gradual tapering over 3 weeks to 0.5 mg/day.
  - Dapsone, clofazamine, chlorambucil, indomethacin, cyclosporine, cyclophosphamide, and sulfapyridine have all been used

- All patients need follow-up with their primary care physician and/or dermatologist within a few days
- With treatment, the eruption clears spontaneously within weeks to months and heals without scarring
- Half of patients experience a recurrence, often at a previously involved site
- Watch for extracutaneous involvement including:
  - Sterile osteomyelitis, which has been observed in children
  - Aseptic meningitis: neutrophils in the cerebrospinal fluid
  - Neurologic and psychiatric problems
  - Proteinuria, less often hematuria or glomerulonephritis
  - Neutrophilic pulmonary infiltrates (culture-negative and corticosteroid-responsive)

ICD-9 Code

695.89

CHAPTER 104

PRIMARY AND SECONDARY SYPHILIS

- The presentation of the patient will vary by stage of disease
  - In primary syphilis, the patient notices an ulcer that is usually painless, most commonly found on the genitalia (penis or vulva), but it may also occur on the vaginal mucosa, cervix, perianal area, thighs, breasts, or oral mucosa
    - The primary lesion, a chancre, usually develops approximately 3 weeks after exposure to an infected person, but the time interval may span 10 to 90 days following exposure
    - Since chancres are often painless, patients may not notice their development or may ignore the spontaneously healing lesion
    - Painful regional lymphadenopathy may be present
  - In secondary syphilis, the patient may note a diffuse rash on trunk, hands, or feet, and hair loss with or without "bumps" or "warts" in the anogenital skin
    - Secondary syphilis symptoms occur 3 to 12 weeks after the chancre appears
- Syphilis is a sexually transmitted disease caused by infection with *Treponema pallidum,* a spirochete
  - The organism may be demonstrated by darkfield microscopy, immunoperoxidase staining, and serology

- Syphilis affects all races equally, and men are more frequently infected than women
- The disease is most frequently diagnosed in sexually active young adults, but it occurs in all ages
- Symptoms referable to various organ systems may be present, including lymphoreticular, ophthalmologic, auditory, respiratory, musculoskeletal, hematologic, neurologic, gastrointestinal, and cardiac systems

Primary Syphilis

- The chancre appears as a well-demarcated, indurated, firm, beefy red, painless ulcer that is usually 0.5 to 3.0 cm in diameter (Fig. 104-1)
  - Most common locations in men are the glans, coronal sulcus, foreskin, and anal mucosa
  - Most common locations in women are the labia, fourchette, urethra, and perineum
  - Other sites at highest risk include the oral mucosa, face, neck, fingers, and breast
- Regional, rubbery, palpable lymphadenopathy (buboes) may be noted

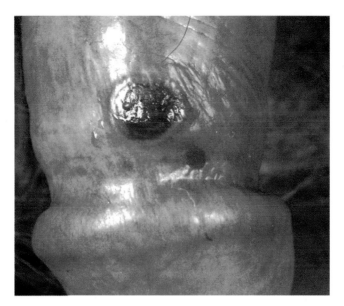

FIGURE 104-1 *Primary syphilis with chancre.*

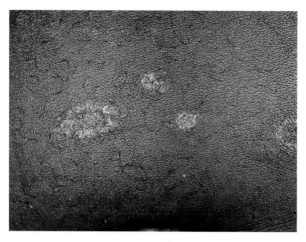

FIGURE 104-2 *Papulosquamous syphilitic eruption.*

Secondary Syphilis

- There are several different appearances, including macular, papular, annular, vesiculobullous, pustular, and nodular lesions (Fig. 104-2)
- Secondary syphilis may clinically mimic a large number of other dermatologic conditions
- The most common appearance is a symmetric, widespread distribution of pink to erythematous scaling lesions on the trunk and extremities
  - Palms and soles often have classic "copper penny" appearance, with hyperpigmented skin
  - The face is usually spared
- Condyloma lata in anogenital and mouth regions appear as soft, moist, flat-topped, red to flesh-colored papules or plaques (Fig. 104-3)
- Patchy, nonscarring, "moth-eaten" alopecia may occur
- Mucous patches are small, slightly elevated papules on the oral or genital mucosa, most commonly on the tongue and lips

DIAGNOSIS

Primary Syphilis

- This is a clinical diagnosis supported by serologic testing (RPR, VDRL, or FTAABS)
- Although examination of serous exudate from chancre by darkfield microscopy may be rapidly diagnostic, this test is now virtually unobtainable outside of high-volume sexually transmitted disease clinics
- Direct immunofluorescence of the serous exudate from chancre may aid the diagnosis

Secondary Syphilis

- This is a clinical diagnosis supported by serologic testing (RPR, VDRL, or FTAABS)
- If the diagnosis is not clear, examination of a skin biopsy with special stains may aid the diagnosis
- Warthin-Starry stain will show beaded, spirochetal rods, and immunoperoxidase staining can be performed on paraffin-embedded tissue specimens

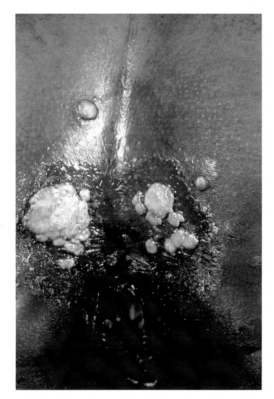

FIGURE 104-3 *Rounded, gray, moist vegetating papules associated with syphilis.*

Primary Syphilis

- Herpes simplex virus infection: groups of umbilicated vesicles, vesicolopustules, or erosions on an erythematous base may be present on any mucocutaneous surface
- Chancroid: a tender erythematous papule first appears that evolves into a pustule, erosion, and then an ulcer with sharp, undermined borders and a friable gray-yellow base of granulation on the external genitalia
- Traumatic ulceration: may occur in any location including the genitalia, and unusual, angular shapes suggesting external causes are found
- Lymphogranuloma venereum: this infection has a painless, nonindurated superficial ulcer in association with painful regional lymphadenopathy
- Granuloma inguinale: presents with one or more painless nodules in the genital areas
- Erythema multiforme: this reaction pattern is often associated with constitutional symptoms, a typical rash of targetoid lesions, and involvement of other mucosal sites such as the oral mucosa and conjunctivae
- Aphthous ulcers: these painful ulcers of the oral or genital mucosa can mimic chancroid, but aphthous ulcers tend to be shallower and have no associated lymphadenopathy
- Crohn's disease: this inflammatory bowel disease may present ulcers that are usually linear and resemble lacerations
- Squamous cell or basal cell carcinoma: these cancers may occur in the anogenital area or anywhere on the body, but they have a chronic, slowly Enlarging course lasting months to years

Secondary Syphilis

- Pityriasis rosea: this condition has no palm or sole lesions, and mucous membranes are normal
  - If there is any confusion, serologic testing for syphilis such as an RPR should be performed
- Drug eruption: drug eruptions can uncommonly present with discreet scaling papules on the trunk and extremities, but there are no palm or sole lesions, and mucous membranes are normal
- Lichen planus: can produce a large number of raised, erythematous to violaceous papules with Wickham's striae in the oral and possibly anogenital mucosae, but palm or sole lesions are generally absent
- Viral exanthem
- Tinea (pityriasis) versicolor: this fungal infection produces scaling and hypopigmentation and hyperpigmentation of the trunk, with sparing of the mucous membranes and palms and soles
- Psoriasis: guttate psoriasis can present with multiple, round, scaling, generalized, erythematous macules and papules, with sparing of the mucous membranes and palms and soles

Primary and Secondary Syphilis

- The treatment of choice is benzathine penicillin G 2.4 million units intramuscularly as a one-time dose
- If the patient is allergic to penicillin, uncomplicated syphilis may be treated with doxycycline 100 mg by mouth bid, tetracycline 500 mg qid by mouth for 28 days, or ceftriaxone 125 mg intramuscularly daily or 250 mg intramuscularly every other day for 10 days
- Consider drawing an HIV test to help guide treatment
- In HIV-positive patients, benzathine penicillin G 2.4 million units intramuscularly per week for 3 weeks is preferred by some physicians
- If the infection occurs in a child, the patient should be evaluated for congenital syphilis
   - If acquired after birth, may use benzathine penicillin G 50,000 units/kg up to 2.4 million units

- Patients need follow-up evaluation with their primary care physician, sexually transmitted disease clinic, or dermatologist within 2 weeks to make certain they have had resolution of their disease
- Patients need reevaluation at 6 and 12 months for clinical and serologic evaluation
   - If patients are HIV-positive, consider reevaluation at 3, 6, 9, 12, and 24 months
- Patients should be re-treated if a fourfold or greater increase in the RPR titer occurs within 6 months
   - Must be evaluated for neurosyphilis if relapse suspected
   - If there is no evidence of neurosyphilis, re-treat with benzathine penicillin G 2.4 million units intramuscularly per week for 3 weeks

ICD-9-CM Codes

091.2   Primary syphilis
091.3   Secondary syphilis

TELOGEN EFFLUVIUM

HISTORY

- A patient of any age presents with diffuse hair loss without associated pain or irritation of the scalp
- Patients may report recent history of systemic illness, hospitalization, change in medication (beta-blockers, female hormones, retinoids, anticoagulants, angiotensin-converting enzyme inhibitors, and chemotherapeutic agents), nutritional disorders, or physical or psychological stress
  - The stressor occurs usually 3 to 4 months before onset of hair loss

PHYSICAL EXAMINATION

- Diffuse thinning on the scalp with decreased number of hair shafts and no scarring (Fig. 105-1)
- No primary lesions or significant erythema are visible on the scalp
- A pull test (attempting to manually remove hairs from scalp with minimal tension between thumb and second finger) is positive, with three or more hairs noted on each pull
- Hair shafts under microscope appears normal, but telogen (club) hairs seen

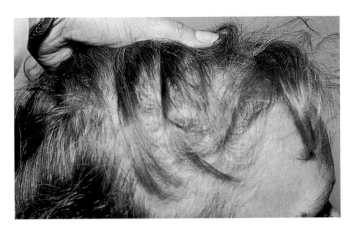

FIGURE 105-1 *Telogen effluvium.*

- This diagnosis is usually made by history and physical exam, especially if an inciting event can be found
- A skin biopsy is rarely necessary to distinguish from other types of alopecia
- Laboratory examination may be necessary to evaluate for causes of telogen effluvium, including complete blood count, as well as thyroid-stimulating hormone and iron studies

DIFFERENTIAL DIAGNOSIS

- Diffuse alopecia areata: may be quite difficult to distinguish from telogen effluvium
  - If telogen effluvium is nonresolving, a skin biopsy may be warranted to distinguish it from alopecia areata
- Tinea capitis: usually has an inflammatory component of the scalp, with scaling and erythema
  - Usually tinea capitis is more localized than telogen effluvium, and KOH preparation examination of the hair shaft will be positive
- Androgenetic alopecia: usually begins in the third and fourth decades of life and has a classic distribution of vertex and frontal involvement with a receding hairline or vertex thinning in men and women
  - The pull test is usually negative
  - Rarely, a skin biopsy will help to distinguish these two
- Hair shaft abnormality: this congenital condition presents with broken-off hairs instead of patchy alopecia, but it may be diffuse like telogen effluvium
  - Microscopic evaluation of the hair shaft shows characteristic abnormalities

- Trichotillomania: patchy alopecia with broken hair shafts of different lengths; the pull test is negative, and trichotillomania has a "moth-eaten" appearance
- Chemical trauma: permanent wave or hair-straightening procedures may cause hair shafts to become quite brittle, breaking off with the pull test mid-shaft

TREATMENT

- No specific treatment is necessary, since it is usually a self-limited process
- Patient reassurance is absolutely required as this may be a very psychologically stressful disease
- Some physicians advocate using topical minoxidil in an attempt to increase the growth of the remaining hairs, but others do not

MANAGEMENT/FOLLOW-UP

- If follow-up is warranted, patients can see their primary care physician or dermatologist nonemergently
- Telogen effluvium will resolve without treatment if the etiology can be determined and removed, but it may take 6 to 12 months for hair volume to return to normal

ICD-9-CM Code

704.02

CHAPTER 106

THROMBOTIC THROMBOCYTOPENIC PURPURA

HISTORY

- The patient presents with diffuse petechiae or ecchymoses that may be accompanied by jaundice, fever, and nonspecific constitutional symptoms such as nausea, abdominal pain, and arthralgias
- This is a condition for which the etiology is unknown, but it is felt that the manifestations are caused by localized platelet thrombi and fibrin deposition
- The major findings, each of which has its own associated signs and symptoms, include thrombocytopenic purpura, microangiopathic hemolytic anemia, fever, renal disease, and central nervous symptoms
- This condition affects all ages, primarily young adults; women are more frequently affected than men
- It is most commonly idiopathic

PHYSICAL EXAMINATION

- The patient may be febrile
- Nonpalpable petechiae and ecchymoses are found diffusely on the extremities and the trunk (Fig. 106-1)
- Yellow discoloration of the sclera and of the skin may be noted, indicating jaundice
- Internally, patients may have renal and neurologic involvement in addition to the hematologic abnormalities that define this disease

DIAGNOSIS

- Made by finding a combination of a hemolytic anemia with schistocytes, thrombocytopenia, fever, and neurologic and renal abnormalities
- Patients generally have normal or only slightly abnormal coagulation tests and fibrin levels
- Examination of a skin biopsy shows arterioles filled with hyaline material, presumably fibrin and platelets; a direct immunofluorescence examination may show immunoglobulin and complement in the arterioles

DIFFERENTIAL DIAGNOSIS

- Idiopathic (autoimmune) thrombocytopenic purpura: occurs both in children (acute form) and adults (chronic form) and presents with petechiae and ecchymoses, gastrointestinal bleeding, menorrhagia, epistaxis, bleeding gums, and possibly intracranial hemorrhage with the presence of antiplatelet antibodies
- Disseminated intravascular coagulation: presents with widespread petechiae and ecchymoses, profuse bleeding from multiple sites, fragmented red blood cells on smear, prolonged prothrombin time and activated partial thromboplastin time, reduced fibrinogen level, and elevated fibrin degradation products

- The treatment is emergent
- The aim of treatment is generally to stabilize the patient hemodynamically, begin initial evaluation, and obtain hematologic consultation to manage the condition
- Treatments that have been used include chemotherapeutic agents, plasmapheresis, glucocorticoids, splenectomy, and antiplatelet drugs

- Patients may die within weeks, so intensive inpatient management is urgently required
- Usually for lasts days to weeks but may continue for months
- Patients should be followed closely by a hematologist and have monitoring of their hematologic parameters

ICD-9-CM Code

446.6

CPT Code

11100 Biopsy

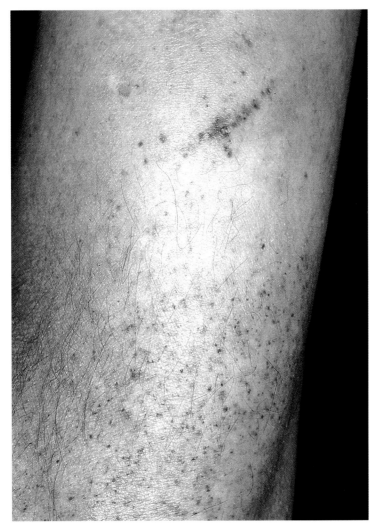

FIGURE 106-1 *Thrombocytopenic purpura. Myriads of petechiae on the upper arm of an HIV -infected 25-year-old male were the presenting manifestation of his disease. A linear arrangement of petechiae with an ecchymosis at the site of minor trauma.*

CHAPTER 107

TINEA CAPITIS

- The patient, usually a young child, presents with hair loss in focal areas on the scalp of weeks' to months' duration
- Tinea capitis is more common in black and Hispanic children
- Since transmission by direct contact, either person-to-person, animal-to-person, or through fomites, patients may recall exposure to an infected person
- Lesions may itch or burn slightly, but if a kerion forms, then there is often associated pain and tenderness
- Tinea capitis is caused by dermatophyte infection, most commonly *Trichophyton tonsurans* in the United States and less commonly *Microsporum canis*

PHYSICAL EXAMINATION

- Ectothrix tinea capitis (the organism lives outside the hair shaft just under the cuticle)
  - Scaly patches of alopecia on the scalp with minimal inflammation and broken-off hairs just above the scalp with a gray, dull appearance (Fig. 107-1)
  - Focal patches may coalesce into larger patches
- Endothrix (the organism lives within the hair shaft)

- "Black dot" lesions are found, in which scaling patches of alopecia contain small, black dots noted at the scalp surface where hairs have broken off, with associated inflammation (Fig. 107-2)
- Lesions are usually poorly circumscribed and can mimic seborrheic dermatitis
- Inflammatory follicle-based pustules may lead to kerion formation (Fig. 107-3)
  - A kerion is an inflammatory mass with surface pustules studded with broken hairs and purulent exudates
  - This condition is usually associated with cervical and occipital lymphadenopathy
  - Favus is another result of inflammation, with the observation of thick, cup-shaped, yellow-colored crusts filled with skin fragments and hyphae associated with scarring

DIAGNOSIS

- The diagnosis usually made by finding a scaling alopecia and is confirmed by KOH preparation examination or fungal culture
  - In ectothrix infection, plucked hairs demonstrate spores surrounding the hair shaft in the cuticle

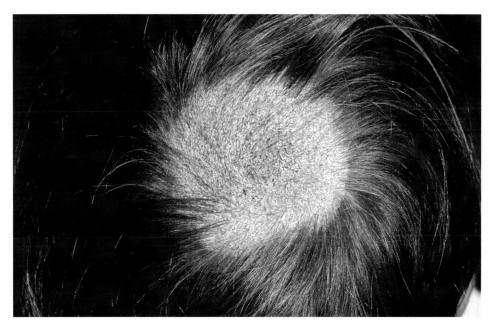

FIGURE 107-1 *Tinea capitis: "gray patch" type.*

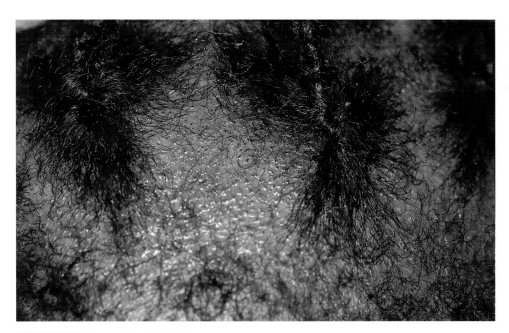

FIGURE 107-2 *Tinea capitis: "black dot" type.*

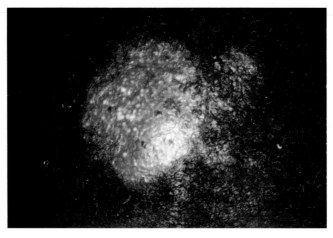

FIGURE 107-3 *Kerion on scalp.*

- In endothrix infection, plucked hairs demonstrate spores within the hair shaft
- In favus, hyphae are present within the hair shaft without associated spores
- Wood's lamp examination possibly useful in *Microsporum* infections, which shows a bright green band of fluorescence above the level of the scalp
- Rarely, a skin biopsy is needed to distinguish from inflammatory processes of the scalp

DIFFERENTIAL DIAGNOSIS

- Psoriasis: may closely mimic tinea capitis, but psoriasis has considerably more erythema than tinea capitis
  - Evidence of psoriasis elsewhere on the body will be helpful in diagnosis, and KOH preparation examination for fungus will be negative in psoriasis
- Atopic dermatitis: usually one will see evidence of atopic dermatitis elsewhere on body, and KOH preparation examination will be negative

- Seborrheic dermatitis: can present very similarly to tinea capitis, but KOH preparation examination is negative for hyphae
  - Evidence of seborrheic dermatitis may be found elsewhere on the body such as on the eyebrows, forehead, and ears
- Alopecia areata: may mimic tinea capitis, but alopecia areata demonstrates no evidence of scaling or black dots, and KOH preparation examination will be negative
- Trichotillomania: patchy alopecia with broken hair shafts of different lengths and a "moth-eaten" appearance; KOH preparation examination will be negative
- Secondary syphilis: black dots are absent, and the "moth-eaten" appearance may be present
  - Syphilis serology may be helpful in distinguishing these two, and KOH preparation examination will be negative

TREATMENT

- The treatment of tinea capitis is nonemergent
- Tinea capitis requires systemic treatment
  - Griseofulvin microsize (Grifulvin®) 10 to 20 mg/kg per day taken with a fatty meal is commonly used in children (maximum dose of 500 mg per day) for 6 to 8 weeks with oral therapy; some physicians advocate checking complete blood count and liver function tests while on therapy, but others believe it is not necessary
  - In adults, griseofulvin microsize (Grifulvin®) 250 to 500 mg by mouth twice per day for 1 to 2 months is the usual dose
- Other treatment options include itraconazole and terbinafine
  - Itraconazole (Sporanox®) 3 to 5 mg/kg/day is recommended for 6 to 10 weeks for children; dose is 200 mg per day for adults; may monitor liver function tests
  - Terbinafine (Lamisil®) 125 mg/day for 4 to 6 weeks in children <40 kg; in adults, 250 mg per day; may monitor liver function tests

- Systemic corticosteroid therapy may be needed in patients with kerion; prednisone 1 mg/kg/day for the first 7 to 14 days of antifungal therapy is usually given
- If secondary bacterial infection is present, systemic antibiotics may also be necessary such as erythromycin, dicloxacillin, or cephalexin

MANAGEMENT/FOLLOW-UP

- Patient will need follow-up with his or her primary care physician or dermatologist in several weeks to assess progress

ICD-9 Code

110.0

CHAPTER 108

TINEA CORPORIS

HISTORY

- Patients present with one or more enlarging, itchy, red areas on their body
- Family members may have similar lesions and may have a new pet in the home
- Tinea corporis is spread mostly by direct contact
- Affects all ages and both sexes equally
- Often patient has tinea pedis as well
- The most common agents are *Trichophyton rubrum, Microsporum canis,* and *Trichophyton mentagrophytes*
- The organism lives in the stratum corneum of the skin, never invading into the deeper dermis, but extension down hair follicles may occur (Majocchi's granuloma)

PHYSICAL EXAMINATION

- Annular, nonscarring plaques with erythematous, scaling, expanding borders and central clearing (Figs. 108-1 and 108-2)
- If hair follicles are involved, one may observe erythematous, follicular-based papules within plaque

DIAGNOSIS

- Diagnosis is usually suggested by physical exam and history, but confirmation with examination of a KOH preparation is helpful
  - A KOH preparation may only be positive in one-third of patients, so fungal cultures can become important as well to confirm the diagnosis
- If a prominent follicle-based component is noted, a skin biopsy may be necessary to evaluate for hair shaft involvement

DIFFERENTIAL DIAGNOSIS

- Granuloma annulare: often has annulae, but these annulae lack scale and have little erythema, and KOH preparation and fungal culture results are negative
- Erythema annulare centrifigum: this rare condition can present with multiple scaling, erythematous, truncal annulae, but the KOH preparation and fungal culture results are negative

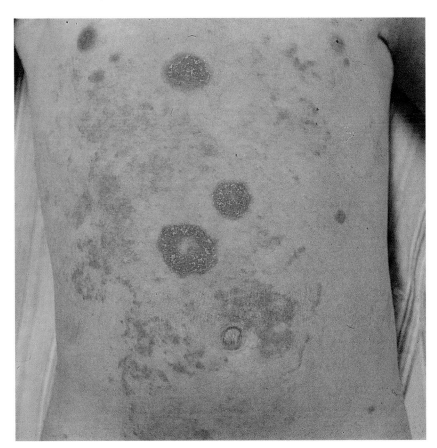

FIGURE 108-1   *Tinea corporis: acute and subacute.*

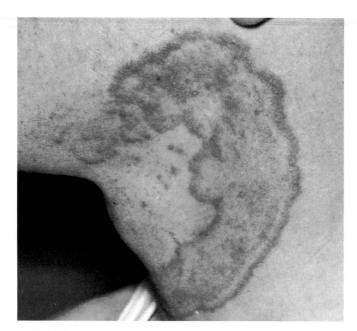

FIGURE 108-2 *Tinea corporis with typical "ringworm-like" configuration.*

- Nummular eczema: does not generally display annulae
- Subacute cutaneous lupus erythematosus: this variant of lupus erythematosus presents with scaling annular plaques of the trunk, associated with many serologic findings of lupus, and KOH preparation and fungal culture results are negative
- Secondary syphilis: generally does not display annulae, and KOH preparation and fungal culture results are negative
- Psoriasis: generally does not display annulae, and KOH preparation and fungal culture results are negative
- Mycosis fungoides: this T-cell lymphoma is a chronic condition that may present with patches and plaques, some of which may be configurate annulae, but KOH preparation and fungal culture results are negative
- Pityriasis rosea

TREATMENT

- Treatment is nonemergent
- For localized, typical plaques that are few in number, topical antifungal agents may be used
- Daily topical treatment with allylamines such as naftifine (Naftin®) cream or terbinafine (Lamisil®) cream or imidazoles such as econazole (Spectazole®) or keto-conazole (Nizoral®) for 1 to 3 weeks
- For more widespread involvement or for patients with follicular involvement, systemic therapy with oral medications in adults, such as itraconazole (Sporanox®) 200 mg qid for 7 to 14 days, or terbinafine (Lamisil®) 250 mg per day for 7 to 14 days (adult dosages)

MANAGEMENT/FOLLOW-UP

- Patients should follow up with their primary care physician or dermatologist after therapy is completed (in 2 to 4 weeks) to be sure that areas have been adequately treated
- Lesions that do not respond to treatment may require a skin biopsy to exclude other disease process

ICD-9-CM Code

110.5

TINEA CRURIS

HISTORY

- Patient presents with itchy rash in the groin, describing the rash as "jock itch"
- Usually occurs in adults and men more commonly than women
- Usually acquired by direct contact but has also been reported to be transmitted indirectly by contact with fomites
- Patient who has tinea cruris will often also have tinea pedis
- Infection is caused by a dermatophyte, most commonly *Epidermophyton floccosum, Trichophyton rubrum, and T. mentagrophytes*
- Occurs more commonly in the summertime and in warm, humid climates

PHYSICAL EXAMINATION

- Erythematous, lichenified, somewhat annular, well-defined, confluent plaques with a raised, papular, scaly border and central clearing in groin area (Fig. 109-1)
- Scrotum is almost always completely spared
- Maceration may be noted, which is related to the nature of the moist area of the groin
- Feet may show evidence of tinea pedis

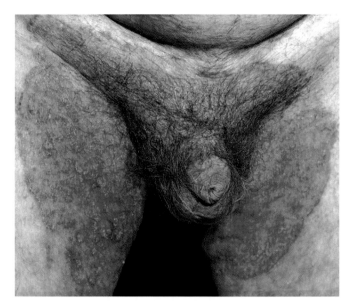

FIGURE 109-1 *Tinea cruris.*

- Diagnosis is usually made by history and physical exam; KOH preparation of scale in the area shows septate, branching hyphae, and fungal culture should be positive
- Sparing of the scrotum and presence of tinea pedis is also a helpful clue
- Biopsy rarely warranted, but may be necessary to rule out some other disease processes

DIFFERENTIAL DIAGNOSIS

- Candidiasis: may mimic tinea cruris closely, but often involves the scrotum and will show pseudohyphae and spores on KOH preparation; pustules may also be seen
- Psoriasis: close mimic of tinea cruris; evidence of classic psoriasis elsewhere on the body may be helpful, and KOH preparation will be negative
- Erythrasma: may be difficult to distinguish from tinea cruris, and may also coexist with it; Wood's lamp examination in erythrasma will show a coral-red fluorescence
- Seborrheic dermatitis: can present very similarly to tinea cruris, but KOH preparation is negative for hyphae, and evidence of seborrheic dermatitis elsewhere on the body is helpful
- Benign familial pemphigus, Langerhans cell histiocytosis, and Darier's disease are other disease processes that may require biopsy to distinguish between them, especially in eruptions unresponsive to antifungal treatments

TREATMENT

- Treatment is nonemergent
- Daily topical treatment with allylamines such as naftifine (Naftin®) cream or terbinafine (Lamisil®) cream or imidazoles such as econazole (Spectazole®) or ketoconazole (Nizoral®) for 1 to 3 weeks
- For more severe or bullous cases, may need systemic therapy with oral medications in adults, such as itraconazole (Sporanox®) 200 mg qid for 7 to 14 days, or terbinafine (Lamisil®) 250 mg per day for 7 to 14 days (adult dosages)
- Topical or oral antibiotic therapy may be necessary to treat secondary bacterial infections
- Keeping areas clean and dry may also be quite helpful
  ○ Absorbent antifungal powders (e.g., Micatin® or Zeasorb AF® powder) may be helpful in maintaining dryness and decreasing the risk of future colonization

MANAGEMENT/FOLLOW-UP

- No specific follow-up is required. In recurrent cases, evaluation for concurrent tinea pedis and treatment may be helpful in management

ICD-9 Code

110.3

CPT Code

None

CHAPTER 110

TINEA PEDIS

- Patient presents with complaints of itching, scaling, and cracking of the feet of months' to years' duration; may be unaware of infection in some cases
- Tinea pedis is spread by direct contact and through contact with infected surfaces
- Hot, humid weather and occlusive footwear are predisposing factors
- Occurs most commonly in the third to fifth decades of life
- There are four main types of infection
  - Interdigital: most common type and is prominent in the web spaces, but is often asymptomatic; commonly caused by *Trichophyton rubrum, T. mentagrophytes,* and *Epidermophyton floccosum*
  - Moccasin type: chronic papulosquamous type that is usually bilateral and most commonly caused by *T. rubrum*; hands and toenails may also be involved
  - Vesiculobullous type: least common form of disease, usually involving the plantar surface; most commonly caused by *T. mentagrophytes* var. *mentagrophytes*
  - Ulcerative type: usually acute and associated with ulceration, maceration, pain, and a pungent odor; usually caused by *T. rubrum, E. floccosum,* and *T. mentagrophytes*
- Frequently, secondary infection with bacteria and/or *Candida* occurs

- Interdigital: scaling, maceration, and fissuring with minimal erythema in the interdigital areas, with lateral toe web spaces being the most common sites of infection (Fig. 110-1)
- Moccasin type: fine white scaling and hyperkeratosis along the lateral borders of the feet, heels, and soles, occasionally with well-demarcated erythema and fine papules; usually affects both feet and may be asymptomatic (Fig. 110-2)
- Vesiculobullous type: vesicles, vesiculopustules, and erythema on the instep and plantar surface of feet
- Ulcerative type: maceration, fissuring, weeping, and denudation spreading onto dorsal and plantar surfaces

- Usually made by history and physical exam, with the help of KOH preparations, which show septate, branching hyphae
- Fungal culture may also be helpful, and biopsy is needed rarely

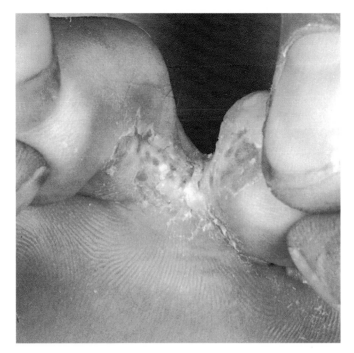

FIGURE 110-1 *Tinea pedis, interdigital.*

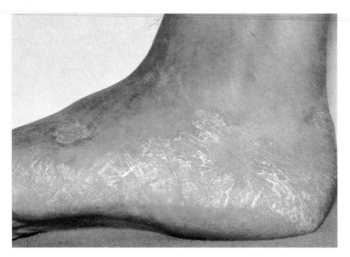

FIGURE 110-2 *Tinea pedis.*

- Candidiasis: may mimic tinea pedis closely; see pseudohyphae and spores on KOH preparation
- Psoriasis: may also mimic tinea pedis, but evidence of classic psoriasis elsewhere on the body helpful in diagnosis, and KOH preparation will be negative
- Erythrasma: may be difficult to distinguish from tinea pedis and may also coexist with it; Wood's lamp examination in erythrasma will show a coral-red fluorescence
- Allergic contact dermatitis and dyshidrotic eczema may be considered in the vesiculobullous variant of tinea pedis; KOH preparation of these diseases will be negative for hyphae

TREATMENT

- Treatment is nonemergent
- Daily topical treatment with allylamines such as naftifine (Naftin®) cream or terbinafine (Lamisil®) cream or imidazoles such as econazole (Spectazole®) or ketoconazole (Nizoral®) for 1 to 3 weeks
- For more severe or bullous cases, may need systemic therapy with oral medications in adults, such as itraconazole (Sporanox®) 200 mg qid for 7 to 14 days, or terbinafine (Lamisil®) 250 mg per day for 7 to 14 days (adult dosages)

- Topical or oral antibiotic therapy may be necessary to treat secondary bacterial infections
- Keeping areas clean and dry may also be quite helpful
  - Absorbent antifungal powders (e.g., Micatin® or Zeasorb AF® powder) may be helpful in maintaining dryness and decreasing the risk of future colonization

MANAGEMENT/FOLLOW-UP

- May be a chronic, recurrent disease process, especially in the elderly, those with diabetes, or immunocompromised patients
- No specific follow-up is necessary; however, treating tinea pedis in patients with diabetes and lymphedema may help prevent cellulitis since tinea pedis may be a portal of entry for bacteria into the skin

ICD-9-CM Code

110.4

CHAPTER 111

TINEA VERSICOLOR (PITYRIASIS VERSICOLOR)

HISTORY

- The patient presents with light or dark scaly patches
- The most common time of onset is the summer, when affected areas do not tan to same extent as normal-appearing skin surrounding the lesions
- This condition may be mildly pruritic or asymptomatic
- The causative organism is *Malassezia furfur,* an organism that is considered normal flora of the skin
- This condition affects males and females equally
- Found in areas of skin where sebum production is greater

PHYSICAL EXAMINATION

- One finds hypopigmented or hyperpigmented patches with a very fine, powdery, superficial scale on truncal areas including the chest, back, abdomen, neck, and proximal extremities (Figs. 111-1 and 111-2)
- Lesion color varies from white to reddish brown, with the lighter color due to metabolites made by *M. furfur* that inhibit tyrosinase in basal keratinocytes

DIAGNOSIS

- A KOH preparation of the scale from the lesion reveals clusters of yeast and short, septate branching hyphae; often called "spaghetti and meatballs" appearance
- Culture and biopsy are not necessary since KOH preparation has the characteristic appearance under microscope
- Wood's lamp examination may show yellowish fluorescence of involved skin

DIFFERENTIAL DIAGNOSIS

- Nummular eczema: usually more erythematous and eczematous in appearance than tinea versicolor, tends to involve extremities more than trunk, and KOH preparation does not reveal yeasts or hyphae
- Pityriasis rosea: can have similar appearance to tinea versicolor but tends to have a "Christmas tree" distribution on the trunk, and KOH preparation of the scale is negative
- Secondary syphilis: the history of this patient is different, such as having a chancre in the past, and serology will help with diagnosis since patient should have a positive RPR

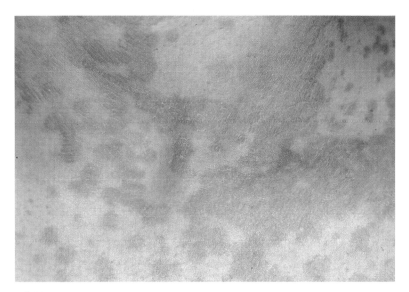

FIGURE 111-1 *Pityriasis versicolor.*

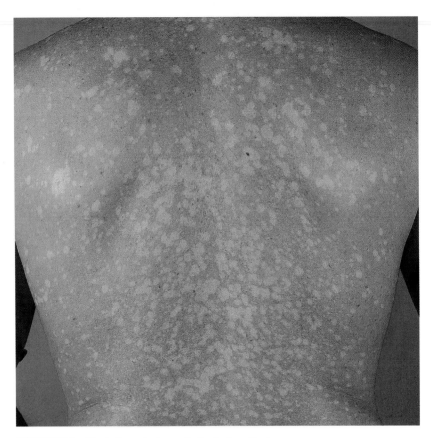

FIGURE 111-2 *Pityriasis versicolor on the back of a patient.*

TINEA VERSICOLOR (PITYRIASIS VERSICOLOR)

- Seborrheic dermatitis: has a different distribution than tinea versicolor, often involving the scalp and perinasal/perieyebrow areas, as well as the central chest and periauricular area.
- Vitiligo: usually begins acrally, not truncally, and comprises depigmented, nonscaling patches as opposed to hypopigmented, scaling patches

TREATMENT

- The treatment of tinea versicolor is non-emergent
- No therapy is curative, and treatments used are suppressive only
- Selenium sulfide (Selsun®) 2.5% lotion or shampoo can be used
  - If using the lotion, should be used once per day for 2 weeks and then once per day for the first 7 days of each month as suppressive therapy
  - If using the shampoo, patient should lather the affected areas liberally, leave on 10 minutes, then rinse, daily for 2 weeks, then once per day for the first 7 days of each month as suppressive therapy

- Ketoconazole (Nizoral®) shampoo can be used in similar manner
- Oral itraconazole (Sporanox®) 400 mg po for 2 days or ketoconazole (Nizoral®) 400 mg po as a one-time dose at initial diagnosis should help clear the skin lesions more quickly than topicals alone
  - Because ketoconazole has poor keratin affinity, patients should exercise 1 to 2 hours later and perspire, which helps to deposit the medication on the skin surface

MANAGEMENT/FOLLOW-UP

- The patient can follow up with the primary care physician or dermatologist on an as-needed basis

ICD-9 Code
111.0

CHAPTER 112

TOXIC EPIDERMAL NECROLYSIS (TEN)

HISTORY

- Patients report the sudden onset of erythema and tenderness of the skin with subsequent detachment of large portions of the epidermis
- Patients may have a variable prodrome of fever, malaise, arthralgia, myalgia, anorexia, nausea, vomiting, pharyngitis, cough, photophobia, and dysuria
- There may be a history of a new medication, including sulfonamide and other antibiotics, anticonvulsant agents, nonsteroidal antiinflammatory drugs, or allopurinol, but more than 100 different drugs have been implicated
- Other reported historic causes may also be reported, including Mycoplasma pneumoniae, vaccination, hepatitis, inflammatory bowel disease, radiotherapy, and malignancy
- Females are twice as likely to develop toxic epidermal necrolysis as males, and the disease is more common in adults than in children
- The incidence of toxic epidermal necrolysis is greatly increased in the HIV-infected population
- Mucosal involvement may make eating and breathing difficult; anogenital involvement may lead to urinary retention
- Conjunctival involvement may present with conjunctivitis, lacrimation, or photophobia
- Respiratory tract mucosal involvement may make breathing difficult, with cough, bronchial obstruction, and bronchopneumonia
- Gastrointestinal tract involvement may produce diarrhea, abdominal pain, bleeding, colonic perforation, and hepatitis
- Dehydration and electrolyte imbalance may lead to pulmonary edema, mental confusion and obtundation, coma, and seizures

PHYSICAL EXAMINATION

- Patients appear ill
- Confluent erythema involving the face and upper body, with rapid spread to involve most body surfaces (erythroderma; Figs. 112-1 and 112-2)
- Atypical target lesions that are flat, irregularly shaped macules and patches with dusky centers; may coalesce
- Large flaccid blisters and erosions develop in involved sites, followed by sheet-like sloughing of the epidermis at pressure points
- Mucous membranes may display painful erosions
  - In one-third of patients, mucous membrane involvement precedes cutaneous involvement by 1 to 3 days

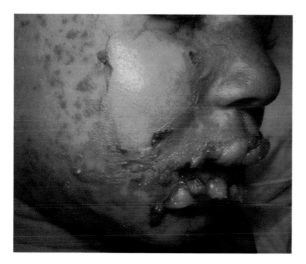

FIGURE 112-1 *Toxic epidermal necrolysis.*

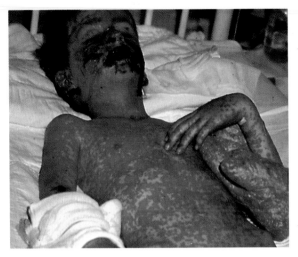

FIGURE 112-2   *Toxic epidermal necrolysis.*

- ○ The mucous membranes become sore and burn, develop erythema, and then vesiculate, leading to erosions covered by grayish-white pseudomembrane or hemorrhagic crust
- ○ Any mucous membrane may be involved, including the eyes, nose, mouth, and anogenital mucosae
- The Nikolsky and Asboe-Hansen signs may be present
  - ○ Nikolsky sign: in patients with active blisters, rubbing the skin with a gloved finger will produce an erosion
  - ○ Asboe-Hansen sign: light lateral pressure on the blister edge spreads the blister into clinically normal skin
- Hypotension and tachycardia may produce fainting and cardiac symptoms

DIAGNOSIS

- This is a diagnosis based on the clinical history and physical exam
- This diagnosis is usually supplemented by emergent examination of a skin biopsy specimen

- Thermal burns: the history provides conclusive help in this differentiation
- Drug eruption: toxic epidermal necrolysis may be a hypersensitivity reaction to a drug, but typical drug eruptions lack painful sheets of erythema that vesiculate and slough
- Erythema multiforme: tends to present with more distinct, individual lesions rather than broad sheets of erythema, but early in the course of both, differentiation may be impossible
- Acute graft-vs-host disease: following a bone marrow or other allograft transplant, patients may present with signs and symptoms that are virtually identical clinically to those of toxic epidermal necrolysis
- Staphylococcal scalded skin syndrome: occurs most commonly in children, whereas toxic epidermal necrolysis occurs most commonly in adults
  - Staphylococcal scalded skin syndrome patients have an infection source of staphylococci
  - Both conditions may present with sloughing painful skin, but the erosions of staphylococcal scalded skin syndrome are more superficial than those of toxic epidermal necrolysis
- Viral exanthem: does not cause painful sheets of erythema that vesiculate and slough

- Treatment is emergent and supportive, and patients need management virtually identical to that of serious thermal burn patients
- If a cause can be identified, it should be withdrawn or treated
- Fluid resuscitation, skin coverage with bland ointments and dressings, and burn intensive care unit protocols are required
  - If widespread disease is present, transfer to a facility with a burn unit may be imperative
- Systemic corticosteroids are controversial and are probably not helpful
- Pulmonary care, ophthalmologic supportive care, urologic care, gynecologic care, and gastrointestinal care may all be required
- Necrotic tissue may require periodic debridement once the disease activity has stopped

- Lengthy burn unit stays are the norm for survivors
- New lesions may develop for days to weeks
- All the sequelae of major thermal burns, from sepsis to scarring, occur

ICD-9-CM Code

695.1

TOXIC SHOCK SYNDROME

HISTORY

- Sudden onset of high fever with multisystemic signs and symptoms: headache, myalgia, diarrhea, nausea, vomiting, pharyngitis
- A common history is that of menses in women using superabsorbent tampons
- Any infection with toxigenic strains of *Staphylococcus* may precipitate toxic shock syndrome (TSS), including postpartum infections, septic abortions, empyema, osteomyelitis, abscesses, and postsurgical wound infections
- Hypotension resulting in fainting, shock, ventricular arrhythmias, disseminated intravascular coagulation, adult respiratory distress syndrome, and renal failure are all potential sequelae

PHYSICAL EXAMINATION

- The patient appears ill and generally has a fever of 38.8°C or higher
- There may be clinical evidence of hypotension, peripheral edema, and muscle tenderness
- On skin examination one finds a flexurally accentuated early macular or maculopapular exanthem that becomes diffuse and may resemble scarlet fever
- The distribution always involves extremities, with erythematous palms and soles
- Erythema of the mucous membranes with conjunctival injection is commonly observed (Fig. 113-1)
- Sheet-like desquamation of the involved skin (usually palms and soles) after 1 to 2 weeks
- Patients may also display reversible alopecia and nail shedding

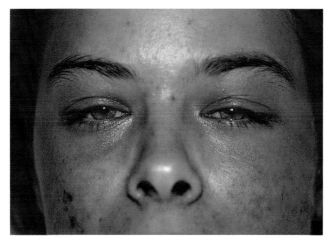

A.

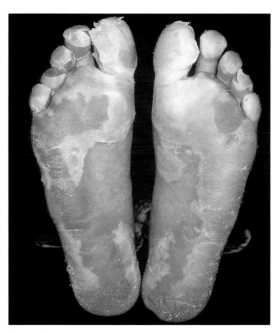

B.

FIGURE 113-1 S. aureus: *toxic shock syndrome.*

- This is a clinical diagnosis made by the combination of high fever and generalized erythematous eruption, followed by desquamation and hypotension, with at least three organ systems involved

DIFFERENTIAL DIAGNOSIS

- Drug eruption: fever, hypotension, and multiorgan involvement are rare in drug eruptions
- Streptococcal toxic shock-like syndrome: may closely mimic staphylococcal TSS and may need emergent treatment

- Scarlet fever: presents with a more typical sandpaper-like eruption and evidence of streptococcal infection
- Rocky Mountain spotted fever: petechiae, especially of the palms and soles, are more common with Rocky Mountain spotted fever
  - Patients also may have a recent history of tick bite, headache, and night sweats
- Acute meningococcemia: petechiae and frank purpura in the appropriate clinical setting are more commonly seen with meningococcemia

- Treatment of this condition is emergent
- Immediate fluid replacement intervention to treat/prevent shock
- Systemic antistaphylococcal antibiotics
  - Nafcillin 10 to 15 g IV q4hr in adults
- Remove any source of local staphylococcal infection (e.g., abscess or tampon)
- Immune globulin (400 mg/kg over 2 to 3 hours) containing antibodies to staphylococcal toxins
- Systemic corticosteroids are of uncertain benefit

- Patients usually require a lengthy hospital stay with close monitoring
- Multisystem involvement may include:
  - Myalgias and rhabdomyolysis
  - Encephalopathy
  - Azotemia
  - Elevated aspartate aminotransferase and serum bilirubin
  - Thrombocytopenia

ICD-9 Code

040.89

URTICARIA

HISTORY

- Patient presents with transient, migratory, pruritic hives
- Individual lesion do not last longer than 24 hours
- Urticaria may occasionally be associated with angioedema symptoms including difficulty in breathing and wheezing
- Urticaria affects 15% to 25% of the population at some point in their lifetime
- Eruption of urticaria is usually acute in onset and lasts less than 6 weeks
  - If urticaria persists longer than 6 weeks, it becomes chronic urticaria
- Occasionally, a trigger, such as an infection, medication, or food, can be pinpointed
- Urticaria is divided into several subtypes: immunologic (IgE-mediated, complement-mediated), physical (dermatographism, cold, solar, cholinergic, vibratory), urticaria related to direct mast cell degranulation (contrast media, narcotics, nonsteroidal antiinflammatory drugs [NSAIDs], etc.), and urticaria associated with autoimmune connective tissue disorders
- Angioedema is similar to urticaria, but it involves deeper dermis and subcutaneous tissues, thus leading to more diffuse, deeper lesions

PHYSICAL EXAMINATION

- Erythematous, urticarial papules and plaques that may be oval to annular in shape, ranging in size from 0.5 to 8 cm (Fig. 114-1)
- Lesions may be found at any location on the body
- Dermatographism, or creation of urticarial wheals by gently stroking the back with a fingernail or other blunt object

DIAGNOSIS

- The diagnosis is based on the history and physical exam
- A skin biopsy is rarely necessary to rule out other disease processes, such as urticarial vasculitis, which is a more serious disease associated with internal manifestations
- Unless evaluation is required for a concurrent condition, no specific laboratory evaluation is needed in acute urticaria
- In cases of chronic urticaria, further systemic evaluation may be necessary including complete blood count with differential and other tests deemed necessary

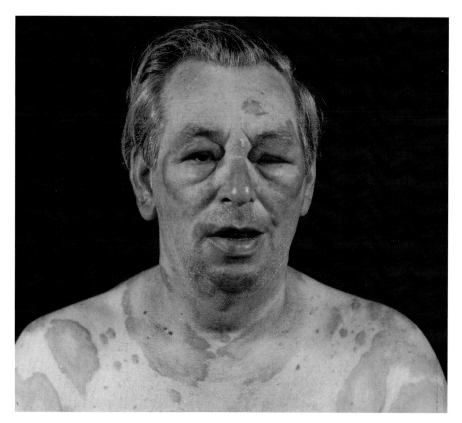

FIGURE 114-1 *Urticaria.*

- For physical urticarias, specific testing to exacerbate the condition, such as cold application to the skin or physical exercise, may be necessary in making the diagnosis

DIFFERENTIAL DIAGNOSIS

- Urticarial vasculitis
- Contact urticaria
- Erythema multiforme
- Bullous pemphigoid
- Insect bites

TREATMENT

- Most cases of acute urticaria last a few weeks and are self-limited
- The mainstay of therapy is oral H_1-blocking antihistamines
- Second-generation antihistamines are less sedating and have longer duration of action
  - Loratadine (Claritin®) 10 to 30 mg daily (adults) or 0.1 to 0.4 mg/kg/day (children)
  - Cetirizine (Zyrtec®) 10 to 30 mg daily (adults) or 0.1 to 0.4 mg/kg/day (children)
  - Fexofenadine (Allegra®) 180 mg daily (adults)
- First-generation antihistamines are more sedating, impair psychomotor function, and require frequent daily dosing
  - Diphenhydramine (Benadryl®) 25 to 50 mg po q6hr (adults) or 0.4 mg/kg po q6hr (children)
    - Diphenhydramine may also be given IM in the emergency department setting for rapid onset of activity
  - Hydroxyzine (Atarax®, Vistaril®) 25 to 50 mg po q8hr (adults) or 0.4 mg/kg po q6hr (children)
- For severe cases of acute urticaria and virtually any patient with respiratory symptoms, oral or intramuscular corticosteroids may be useful when combined with antihistamines
  - Prednisone 0.5 to 1 mg/kg/day in divided daily doses for 1 to 2 weeks
  - Triamcinolone acetonide (Kenalog®) 0.5 to 1 mg/kg IM

- Injectable epinephrine pens should be prescribed to patients with symptoms of respiratory compromise associated with acute urticaria

- Follow-up with the primary care physician or dermatologists is recommended within 1 week for acute urticaria
- Patients with chronic idiopathic urticaria should be followed by their primary care physician or dermatologists

- Avoidance of trigger factors is key in preventing recurrent bouts of acute urticaria; patient should avoid direct mast cell degranulators, such as NSAIDs and narcotics (morphine, codeine)

ICD-9 Code

708.9

CPT Code

11100   Skin biopsy

CHAPTER 115

URTICARIAL VASCULITIS

HISTORY

- Approximately 70% of patients with this disorder are female
- Characteristic purpuric wheals, which usually last longer than 24 hours
  - Urticarial wheals always last less than 24 hours
- Although most patients have idiopathic disease, there may be a prior history of associated conditions like autoimmune disorder (such as systemic lupus erythematosus, dermatomyositis), serum sickness reactions to drugs (penicillins, sulfonamides, thiazides, allopurinol, phenytoins, nonsteroidal antiinflammatory drugs [NSAIDs]), physical urticarias (cold urticaria, solar urticaria, exercise-induced urticaria, delayed pressure urticaria), IgM paraproteinemia, or viral infection (such as hepatitis and infectious mononucleosis), or it may be seen in association with cancer
- History of either characteristic cutaneous eruption or visceral symptoms of headache, fever, malaise, and myalgias
- Gastrointestinal symptoms may include abdominal pain, bleeding, intussusception, and diarrhea
- Musculoskeletal symptoms of episodic arthralgias and stiffness of the elbows, wrists, fingers, knees, ankles, and toes

PHYSICAL EXAMINATION

- Erythematous, sometimes indurated wheals or papules with or without associated angioedema; these wheals, which may have a burning quality, last for more than 24 hours; they sometimes heal with postinflammatory hyperpigmentation or become ecchymotic (Fig. 115-1)
- Other manifestations include livedo reticularis and nodules, occasional hepatosplenomegaly, and lymphadenopathy

DIAGNOSIS

- Clinical history and examination, combined with results from a skin biopsy, is required to make a definitive diagnosis

DIFFERENTIAL DIAGNOSIS

- Urticaria: usually lacks purpura found in urticarial vasculitis, and urticarial lesions always last less than 24 hours
- Thrombocytopenia: may cause purpura, but the lesions lack urticarial qualities
- Septic emboli: generally found in febrile patients with other signs and symptoms of systemic illnesses, and skin lesions tend to be distal
- Disseminated intravascular coagulation: generally presents with widespread purpura in the appropriate clinical setting and lacks urticarial features
- Panniculitis: deep, painful nodules characterize this condition
- Other systemic vasculitides may directly mimic this condition, and other laboratory findings and skin biopsy results help differentiate urticarial vasculitis from other vasculitides

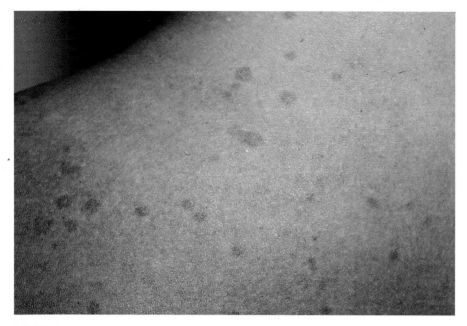

FIGURE 115-1 *Urticarial vasculitis.*

TREATMENT

- If treatment is needed emergently, systemic corticosteroids such as prednisone at 1 mg/kg/day may be initiated for 1 week combined with H_1 antihistamines such as loratidine or cetirizine at 10 to 20 mg per day (adults)
- Treatment beyond this is geared toward treatment of the underlying process if this process is identifiable
  - Offending drugs in drug-hypersensitivity vasculitis should be withdrawn
  - Identified infections should be treated
- Other reported treatments that are not appropriate for the emergency setting have included:
  - NSAIDs
  - Antimalarial agents such as hydroxy-chloroquine
  - Colchicine
  - Dapsone
  - Pentoxifylline
  - Methotrexate
  - Azathioprine
  - Cyclophosphamide
  - Cyclosporine
  - Plasmapheresis

MANAGEMENT/FOLLOW-UP

- May recur for years
- Patients need long-term monitoring for evidence of obstructive pulmonary disease, interstitial lung disease, diffuse glomerulitis, and glomerulonephritis
- Idiopathic cases may evolve into connective tissue diseases

ICD-9 Code

287.0

CHAPTER 116

VARICELLA (CHICKEN POX)

HISTORY

- Patients complain of the sudden appearance of skin lesions that begin on the face and move to the trunk and extremities over a few days
- The eruption may or may not be preceded by a prodrome, including fever, myalgia, and headache
- Varicella most commonly occurs in children under the age of 10 but can occur in any age group
- Patients often will report a recent history of exposure to chickenpox
- Immunization (Varivax®) is now given to many children born in the United States, but its use is not universal
  - Breakthrough varicella may occur that is typically more mild than varicella

PHYSICAL EXAMINATION

- Patient may be febrile and/or ill-appearing
- Individual lesions begin as erythematous papules, which quickly evolve to vesicles and then pustules within 24 hours; the individual lesions then crust over and are no longer infectious
- Characteristic "dew drop on a rose petal" appearance describes the vesicular stage with surrounding erythema (Fig. 116-1)
- Lesions appear in crops; thus a patient will have lesions in different stages of evolution at any given time
- Lesions begin on face and scalp and spread inferiorly to the trunk and extremities; mucosal lesions often present as erosions (Fig. 116-2)

DIAGNOSIS

- Diagnosis is made by history and clinical exam
- A Tzanck preparation can be performed to confirm that a viral infection is present, but it cannot distinguish between various viruses
  - Using a #15 scalpel blade, unroof the skin of an intact blister
  - Using either the scalpel blade or a sterile cotton-tipped applicator, either obtain the fluid from the blister or scrape the base of the blister and apply directly to a dry glass slide
  - Allow the specimen to air dry on the slide and then prepare with Wright's, Giemsa, or a similar stain
  - Multinucleated giant cells indicate a positive finding
  - Interpretation of a Tzanck smear can be quite difficult; an experienced individual should interpret the slide, and other tests can be performed to confirm infection
  - A negative Tzanck smear does not rule out varicella infection

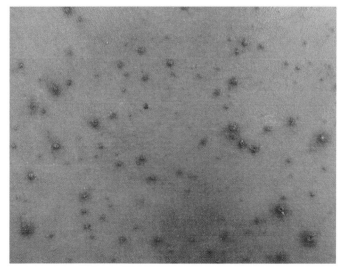

A.

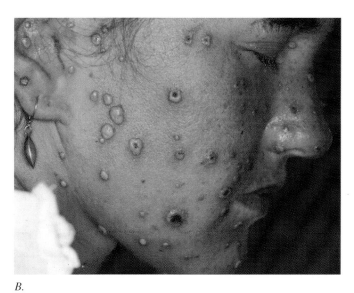

B.

FIGURE 116-1 *Varicella: a wide range of lesions.*

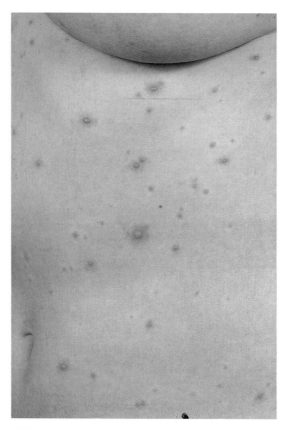

FIGURE 116-2 *Varicella-zoster virus infection: varicella.*

DIFFERENTIAL DIAGNOSIS

- Disseminated herpes simplex virus infection: also in the herpes family of viruses, this infection remains localized in immunocompetent individuals; however, immunosuppressed patients may have disseminated infection; presents as vesicles, pustules, and/or erosions, with some lesions concentrated at the site of the primary or recurrent herpes infection
- Disseminated zoster infection: secondary to the same virus that causes varicella (varicella-zoster virus); widespread lesions of zoster may be indistinguishable from varicella; the lesions usually begin in a dermatome, with rapid dissemination in an immunocompromised patient

- Eczema herpeticum: acute eruption, over a period of a few days to a week, of vesicles and erosions in areas of preexisting skin disorders, such as atopic dermatitis or Darier's disease
- Bullous impetigo: vesicles, bullae, and/or erosions located on otherwise normal-appearing skin; contains clear to yellow colored fluid; usually lesions are scattered and occur on trunk, face, hands, and intertriginous sites

- The treatment of varicella is nonemergent unless there is clinical evidence of major internal organ involvement (e.g., varicella pneumonia)
- Varicella treatment varies depending on the immune status of the patient
  - Immunocompetent patients
    - Neonate: acyclovir (Zovirax®) 500 mg/m² q8hr × 10 days
    - Child: either symptomatic treatment alone, with calamine lotion or cool compresses, or acyclovir (Zovirax®) 20 mg/kg po for each dose qid × 5 days
    - Adolescent or adult: acyclovir (Zovirax®) 800 mg po 5×/day × 7 days; or valacyclovir (Valtrex®) 500 mg po bid for 5 days; or famciclovir (Famvir®) 250 mg po bid for 5 days
    - Varicella pneumonia or pregnancy: acyclovir (Zovirax®) 800 mg po 5×/day × 7 days or acyclovir 10 mg/kg IV q8hr × 7 days
  - Immunocompromised patients
    - Mild varicella: acyclovir (Zovirax®) 800 mg po 5 ×/day × 7 days; or valacyclovir (Valtrex®) 500 mg po bid × 5 days; or famciclovir (Famvir®) 125 mg po bid × 5 days
    - Severe varicella: acyclovir 10 mg/kg IV q8hr × 7 days
    - Acyclovir-resistant varicella or advanced AIDS: foscarnet 40 mg/kg IV q8hr until healed
- Supportive care consists of application of cool compresses to lesions, shake lotions such as calamine lotion, oatmeal baths, and topical anesthetics (e.g., Sarna® lotion, Lanacane® Creme, Aveeno® Anti-Itch cream)

- Patients should be told that their lesions are contagious until the last lesion has crusted over; they should remain home from school and/or work until the lesions are all crusted
- Although both varicella and zoster are caused by the same virus, patients cannot get shingles from someone with chickenpox, but they can get chickenpox from someone with shingles
- Avoid contact with pregnant females or immunosuppressed individuals
- Avoid aspirin in these patients because of the association with Reyes' syndrome

- Immunocompetent patients should follow up with a primary care physician only if needed
- Immunosuppressed patients, if not admitted for intravenous therapy, should follow up with their primary care physician within a few days

ICD-9-CM Code

052.9

CHAPTER 117

VIRAL COMMON WARTS

HISTORY

- A patient usually presents with asymptomatic growths anywhere on his/her body that may have been present for weeks, months, or years and is often aware that the lesion is a wart; plantar warts may be painful
- Warts are caused by the human papillomavirus (HPV); the clinical morphology and location often depend on the type of HPV virus
- Warts are spread by direct contact with an infected source

- Immunocompromised patients have an increased incidence of cutaneous warts
- May affect any person at any age

PHYSICAL EXAMINATION

- Common wart: flesh-colored, round, painless, firm papules on hands, fingers, and knees, although may be seen in other locations; small, red-black dots may be seen within that are indicative of thrombosed capillaries (Fig. 117-1)

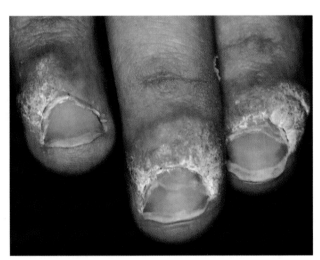

A.

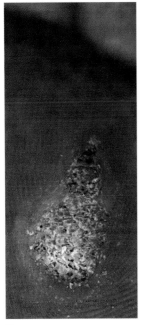

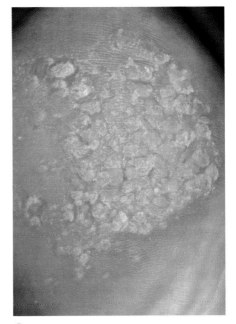

B.   C.

FIGURE 117-1 *Common warts.*

- Plantar warts: flesh-colored, tender plaques with small, red-black dots within lesion on soles of feet with a notable loss of skin lines (dermatoglyphics)
- Flat warts: well-demarcated, flesh-colored, very thin, numerous flat-topped papules clustered together on the legs and face
- Anogenital warts (condyloma): cauliflower-like, flesh-colored, moist papules noted around the genitalia and perianal area (see Condyloma Acuminatum)

DIAGNOSIS

- The diagnosis is usually made clinically by history and appearance
- If clinicians are unsure of the diagnosis or the lesion does not respond to appropriate treatment, a skin biopsy may be helpful

DIFFERENTIAL DIAGNOSIS

- Common wart: seborrheic keratosis (flesh-colored), acrochordons, molluscum contagiosum, squamous cell carcinoma
- Plantar warts: corn, squamous cell carcinoma
- Flat warts: syringomas, lichen nitidus, molluscum contagiosum, lichen planus

TREATMENT

- The treatment of all warts is nonemergent
- Numerous treatments are available, but patients should be informed that wart treatment is a process rather than an event

- Acid application
  - Acids may be applied by clinicians (trichloroacetic acid or bichloroacetic acid) or by patients (salicylic acid, e.g., Occlusal®, Compound W®, DuoFilm®)
  - When patients apply products at home, the process of destruction of warts may take 2 to 12 weeks
  - Acid products work more effectively if a bandage is applied after application
  - Acids should not be used on the face
- Cryotherapy with liquid nitrogen can be an effective modality
  - The efficacy of this approach and all destructive approaches is operator-dependent
  - This can be quite painful and is certainly difficult to use in children
  - Cryotherapy may cause scarring, hypopigmentation, and depigmentation
- Curettage and electrodesiccation
  - The efficacy of this approach and all destructive approaches is operator-dependent
  - This approach requires local anesthesia
  - This can be quite painful and certainly difficult to use in children
  - Curettage and electrodesiccation may cause scarring, hypopigmentation, and depigmentation
- Surgical excision
  - The efficacy of this approach and all destructive approaches is operator-dependent
  - This approach requires local anesthesia
  - This can be quite painful and certainly difficult to use in children
  - Surgical excision may cause scarring, hypopigmentation, and depigmentation
- CO_2 laser destruction
  - The efficacy of this approach and all destructive approaches is operator-dependent
  - This approach requires local anesthesia
  - This can be quite painful and certainly difficult to use in children
  - CO_2 laser destruction may cause scarring, hypopigmentation, and depigmentation
- Cantharidin, an extract of the green blister beetle, can be applied; it causes a blister at the site of application and focal destruction of the cells
  - Cantharidin application is painless at the time of application
  - This agent requires multiple applications 2 or more weeks apart
  - Cantharidin is hazardous, and every effort should be made to avoid all contact with the eyes

- Intralesional bleomycin may also be used, but it carries a significant risk of extensive tissue necrosis
  - The efficacy of this approach and all destructive approaches is operator-dependent
  - This is quite painful and virtually impossible to use in children
  - Bleomycin may cause scarring, hypopigmentation, and depigmentation
- Imiquimod (Aldara®) is an immuno-modulatory medication indicated for anogenital warts, but it may have utility for treating other warts
  - This medication may be applied from three times per week to daily on lesions
  - Because percutaneous penetration is limited, combining this approach with topical OTC acid treatment may be beneficial
- Regardless of the modality of treatment chosen, multiple treatments are usually required to remove the warts entirely

- Patients should follow up with their primary care physician or dermatologist on a monthly basis until lesions have resolved, which may take several months; the response to therapy is somewhat dependent on the size of the wart being treated

ICD-9 Code

078.10   Common warts

CPT Code

17000   Benign destruction (1 lesion)
17003   Benign destruction (2 to 14 lesions)

CHAPTER 118

VIRAL EXANTHEM

HISTORY

- The patient, who is usually younger than 20 years of age, presents with a diffuse, somewhat pruritic or asymptomatic rash, often in association with other symptoms suggestive of a viral infection, such as fever, malaise, sore throat, coryza, or diarrhea
- The eruption is usually acute in onset, beginning around the time of onset of the viral illness
  - The exanthem may also begin at the end of a viral infection course
- The chronologic time frame from onset of symptoms and eruption is important in defining some viral syndromes
- Many different types of viral infections cause exanthems, such that it is not specific for any one virus
  - Only a few viral infections have a very typical appearance that allows for clinical diagnosis including erythema infectiosum, rubella, rubeola, and varicella
- Many viral exanthems are associated with mucous membrane involvement (enanthems)
- Make certain that there is no suggestion of a recent drug ingestion that could cause a morbilliform (maculopapular) drug eruption

PHYSICAL EXAMINATION

- Pink to erythematous, blanchable macules and papules diffusely on the skin, with prominent involvement in a central body distribution (Figs. 118-1 and 118-2)
- Palms and soles are usually spared, but mucous membranes may be involved; lymphadenopathy and hepatosplenomegaly may be seen

DIAGNOSIS

- The diagnosis is usually made by history and physical exam

DIFFERENTIAL DIAGNOSIS

- Morbilliform drug eruption: may present as a maculopapular or measles-like erythroderma, and a history of recent drug exposure is obtained
- Erythema multiforme

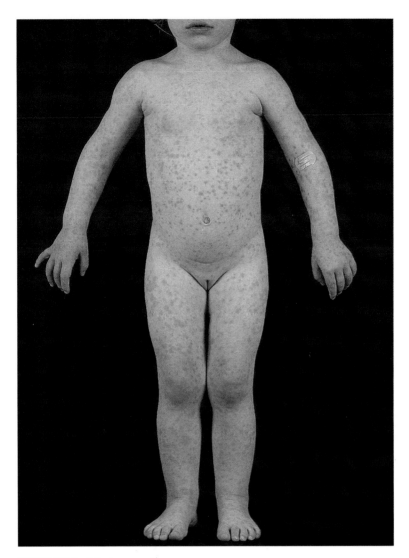

FIGURE 118-1 *Infectious exanthem.*

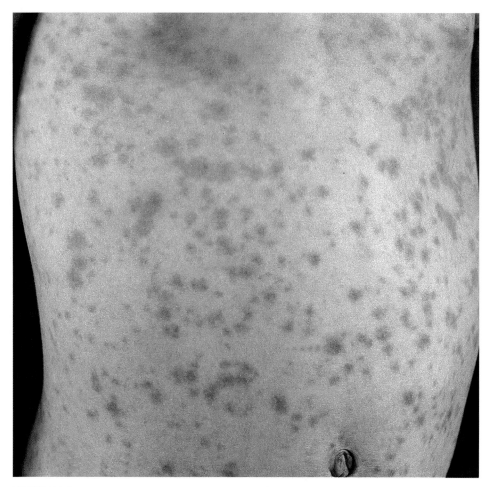

FIGURE 118-2 *Infectious exanthem.*

- Kawasaki's disease: five of the six major criteria are generally present, including 1) presentation with 5 days or more of a spiking fever up to 40°C in infants and children; 2) acute nonsuppurative cervical lymphadenopathy; 3) changes in peripheral extremities, including edema and erythema, progressing to desquamation; 4) bilateral conjunctival injection; 5) oral mucosal disease, including oropharyngeal erythema, erythematous to fissured lips, and "strawberry" tongue; 6) scarlatiniform eruption
- Scarlet fever: presents with a more typical sandpaper-like eruption and evidence of streptococcal infection
- Roseola infantum: the eruption of roseola does not have a sandpaper-like characteristic, there are no oropharyngeal findings suggestive of streptococcal infection, and patients with roseola are usually feeling better at the time of the skin eruption
- Rubella: the exanthem begins on the face as pink macules that become confluent and spreads centrifugally, downward to the trunk and extremities, associated with lymphadenopathy in the suboccipital, postauricular, anterior, and posterior cervical nodes; pinpoint petechiae may be present on the soft palate
- Rubeola: erythematous macules and papules that begin at the forehead and behind ears and then spread cephalocaudally to the neck, upper extremities, trunk, and then the lower extremities, with buccal and labial mucosa erythema; Koplik spots in the oral mucosa, usually opposite the second molars

- Most nonspecific viral exanthems are self-limited; they last for 2 to 10 days, and reassurance is needed
- Symptomatic treatment, such as antihistaminic agents, may help
  - Hydroxyzine (Atarax®, Vistaril®): adults: 10 to 50 mg qhs; children: 0.3 mg/kg/day of a 10 mg/5 ml suspension
  - Diphenhydramine (Benadryl®): adults: 25 to 50 mg qhs; children: 0.3 mg/kg/day of a 10 mg/5 ml suspension
- Topical corticosteroids, such as hydrocortisone 2.5% cream to the face or triamcinolone (Aristocort®) 0.1% cream to the trunk bid for 7 to 10 days may be helpful as well

- No specific follow-up is required

ICD-9-CM Code
057.9

CPT Code
11100   Skin biopsy

CHAPTER 119

VITILIGO

HISTORY

- The patient presents with complete loss of skin color that may have been ongoing for several months to years
- Vitiligo is thought to be an autoimmune condition that results in destruction of melanocytes, leading to depigmentation of skin
- It is uncommonly associated with other diseases, such as thyroid disease, diabetes mellitus, Addison's disease, alopecia areata, and pernicious anemia
- Vitiligo may be a heritable disease in some patients
- All races are affected, and sex predilection is equal, but lesions are much more obvious in dark-skinned races
- May occur at any age, but peak onset is between 10 and 30 years old

PHYSICAL EXAMINATION

- Typical lesion is a depigmented, milky-white macule without significant scaling or erythema
- Numerous lesions may coalesce into patches with slightly brushed to distinct borders and residual pigmentation around hair follicles within the patches noted (Fig. 119-1)
- Three general patterns of depigmentation exist: focal (one or a few spots), segmental (usually a band-like distribution in one area of the body), and generalized

- ○ Generalized is the most common type and has a predilection for acral sites, around the eyes, mouth, digits, elbows, knees, nipples, and groin
- Prematurely gray or white hair may be noted, not necessarily in association with an underlying vitiliginous macule
- Visual acuity and hearing are normal
- Skin cancers have been reported within depigmented areas with repeated exposure to UV radiation

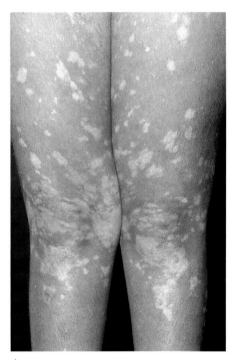

A.

FIGURE 119-1 *Vitiligo.*

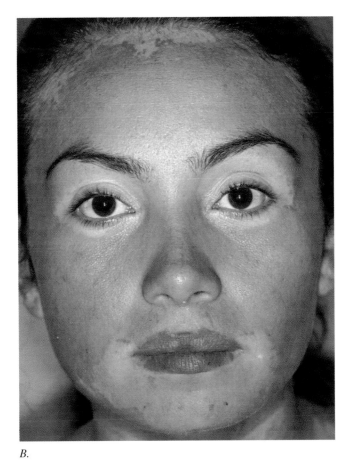

B.

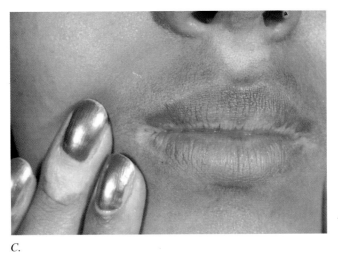

C.

DIAGNOSIS

- Usually made clinically by history and physical exam
- A skin biopsy is rarely necessary
- Wood's lamp inspection of the lesions may define them more accurately and help the physician to decide whether the macules are depigmented or hypopigmented, which is often the question that must initially be answered

DIFFERENTIAL DIAGNOSIS

- Is quite extensive:
  - Pityriasis alba: this atopic dermatitis variant often has overlying scale, hypopigmentation, and few lesions
  - Piebaldism: a congenital condition that has a different distribution and a white forelock; it is a congenital absence of melanocytes
  - Chronic cutaneous lupus: evident scarring, scale, and erythema
  - Tinea (pityriasis) versicolor: overlying scale that on KOH examination reveals spores and hyphae
  - Postinflammatory hypopigmentation: patients generally present with a history of a previous skin inflammatory condition, and the resultant macules are hypopigmented, not depigmented as in vitiligo
  - Chemical leukoderma: this vitiligo mimic is quite difficult to distinguish from vitiligo, except by history of exposure to phenol-containing compounds and photographic chemicals
  - Nevus depigmentosus: a congenital and hypopigmented nevoid condition
  - Tuberous sclerosis: patients have confetti-shaped macules that are hypopigmented, not depigmented as in vitiligo
  - Leprosy: anesthetic macules that are off-white in color; patient has had a history of travel to an endemic area

TREATMENT

- The treatment of vitiligo is nonemergent
- Numerous treatments have been used for vitiligo, but none routinely works well
- Advise patients to wear protective clothing, hats, and sunscreens on depigmented areas since these areas are devoid of melanin and ultraviolet protection and have an increased risk of skin cancer
- Cosmetic approaches using liquid and heavy cover-up makeups are reasonable approaches
- Repigmentation techniques
  - Topical corticosteroids, such as hydrocortisone 2.5% cream for delicate areas of face and intertriginous zones or a medium-potency agent such as triamcinolone 0.1% (Aristocort®) or prednicarbate (Dermatop®) 0.1% cream to other areas of body twice per day for 3 weeks, then skip a week, then repeat
    - If no evidence of repigmentation is seen after 2 months, treatment should be stopped since the patient is unlikely to respond; however, if the patient responds to treatment, monitoring of the skin every 2 months should be performed to evaluate for atrophy
    - An alternative would be to try noncorticosteroidal tacrolimus (Protopic®) 0.1% ointment bid for a trial of several months
  - PUVA (psoralen + UVA light) photochemotherapy is available in both topical and oral forms, but treatment must be given in a dermatologist's office

- PUVA requires significant commitment from the patient since he or she will have to travel to dermatologist's office two to three times per week for treatment
- Psoralen therapy makes the skin extremely sensitive to UV radiation, and care must be taken to avoid other sunlight exposure on days of treatment
- Protective eyewear while outside must be worn for the 24-hour period after the psoralen is ingested
- Side effects and risks include nausea, severe sunburn, photoaging, increased risk of skin cancer, and cataracts
  ○ Surgical manipulation has been disappointing
  ○ Permanent, elective depigmentation of normally pigmented skin by applying monobenzylether of hydroquinone (Benoquine®) 20% is often a last-resort therapy in patients who do not respond

to other treatments and find their disease process intolerable
- This treatment should only be undertaken after extensive discussion between the patient and the dermatologist; the end result will take months to years to achieve

- Patients should be monitored by their primary care physician or dermatologist every 2 months while under topical corticosteroid therapy
- Patients should be referred for ongoing care

ICD-9-CM Code
709.01

WEGENER'S GRANULOMATOSIS

HISTORY

- Middle-aged person presents with upper airway disease and nonspecific systemic symptoms of fever, malaise, and weight loss
- Airway disease is variable; can include sinusitis, rhinorrhea, cough, chest pain, hemoptysis, and otitis media
- Can affect the skin in 50% of patients, as well as other organs, such as the kidney, heart, and nervous system
- Ocular involvement occurs in 30% to 50%, with corneal and scleral ulcerations, conjunctivitis, and proptosis

PHYSICAL EXAMINATION

- Symmetric distribution, usually on the extremities and buttocks, consisting of papules and plaques, some of which may ulcerate (Fig. 120-1)
- Petechiae and purpura, subcutaneous nodules, vesicles, and urticarial wheals have been described
- Saddle nose deformity and nasal mucosal ulceration from involvement of the nasal septum and nasal mucosa (Fig. 120-2)

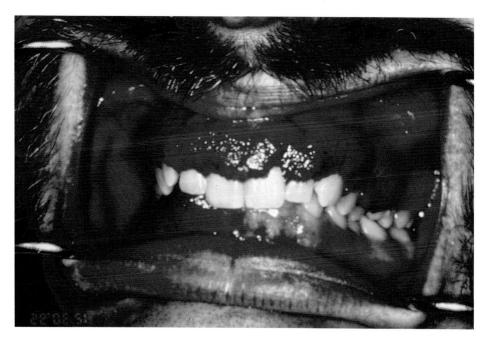

FIGURE 120-1 *Wegener's granulomatosis.*

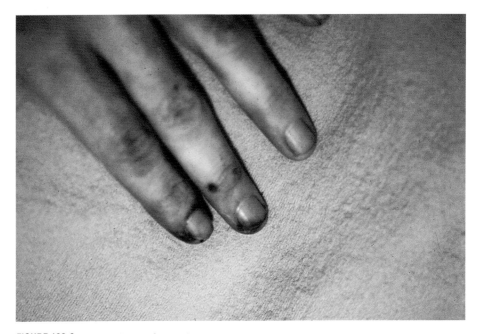

FIGURE 120-2 *Wegener's granulomatosis.*

DIAGNOSIS

- Skin biopsy demonstrating necrotizing granulomas of the respiratory tract, necrotizing granulomatous inflammation of the small arteries and veins of the skin, and/or glomerulonephritis (usually focal segmental) of the kidney
- C-ANCA 96% sensitive
- Chest x-ray with interstitial pattern

DIFFERENTIAL DIAGNOSIS

- Other diseases with vasculitis should be considered in the differential diagnosis, including:
  - Allergic angiitis
  - Goodpasture's disease
- A variety of infectious conditions should also be considered, including:
  - Old World leishmaniasis
  - Lymphomatoid granulomatosis
  - Midline granuloma
  - Rhinoscleroma

TREATMENT

- If organ compromise is evident, treatment may be emergent
- Consultation with a rheumatologist, dermatologist, and other specialists as needed may be indicated
- Systemic glucocorticoids may be required in IV form or orally
- Immunosuppressive therapy is often required with agents such as methotrexate and cyclophosphamide, but it is nonemergent

MANAGEMENT/FOLLOW-UP

- Patients who appear gravely ill may require hospital admission, but most patients require expedited evaluation with a rheumatologist, dermatologist, or other specialists as needed over the next several days

ICD-9 Code

446.4

APPENDIX: DERMATOLOGIC DEFINITIONS AND DIAGNOSES

DEFINITIONS

Alopecia: loss of hair

Aphthous ulcer: a superficial ulcer of the mucosa with an erythematous base

Bulla: a vesicle that is greater than 1 cm in diameter

Cyst: an epithelium-lined sac contining liquid or solid

Depigmentation: complete loss of pigmentation

Ecchymosis: purpura greater than 1 cm in diameter

Edema: excess fluid in the skin

Erythema: a red area of skin that blanches with pressure

Flaccid: lacking firmness, soft

Hyperpigmentation: abnormally increased pigmentation

Hypopigmentation: abnormally decreased pigmentation

Koebner phenomenon: lesions of the skin disease are induced by skin trauma, e.g., psoriasis or lichen planus

Lichenoid: flat-topped, polygonal, grouped papules

Livedo: mottled blue discoloration of the skin in a net-like pattern

Macule: a well-circumscribed flat area of skin that differs from the surrounding skin because of its color; less than 1 cm in diameter

Nevus: a hamartomatous skin lesion with an excess or deficiency of normal epidermal, connective, adnexal, nervous or vascular tissue

Nodule: a deep, firm area of skin

Panniculitis: inflammation of the subcutaneous fat

Papule: a small, firm, elevated area of skin that is less than 1 cm in diameter

Patch: a macular lesion that is greater than 1 cm in diameter

Petechia: purpura usually far less than 1 cm in diameter

Plaque: an elevated firm area of skin that is greater than 1 cm in diameter; often formed by the confluence of many papules

Poikiloderma: pigmentary and atrophic changed of the skin causing a mottled appearances

Purpura: nonblanchable, purple discoloration of the skin that may be palpable or nonpalpable

Pustule: an elevated skin papule containing pus

Rash: a skin eruption (please do not use "skin rash" as rashes occur only in the skin)

Telangiectasia: dilation of a small group of blood vessels

Ulcer: a local defect on the surface of skin or mucous membrane caused by sloughing or necrosis

Vasculitis: necrotizing inflammation of blood vessels

Vesicle: a well-circumscribed, thin-walled, elevated area of skin that contains fluid and is less than 1 cm in diameter

Wheal: a red, edematous area of skin usually associated with pruritus

Xerosis: abnormal dryness or rough scaliness of the skin

DIAGNOSES

Generalized red macules/papules

- Drug eruption
- Erythema multiforme/Stevens-Johnson syndrome
- Fifth's disease
- Kawasaki's disease
- Measles
- Rocky Mountain spotted fever
- Roseola
- Rubella
- Scarlet fever
- Staphylococcal scalded skin syndrome
- Sunburn
- Toxic epidermal necrolysis
- Toxic shock syndrome
- Viral exanthem

Red scaly patches/plaques

- Actinic keratoses
- Asteatotic dermatitis
- Asteatotic eczema
- Atopic dermatitis
- Basal cell carcinoma
- Gandidiasis
- Cellulitis
- Contact dermatitis
- Dermatomyositis
- Diaper rash
- Drug eruption
- Erythrasma
- Exfoliative erythroderma
- Lichen simplex chronicus
- Lupus erythematosus
- Necrobiosis lipoidica diabetacorum
- Nummular eczema

- Parapsoriasis
- Pityriasis rosea
- Pityriasis rubra pilaris
- Psoriasis
- Rosacea
- Sarcoidosis
- Seborrheic dermatitis
- Seborrheic infantile dermatitis
- Sweet's syndrome
- Syphilis
- Tinea corporis
- Tinea cruris
- Tinea pedis

Red scaly papules

- Acne vulgaris
- Actinic keratoses
- Dermatomyositis
- Eruptive xanthoma
- Granuloma annulare
- Impetigo
- Lupus erythematosus
- Nummular eczem
- Pediculosis
- Perioral dermatitis
- Pityriasis rosea
- Pityriasis rubra pilaris
- Psoriasis
- Rosacea
- Scabies
- Syphilis
- Tinea corporis
- Tinea cruris
- Tinea pedis

Red dermal papules/plaques

- Capillary hemangioma
- Erythema multiforme/Stevens-Johnson syndrome
- Granuloma annulare
- Hidradenitis
- Polymorphous eruption of pregnancy
- Polymorphous light eruption
- Sarcoidosis
- Sweet's syndrome
- Urticaria
- Urticarial vasculitis

Tender red nodules

- Abscess
- Acne vulgaris
- Basal cell carcinoma
- Carbuncle
- Cellulitis
- Epidermal inclusion cyst
- Erythema nodosum
- Furuncle
- Hidradenitis
- Keratoacanthoma
- Malignant melanoma
- Pyogenic granuloma
- Rosacea
- Squamous cell carcinoma
- Sweet's syndrome
- Wegener's granulomatosis

Flesh-colored papules/nodules

- Calluses
- Corns
- Epidermal inclusion cysts
- Granuloma annulare
- Keloid
- Keratoacanthoma
- Lichen nitidus
- Molluscum contagiosum
- Squamous cell carcinoma
- Warts

Yellow red papules/nodules

- Eruptive xanthoma
- Molluscum contagiosum

Red pustules

- Acne vulgaris
- Candida
- Disseminated gonococcus
- Folliculitis
- Impetigo
- Pyoderma gangrenosum
- Rosacea
- Sweet's syndrome

Tense bullae/vesicles

- Bullous pemphigoid
- Contact dermatitis
- Dyshidrotic eczema
- Herpes gestationis
- Porphyria cutanea tarda

Erythematous, flaccid vesicles/bullae

- Dyshidrotic eczema
- Erythema multiforme/Stevens-Johnson syndrome
- Herpes simplex virus
- Orf
- Pemphigus vulgaris/foliaceus
- Prickly heat
- Scabies
- Tinea pedis
- Varicella
- Zoster

Atrophic patches/plaques

- Lichen sclerosis
- Lupus erythematosus
- Morphea
- Necrobiosis lipoidica diabetacorum
- Scleroderma
- Striae atrophicae

Purpuric papules/plaques

- Disseminated intravascular coagulation
- Hypersensitivity vasculitis
- Pigmented purpuric eruption
- Urticarial vasculitis

Nonpalpable purpuric macules

- Disseminated gonococcus
- Meningococcemia
- Rocky Mountain spotted fever
- Thrombotic thrombocytopenic purpura

Erosions

- Abrasions
- Ecthyma
- Hand-foot-and-mouth disease
- Pemphigus vulgaris and pemphigus foliaceus
- Staphylococcal scalded skin syndrome
- Toxic epidermal necrolysis

Palmoplantar pits

- Pitted keratolysis

Lichenoid papules

- Lichen nitidus
- Lichen planus

Hyperkeratotic palms/soles

- Acquired keratoderma
- Calluses
- Corns

Livedo

- Calciphylaxis
- Dermatomyositis
- Disseminated intravascular coagulation
- Hypersensitivity vasculitis
- Urticarial vasculitis
- Wegener's granulomatosis

White or hypopigmented macules/patches

- Lichen planus
- Lupus erythematosus
- Raynaud's phenomenon
- Sarcoidosis
- Syphilis
- Tinea versicolor
- Vitiligo

Hyperpigmented or brown nodules/plaques

- Acquired acanthosis nigricans
- Drug eruption
- Keloid
- Keratoacanthoma
- Lichen planus
- Malignant melanoma
- Prurigo nodularis
- Scabies
- Seborrheic keratoses
- Syphilis

Ulcers

- Aphthous stomatitis
- Aphthous vulvitis
- Calciphylaxis
- Chancroid
- Chronic ulcer of the leg
- Ecthyma
- Neurotic excoriations
- Pressure ulcers
- Pyoderma gangrenosum
- Stasis ulcers
- Wegener's granulomatosis

Nonscarring alopecia

- Alopecia areata
- Pediculosis
- Telogen effluvium
- Tinea capitis with kerion

Scarring alopecia

- Lupus erythematosus
- Tinea capitis with kerion

Normal skin

- Pruritus ani

Sweet's syndrome (acute febrile neurotrophilic dermatosis), 304, 368, 370–371, 369*f*
Syphilis
  diagnosis, 374
  primary
    differential diagnosis, 68, 376
    history, 372
    physical examination, 372, 373*f*
  secondary
    chancre, 240, 299
    clinical characteristics, 42
    condyloma lata, 42, 76, 83, 292, 299
    differential diagnosis, 376
    distribution, 16, 42, 83, 234, 240
    hair loss, 24
    KOH preparation, 384, 389
    physical examination, 374, 374*f,* 375*f*
    serology, 267, 396
    treatment/follow-up, 377
Systemic sclerosis, 338

T
T-cell lymphoma, cutaneous, 127. *See also*
  Mycosis fungoides
Telogen effluvium, 24, 378–379, 378*f*
TEN. *See* Toxic epidermal necrolysis
Thermal burns, 284, 403
Thrombocytopenia
  differential diagnosis, 97, 168, 260, 412
  drug-induced, 96
  idiopathic, 96
Thrombocytopenic purpura
  idiopathic autoimmune, 380
  thrombotic, 380–381, 381*f*
Tick bites, 33, 34
Tinea capitis
  diagnosis, 382, 384
  differential diagnosis, 24, 342, 346,
    379, 384
  history, 382
  physical examination, 382, 383*f,* 384*f*
  treatment/follow-up, 385
Tinea corporis
  differential diagnosis, 267, 299, 346,
    386, 389
  history, 386
  physical examination, 386, 387*f,* 388*f*
  treatment/follow-up, 389
Tinea cruris, 292, 390–391, 390*f*
Tinea facei, 342

Tinea pedis
  bullous, 104
  diagnosis, 392
  differential diagnosis, 262, 395
  history, 392
  physical examination, 392, 393*f,* 394*f*
  treatment/follow-up, 395
Tinea versicolor. *See* Pityriasis versicolor
Toxic epidermal necrolysis (TEN)
  diagnosis, 402
  differential diagnosis, 120, 127, 359, 403
  history, 400
  physical examination, 400, 402,
    401*f,* 402*f*
  treatment/follow-up, 403
Toxic shock syndrome
  diagnosis, 406
  differential diagnosis, 321, 324, 336,
    359, 406
  history, 404
  physical examination, 404, 405*f*
  treatment/follow-up, 407
Transient and persistent acantholytic
  dermatosis (Grover's disease), 137
Trauma
  chemical, 379
  purpura from, 260
Treatment. *See under specific dermatologic
  conditions*
Trichotillomania, 24, 379, 384
Tuberous sclerosis, 428
Tzanck preparation, 153–154, 158,
  160, 414

U
Ulcers
  chronic leg, 72, 74–75, 73*f,* 74*f*
  decubitus. *See* Pressure ulcer
  infectious, 284
  traumatic, 154, 376
  vasculitic, 284
Urticaria
  diagnosis, 408, 410
  differential diagnosis, 120, 274, 410, 412
  drug-induced, 98
  history, 408
  papular, 332
  physical examination, 408, 409*f*
  treatment/follow-up, 410–411
Urticarial vasculitis, 120, 412–413, 413*f*

95

returned on or before
stamped below.

Mode 17 APR 2008

12 APR 2010

Mode

The Present and the Past
General Editors: Michael Crowder and Juliet Gardiner

This new series aims to provide the historical background necessary for a proper understanding of the major nations and regions of the contemporary world. Each contributor will illuminate the present political, social, cultural and economic structures of his nation or region through the study of its past. The books, which are fully illustrated with maps and photographs, are written for students, teachers and general readers; and will appeal not only to historians but also to political scientists, economists and sociologists who seek to set their own studies of a particular nation or region in historical perspective.

Australia *John Rickard*
*China *Edwin E. Moise*
France *Jolyon Howorth*
Ireland *J. J. Lee*
Japan *Janet E. Hunter*
Mexico *A. S. Knight*
Russia *Edward Acton*
Southeast Asia *David P. Chandler*
Southern Africa *Neil Parsons*

*Already published